Wound Healing - Recent Advances and Future Opportunities

Edited by Ana Colette Maurício, Rui Alvites and Müzeyyen Gönül

Published in London, United Kingdom

Wound Healing - Recent Advances and Future Opportunities
http://dx.doi.org/10.5772/intechopen.101005
Edited by Ana Colette Maurício, Rui Alvites and Müzeyyen Gönül

Contributors
Elizabeth Concannon, John E. Greenwood, Lindsay Damkat Thomas, Patrick Coghlan, Jeffrey P. Louie, Katie VanDerhoef, Thi Huyen Tran, Marcelo Fonseca Canteros, Aldo Cañete Soto, Dino Ibaceta Orlandini, Jennifer Gómez Aguilera, Paulina Acuña Salazar, Luana Mandriaza Muñoz, Catalina Buchroithner Haase, Manuel Moya Delgado, Giovanni Vivas Rosales, Nicolle Delgado Cárcamo, Florencia Disi Parga, María Belén Larrea Aguilar, María José Pulgar Leyton, Ozlem Su Kucuk, Nazan Taşlıdere, Sourabh Soni, Rubbel Singla, Yogendra S. Padwad, Shalini Sanyal, Qingliang Zhao, Lin Chen, Vesna Karanikolic, Aleksandar Karanikolic, Bidhan Pramanick, Aishwarya G. Patil, Liza G. Gretchen Ovington, Müzeyyen Gönül, Gamze Taş Aygar, Ana Colette Maurício, Carolina Mesquita, Bruna Lopes, Ana Catarina Sousa, Rui Damásio Alvites, Patrícia Sousa, Ana Lúcia Luís, Mariana Branquinho

First published in London, United Kingdom, 2023 by IntechOpen
IntechOpen is the global imprint of INTECHOPEN LIMITED, registered in England and Wales, registration number: 11086078, 5 Princes Gate Court, London, SW7 2QJ, United Kingdom

British Library Cataloguing-in-Publication Data
A catalogue record for this book is available from the British Library

Additional hard and PDF copies can be obtained from orders@intechopen.com

Wound Healing - Recent Advances and Future Opportunities
Edited by Ana Colette Maurício, Rui Alvites and Müzeyyen Gönül
p. cm.
Print ISBN 978-1-80356-224-7
Online ISBN 978-1-80356-225-4
eBook (PDF) ISBN 978-1-80356-226-1

For EU product safety concerns:
IN TECH d.o.o., Prolaz Marije Krucifikse Kozulić 3, 51000 Rijeka, Croatia,
info@intechopen.com or visit our website at intechopen.com.

Meet the editors

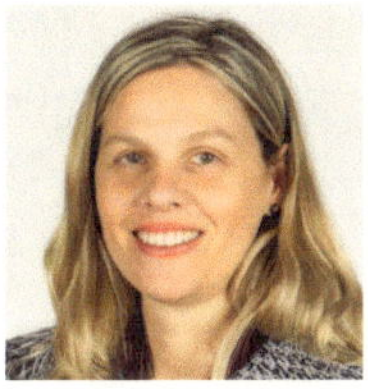

Ana Colette Maurício obtained a DVM and a Ph.D. in Veterinary Sciences from the Faculty of Veterinary Medicine, University of Lisbon, Portugal, in 1995 and 1999, respectively. She obtained a Habilitation in Veterinary Sciences from the Abel Salazar Institute of Biomedical Sciences (ICBAS), University of Porto, Portugal in 2011. Dr. Maurício is a full professor in the Veterinary Clinics Department, University of Porto. She is a member of the Scientific and Representatives Council, director of the Veterinary Sciences Doctoral Programme at ICBAS, scientific coordinator of the Regenerative Medicine/Experimental Surgery sub-unit of the Center for Study in Animal Science, Institute of Sciences, Technologies and Agroenvironment (CECA-ICETA), University of Porto, and of the Associate Laboratory for Animal and Veterinary Science (AL4AnimalS). For the past 15 years, she has coordinated a multidisciplinary research group in experimental surgery/regenerative medicine, developing biomaterials and cell-based therapies. She is the supervisor of several Ph.D., post-doctoral, and master's students. She is the co-author of numerous scientific articles and book chapters, editor of six books, and inventor of five international patents. She is a principal researcher and member of several national and international scientific projects.

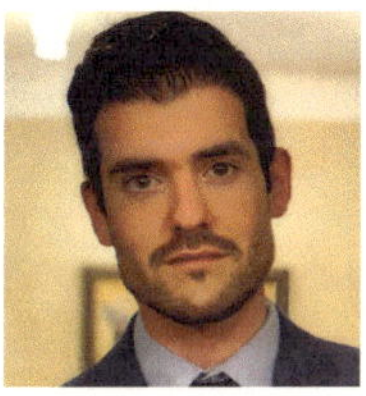

Rui Alvites is a researcher at the Institute of Sciences, Technologies and Agroenvironment, University of Porto, Portugal. He is also an external collaborator at the Abel Salazar Institute of Biomedical Sciences, University of Porto, and a guest assistant professor at Cooperativa de Ensino Superior Politécnico e Universitário, Portugal. He is a junior member of the European Society for the Study of Peripheral Nerve Repair and Regeneration Board and a member and representative of Postdoctoral Researchers at the Associate Laboratory for Animal and Veterinary Science (AL4AnimalS). He obtained a master's degree in Veterinary Medicine from the University of Trás-os-Montes and Alto Douro, Portugal, in 2015 and a Ph.D. in Veterinary Sciences from the Abel Salazar Institute of Biomedical Sciences (ICBAS), University of Porto in 2021. His research interests include regenerative medicine, biomedical and veterinary sciences, and using mesenchymal stem cells, biomaterials, and animal models for the development of new regenerative therapies from a One Health perspective. He is the author and co-author of multiple journal articles and book chapters. He is also a co-author of internationally registered patents Dr. Alvites is a supervisor and co-supervisor of master's and doctoral students in veterinary sciences and regenerative medicine.

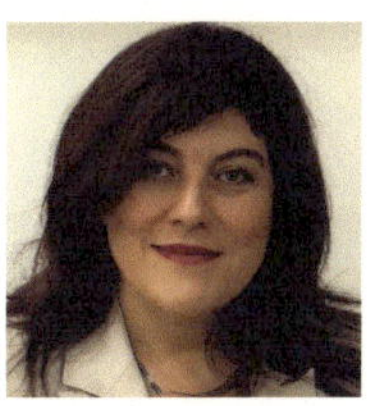

Müzeyyen Gönül graduated from Ankara University School of Medicine, Turkey. Currently, she is a professor in the Department of Dermatology, Health Science University, Etlik City Hospital, Turkey. She has 250 journal articles to her credit. Her research interests are psoriasis, urticaria, autoimmune bullous disorders, and Bechet's disease.

Contents

Preface

Wound Healing - Recent Advances and Future Opportunities is divided into three sections: "Clinical and Physiology Reviews", "Treatment and Management of Specific Skin Conditions", and "Innovative Technologies and Therapies for Wound Healing". It discusses the physiology and pathophysiology of skin conditions as well as treatments and novel approaches for skin regeneration and restoration in terms of structure and function.

Each year, worldwide healthcare systems face an increasing number of patients suffering from skin wounds that result from the breakdown of anatomical continuity and integrity of the epidermis, with consequent functional changes. Skin wounds can vary from acute superficial injuries such as surgical wounds to challenging-to-treat wounds like full-thickness and chronic wounds, burns, and ulcers that require different medical and/or surgical treatments. The treatments currently available to accelerate skin regeneration in full-thickness wounds are based on skin grafting therapies and cell suspensions, which are expensive, inaccessible, and require a donor. They are also associated with a risk of rejection. For this reason, dressings are considered an easy and effective alternative. However, to treat wounds with demanding requirements, dressings also must present advanced functionalities such as antibacterial, anti-inflammatory, or angiogenic properties.

Therapeutic advances based on new and innovative therapeutic options, medical devices, and biomaterials to promote wound healing are being explored and studied by the scientific and clinical community. This book discusses these advances in human and veterinary medicine. It describes advances in surgical wound closure devices and how they impact and support surgical wound healing by minimizing complications such as infection, dehiscence, and incisional hernia. It also reviews new technologies such as cell-based therapies, biomaterials, and medical devices from the World Health Organization's One Health perspective, which is a collaborative approach to achieving optimal health for humans, animals, and the environment. The book also discusses some important dermatological pathologies and skin conditions with the aim of creating a theoretical and practical reference for future research on chronic wound healing.

The editors would like to thank the team at IntechOpen for their assistance and support throughout the publication process.

Ana Colette Maurício
Full Professor,
Department of Veterinary Clinics,
Instituto de Ciências Biomédicas Abel Salazar (ICBAS),
University of Porto (UP),
Porto, Portugal

Rui Alvites
Researcher,
Institute of Sciences,
Technologies and Agroenvironment of the University of Porto (ICETA),
Porto, Portugal

Müzeyyen Gönül
Professor,
University of Health Science,
Dışkapı Yıldırım Beyazıt Education and Research Hospital,
Dermatology Clinic,
Ankara, Turkey

Section 1

Clinical and Physiology Reviews

Chapter 1

Application of Cell-Based Therapies in Veterinary Dermatology

Carolina Mesquita, Bruna Lopes, Patrícia Sousa, Mariana Branquinho, Ana Catarina Sousa, Ana Lúcia Luís, Rui Alvites and Ana Colette Maurício

Abstract

Stem cells have been extensively studied in the field of veterinary medicine due to their unique characteristics. The last are undifferentiated cells with self-renewal, anti-inflammatory, and immunomodulatory capacity. Mesenchymal stem cells (MSCs) are widely used due to its simple isolation and expansion, being collected from different sources such as adipose tissue, bone marrow, peripheral blood, and umbilical cord. For that reason, MSCs have been studied and used as innovative therapies in the treatment of several diseases, such as tendinitis, bone regeneration, osteoarthritis, neuromuscular diseases, heart diseases, respiratory diseases, kidney disorders, ophthalmology, oncology, and dermatology. Concerning dermatological problems, the number of skin diseases in animals has been increasing in recent years. Skin diseases may be related to genetic conditions, external aggressions, or immunological disorders. Many of these skin pathologies are chronic, reason why the animals are subjected to long-term therapies, which can have deleterious side effects. This review aims to highlight the importance of cell-based therapies, using MSCs from different origins and their secretome, in the field of veterinary dermatology and in immune-mediated diseases such as atopic dermatitis, furunculosis, anal vasculitis, and scar tissue regeneration. These approaches should be further explored, as they have revealed promising results in the search for novel therapies.

Keywords: cell-based therapy, mesenchymal stem cells, skin diseases, veterinary dermatology, wound healing

1. Introduction

In the last years, regenerative medicine has been developing in fields such as wound healing and skin regeneration. The skin acts as a protective barrier that isolates the body from harmful agents and injuries. In addition, the skin also contributes to homeostatic maintenance, regulating the body's temperature and internal integrity. Age, tumors development, congenital defects, and degenerative diseases are some of the factors associated with difficulties in wound healing, reason why regenerative medicine can be very helpful in the achieving better results [1]. The skin can be frequently injured because of both chronic and acute wounds (burns, diabetic ulcers, and atopic dermatitis), and these patients experience mental, physical and health constrains that can lead to a huge socioeconomic burden [2]. Recently, MSCs started to be used as therapeutic agents capable of regenerating damaged tissues and organs [3]. For that reason, new cell-based therapies have received attention in both human and veterinary medicine. MSCs are multipotent cells that derive from the embryonic layer of the mesoderm. Besides, under the right *stimulus*, these cells can differentiate into different lineages, such as osteoblasts, myocytes, chondrocytes, among others [3–5]. MSCs are undifferentiated cells with specific characteristics such as self-renewal capacity, originating cells with identical characteristics, and the potential or ability to differentiate from cells in mature tissues, which gives them the ability to repair tissues and organs [6, 7]. There are numerous clinical studies demonstrating the therapeutic potential of MSCs in various fields of veterinary medicine [3]. Moreover, it is known that conventional treatments, based on medical drugs, are often associated with unwanted side effects due to the re-use of these drugs. Nevertheless, despite the capacity of MSCs in wound repair and cutaneous regeneration, there are some limitations, such as the heterogenicity in the delivery protocols, site of delivery, and the lack of information concerning MSCs functional properties and phenotype [2].

Several dermatological problems have a congenital origin and a chronic/recurring nature, forcing these animals to receive repeated and prolonged drug treatments with the consequent development of side effects. Furthermore, skin diseases require a lot of attention, since they are associated with expensive treatments that are usually ineffective [1]. Studying the use of cells as a therapeutic agent instead of conventional drugs, for the control of these patients with dermatological problems, is therefore of special interest.

This review analyzes the most relevant stem cell types in skin regeneration and specific dermatological that may benefit from treatment with this new therapeutic approach.

2. The skin and the wound healing process

The skin is the main barrier that protects the body from the external environment, maintaining the homeostasis and with self-healing capacity. It is a complex organ, with different layers (epidermis, dermis, and hypodermis), that upon the loss of integrity, whether due to a disease or a lesion, needs to re-establish its function [1].

The wound healing process is a complex cascade of events that must occur in sequence and at the adequate time, in order to be successful. It has four overlapping phases: hemostasis, inflammation, proliferation, and remodeling. After a lesion, the first reaction of the body is to prevent blood loss, using the platelets to form a blood clot (hemostasis). Then, the inflammatory phase starts by recruiting inflammatory cells into the lesion site that will produce growth factors, cytokines and enzymes, increasing the temperature, redness, swelling, and local pain. If this phase extends in time, there will be a chronic inflammation that will harm the wound healing. The next phase is the proliferative, which consists in covering and filling the void space created by the lesion. For this, wound contraction occurs by local fibroblasts that differentiate into myofibroblasts. In addition, endothelial cells proliferate and migrate to form

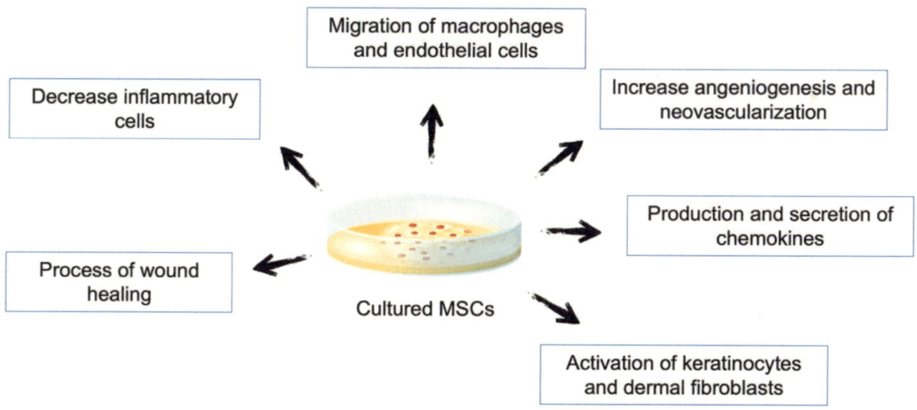

Figure 1.
Wound healing cascade and scar formation.

new blood vessels at the lesion site. It starts in the 4th day post-injury and can last for 2 weeks. Then, the fourth phase (remodeling) occurs and extracellular matrix deposits, promoting the re-epithelization and neovascularization, as the collagen fibers change from type III to type I, helping the tissue to remodel and regain its flexibility and tensile strength. This phase begins 2–3 weeks post-lesion and can last for several years [1, 8, 9].

The wound healing process can sometimes fail and, although the process is not fully understood, the prolonged chronic local inflammation is associated with an abnormal regeneration, as it supports the formation of scars, as demonstrated in **Figure 1**. There are also several factors that increase the risk of inappropriate wound healing, such as smoking, malnutrition, infections, age, metabolic diseases, medications, and even radiation [1, 8]. Tissue engineering, using stem cell-based therapies is being explored in various research fields obtaining good outcomes. Stem cells have gained a lot of attention because of some of their capacities, such as differentiation and the ability to aid tissue regeneration [10].

3. Types of stem cells

Depending on their potential, stem cells can be classified into three types: totipotent (cells have the ability to originate all types of cells from the three germ layers—endoderm, mesoderm, and ectoderm and extra-embryonic tissues); pluripotent (cells can originate cells from the three germ layers but not cells from extra-embryonic tissues), and multipotent (cells can originate cells from several types of tissues but only from one of the germ layers) [3]. Furthermore, stem cells can be collected from two major types of tissues, namely embryonic tissues and adult tissues. Their collection using biotechnology is a complex and costly process [11].

Embryonic stem cells (ESC) can be obtained from the inner cell mass of an early embryo. When removed, these cells can be cultured *in vitro* and have immortal characteristics. In addition, ESC may be induced to originate various cell/tissue types. For these reasons, ESCs are studied to better understand the mechanisms of organ formation and healing. Despite this, these cells can promote the formation of teratomas and can be rejected, when implanted into a patient, and there is some ethics controversy about the use of embryos in science [12].

Characteristics	Adult stem cell	Embryonic stem cell
	BM-MSCs, ADSCs, UC-MSCs	Inner cell mass of an early embryo
Teratomas formation	✗	✓
Rejected as foreign tissue	✗	✓
Differentiation ability	✓	✓
Self-renewal	✓	✓
Immortal cell lines	✗	✓

Table 1.
Summary of Adult Stem cells and Embryonic Stem cells and general characteristics.

Adult stem cells (ASC) can be found in almost every tissue, including adipose tissue, skin, bone marrow, muscle, among others. Some ASC, especially MSCs, can produce growth factors and can differentiate into many lineages. As opposed to ESC, ASCs do not lead to the formation of teratomas, unless there has been some damage prior to its implantation. These different characteristics between ESC and ASCs are compared in **Table 1**. Neonatal stem cells from the amnion, placenta, and umbilical cord are commonly considered as ASCs [12].

Among all these sources, bone marrow-derived MSCs (BM-MSCs) and adipose-derived MSCs (ADSCs) are the most studied and used in veterinary medicine due to the ease of obtaining, abundance of tissue of origin, and lack of moral restrictions [13].

4. Mesenchymal stem cells

MSCs were firstly characterized by Friedenstein's group as being phenotypically identical to fibroblasts and capable to adhere to plastic surfaces [1]. These cells are defined by the International Society for Cellular Therapy as cells that express specific surface markers (CD73, CD90, and CD105), do not exhibit the hematopoietic markers (CD45, CD34, CD14, CD19, CD11b, CD79a, and others), and have the ability to adhere to plastic surfaces when in culture and multipotential ability to differentiate in at least osteoblasts, chondrocytes, and adipocytes under specific *in vitro* conditions [14]. MSCs can be isolated from various sources such as adipose tissue, bone marrow, umbilical cord, dental pulp, olfactory mucosa, and muscle [15, 16].

In addition to their ability to differentiate into various types of tissues, MSCs can be used to produce secretome, which is composed by a wide variety of secreted bioactive substances such as proteins, cytokines, growth factors, antioxidants, proteosomes, and exosomes that interact in an autocrine and paracrine way. MSCs secretome is an alternative therapeutic option and can help solving some limitations related to the use of living cells, such as tumorigenicity, immune compatibility, and infection transmission [10].

Among the numerous performance capabilities of MSCs, it is important to highlight their high capacity to differentiate into various cell types such as osteoblasts, chondrocytes, adipocytes, hepatocytes, myocardial cells, endothelial, neuronal, and epithelial cells, helping in the regeneration of damaged tissues. The potential to secrete cytokines and growth factors can promote angiogenesis and neo-vascularization, thereby increasing tissue blood flow, and the anti-apoptosis characteristics through the production of cellular factors that promote cellular survival prevent apoptosis or programmed cell death. In addition, MSCs can migrate to damaged areas of the body where they can act in tissue repair, which allows its local application directly *in situ* or *via* systemic administration. Their anti-inflammatory action and the inhibition of pro-inflammatory factors, as well as the immunomodulatory potential, make these cells good candidates to the treatment of dermatological disorders, as described in the characteristics in **Figure 2** [3, 14, 17, 18].

4.1 Immuno-modulating capacity of MSCs

MSCs act on different types of cells of the immune system by releasing more than 200 bioregulatory substances with antifibrotic, antiapoptotic, antimicrobial, chemoattraction, stem cell support, hematopoietic, angiogenesis, mitogenesis and neuroprotector properties [7]. In addition, MSCs have two fundamental effects on the immune system, which are an immune-enhancing and anti-inflammatory response [3]. These cells interact with T cells, B cells, natural killer (NK) cells, dendritic cells (DCs) macrophages, monocytes, and neutrophils, exerting immunoregulatory action on the innate and adaptive immune response [17].

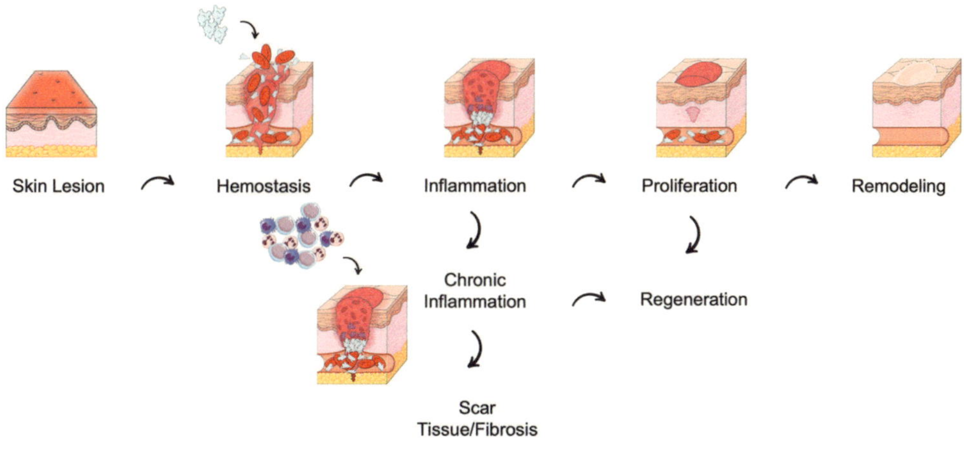

Figure 2.
MSCs role in the wound healing process.

The immunoregulatory potential of MSCs depends on several factors, such as their tissue of origin, MSC dose, administration time, MSC activation, and their contact with immune system cells.

4.2 Mechanism of action of MSCs under the innate immune response

The innate immune response is the body's first line of defense against any external action produced by pathogenic agents such as bacteria, fungi, and virus. It is a fast-acting and nonspecific response to those pathogens. This defense process causes tissue inflammation through the activation of immune system cells such as neutrophils, macrophages, monocytes, natural killer and dendritic cells, and the release of enzymes that form the complement system [19].

MSCs secrete prostaglandin E2 (PGE2), transforming growth factors (TGF-B), and indolamine2,3-dioxygenase that can modulate NK, inhibiting their proliferation, cytokine release, and cytotoxicity. This mechanism can also be exerted through cell-to-cell contact. In addition, MSCs also act on monocytes and macrophages. PGE2, TGF-B, hepatic growth factor, interleukin 6 released by MSCs, reprogram macrophages with a pro-inflammatory M1 phenotype to an anti-inflammatory M2 phenotype with increased production of interleukin-10, and decreased production of tumor necrosis factor and gamma interferon [20–22].

The release of these same soluble factors (PGE2, TGF-B, and interleukin 6) acts on monocytes by inhibiting their differentiation into dendritic cells. Dendritic cells are antigen-presenting cells, when their maturation is inhibited, the correct expression of presenting and co-stimulatory molecules does not occur, which results in a lack of response on the part of T cells [3, 23]. Furthermore, MSCs have the capacity to inhibit the infiltration of monocytes, macrophages, and neutrophils into sites of inflammation, dependent on the tumor necrosis factor stimulated gene 6 protein (TSG6). Similarly, MSCs can also enhance the infiltration of the cells into tumors in a chemokine-dependent manner. In this case, MSCs can promote tumor progression, metastasis, and treatment resistance. For instance, the stimulation of chemokine production may stimulate the capacity of MSCs to attract macrophages, monocytes, and neutrophils. Conversely, an inflammation stage might activate the expression of indoleamine-2,3-dioxygenase (IDO) produced by MSCs that can cause immunosuppressive consequences on myeloid cell migration. For these reasons, it is hard to predict whether the immunomodulatory response of MSCs is expected to be negative or positive, because of MSCs complex innate immune cell interactions [23].

4.3 Mechanism of action of MSCs under the adaptive immune response

The adaptive immune response develops a defense mechanism specific for each pathogen. Therefore, a memory effect is created for each antigen after the first contact, in order to develop a faster and more effective response the next time the organism is in contact with the same antigen [3].

The immune system acts through two pathways, the cellular immune response composed of T lymphocytes that directly attack the pathogens that invade the organism and the humoral immunity response composed of antibodies against pathogenic antigens produced by B lymphocytes [22].

One of the major mechanisms of action of MSCs is their ability to regulate T cells through cell-to-cell interaction or secretion of inflammatory components. In this environment, MSCs can change from T-helper 1 (Th1) phenotype (proinflammatory) into a T-helper 2 (Th2) phenotype (anti-inflammatory) [3]. There is some contradiction about the effects of MSCs on B cells, although there is clear evidence that MSCs have close interaction with these cells. Thus, MSCs are capable of inhibiting B cell proliferation through cell-to-cell contact and with the arrest in the cell cycle. MSCs can regulate immune responses, but their immunomodulatory capacity is not yet fully understood.

This anti-inflammatory and immunomodulatory capacity of MSCs is very promising for the treatment and recovery of skin tissue [14].

5. Application of cell-based therapies in veterinary dermatology

Slow wound healing or persistent wounds are a challenge for clinicians, in both veterinary and human medicines. These wounds can result in inadequate tissue reorganization, culminating in a long period of incapacity and unsatisfactory outcomes [24]. These conditions can be related to various pathological conditions, such as autoimmune diseases, diabetes, and venous stasis, for which no definitive therapies are currently available [25]. Due to this situation, the use of MSCs in veterinary medicine has been increasing in the recent years in different fields. Regarding their application in dermatology, these cells can be used for skin tissue regeneration and for the control of dermatological pathologies, in which the immune system intervenes [14]. Due to their capacity for regeneration, differentiation, revascularization, as well as, their anti-inflammatory and immunomodulatory properties, MSCs have been used as promoters of regeneration on tissues that suffered some damage [1]. However, there are still some questions regarding the use of MSCs, such as their immunomodulation mechanism that is not fully understood. In addition, there are different routes of administration that can result in different risks for the patient. For instance, systemic administration can lead to the entrapment of MSCs in the lung or microvasculature that can cause side effects, such as pulmonary emboli. In addition, almost 90% of the cells are lost, once administered, because of hypoxia, inflammation, physical stress, or immunogenic rejection. For this reason, to reach a therapeutic efficacy, a huge number of cells may be needed, increasing the risk of teratoma formation. Therefore, new studies are needed to achieve more cost-effective treatments to overcome these obstacles [3]. Despite these, this review demonstrates the positive effects of using MSCs therapies and the need to standardize protocols.

There are several skin diseases that can produce chronic and recurring wounds, such as canine atopic dermatitis (CAD), pemphigus foliaceus (PF), and perianal fistula. The conventional treatment for the skin diseases consists in glucocorticoids, cyclosporine, and oclacitinib, which are used due to their immunomodulatory effect. However, their repeated use has several side effects, such as polydipsia, polyuria, polyphagia, vomiting, and diarrhea. It can also require increasing doses of medication over time due to drug habituation [3, 26].

5.1 Application of MSCs in tissue repair and chronic non-healing wounds

A wound is a disruption of the functional integrity and anatomic structure of the skin, so wound healing is a highly ordered process. The skin tissue repair steps need to occur in consecutive order and timing, to be successful; otherwise, the healing process will fail and cause complications, such as chronic non-healing wounds [1].

There are various types of non-healing wounds, such as bed sores, diabetic foot, and trophic ulcers of many etiologies. For instance, ulcer treatment requires necrotic tissue debridement, wound cleansing, amelioration of damaging factors (infection), improvement of arterial blood circulation, and medical management to aid with the comorbidities. Nonetheless, chronic wounds take a long time to heal and often recur after healing with extensive and intensive treatment. Thus, a great possibility in the treatment of chronic wounds is associated with cell-based therapies [27].

The use of MSCs in wound healing is due to their ability to remove necrotic and dead cells, improve vascularization and re-epithelization, and diminish scar formation and wound contraction. Transplanted MSCs release several growth factors that help coordinate different repairing activities. Fibroblasts, endothelial cells, and local stem cells are triggered to aid in tissue repair, by increasing angiogenesis, restraining leukocyte transmigration, and stimulating the proliferation, migration, and differentiation of keratinocytes and fibroblasts. MSCs also release immunosuppressive factors, helping to suppress the proliferation of immune cells, reducing inflammation, and, consequently, reducing scar formation [1].

Kuperman *et al.* demonstrated that the local application of mouse oral mucosa stem cells (mOMSCs) increased the wound healing rate and re-epithelialization and led to a larger area of granulation tissue in diabetic mice compared to the control group [28].

Gorecka *et al.* applied human-induced pluripotent stem cell-derived smooth muscle cells (hiPSC-SMCs) embedded into 3D collagen scaffolds in diabetic mice, promoting angiogenesis and accelerating diabetic wound healing [29].

A study in rabbits showed that wounds treated with a combination of plasma rich in growth factors and adipose-derived mesenchymal stem cells (PRGF+ADSCs) have higher wound healing and epithelization rates, less inflammation and scar tissue, greater collagen deposits, and better angiogenesis compared to the control group. Furthermore, the group treated with the combination PRGF+ADSCs showed a faster recovery of the damaged tissue [30].

Several studies in rodent models have demonstrated that MSCs applied subcutaneously, topically, or intravenously can improve wound healing [12, 31–33].

In a study focusing on skin wounds in dolphins, the animals were treated with autologous ADSCs in a blinded clinical study and the group treated with ADSCs showed improved wound healing [12].

The use of secretome is an alternative treatment when dealing with chronic skin wounds. Sue *et al.* used a rat skin excisional wound healing model to demonstrate that the subcutaneous injection of ADSCs secretome around the wound could accelerate cutaneous wound healing [34].

Park *et al.* investigated if ADSCs secretome could accelerate wound healing using nude mice. In this study, a full-thickness excisional skin wound was created bilaterally on the dorsal surface of the animal. Then, the secretome was used topically in the wounds and covered with a transparent dressing. The evaluation of the lesions demonstrated that the treatment using secretome was able to stimulate angiogenesis, skin thickening, and the recruitment of immune cells, therefore enhancing the wound healing process [35].

5.2 Application of MSCs in immune-mediated diseases

CAD is a complicated disease that results from environmental factors (allergens) and a genetic predisposition (filaggrin mutation) that alter the immune response and culminate in a skin barrier dysfunction [36]. It is a common multifactorial inflammatory and pruritic skin disease in dogs, associated with the production of IgE antibodies [37]. Its prevalence is around 10–15%, and the management of these patients is a real challenge for tutors and veterinarians [38]. During the acute phase of CAD, there is an activation of Th2 cells caused by the immune dysregulation, which culminates in the production of numerous pro-inflammatory cytokines. Over time, the chronicity of the pathology is maintained by a broader roster of T helper variations. Pharmacological treatments consist in corticosteroids (less specific) and cyclosporine A (more specific), and some new approaches used to achieve the most target agents, such as lokivetmab and oclacitinib. Despite the newest therapies, approximately 25–40% of dogs with CAD endure clinical signs and do not reach a full resolution of the pathology [39]. For that reason, the use of MSCs would be a good alternative therapy, since their use in an inflammatory environment, can alter the cytokine profile of T cells and dendritic cells, which can lead to an anti-inflammatory environment [12].

In 2018, a study gathered 26 animals diagnosed with CAD refractory to conventional treatments to which an intravenous dose of 1.5×10^6 ADSCs/kg bodyweight was administered. Pruritus was evaluated using the Canine Atopic Dermatitis Extent and Severity Index, version 4 (CADESI-4), and a decrease in pruritus within a time span of 1 week to 1 month was observed, with the animals being controlled for a period of 6 months. Owners reported improvement of the animals with a satisfactory global assessment of the treatment without the occurrence of adverse events [40].

In 2019, a group of 12 canine patients diagnosed with CAD were intramuscularly inoculated with 0.5×10^6 of cryopreserved ADSCs. Injections were repeated weekly for 6 weeks. During this period, the effectiveness of the treatment was evaluated by the pruritus index and by the CAD Lesion Index (CADLI) test, and a notable reduction in both was observed. The animals were monitored at all times, and no systemic side effects or changes at the injection site were observed [41].

In 2020, a group of 16 animals diagnosed with CAD was evaluated with CADESI-4 and divided into three groups, namely mild, moderate, and severe according to the severity of their injuries. For 82 days, $2x10^6$ MSCs were inoculated intravenously every 21 days to all animals. At the end of the 82 days, skin biopsy histopathology analysis was performed, observing a significant reduction in epidermal thickness in the moderate and severe groups. The results demonstrate that MSCs attenuated the clinical signs of CAD resulting in a safe therapy and causing no adverse effects [42].

In 2021, a double-blind study divided patients with CAD into three groups, a control group that received PBS solution, one group that received low-dose ADSCs (5×10^5 cells/kg), and the third group received a higher dose (5×10^6 cells/kg) of MSCs. Three subcutaneous treatments were performed at 4-week intervals. Pruritus was assessed by tutors using the pruritus visual analog scales (PVAS) and by veterinarians using CADESI-4. Both observed a decrease in pruritus during the 30 days following injections in the group receiving higher dose of MSCs. The animals were monitored throughout the study and did not manifest adverse side effects [43].

Recently, in 2022, a study evaluated the immunomodulatory effect of cADSCs and extracellular vesicles derived from cADSCs (cADSC-EVs) demonstrating that these cells have a beneficial effect in atopic animals. The cASCs and cADSC-EVs affect the expression levels of epidermal differentiation proteins, such as keratin1, filaggrin, loricrin, and involucrin promoting the recovery of the deficient skin barrier in these atopic animals. With the recovery of the skin barrier, it was possible to reduce the loss of water and prevent the entry of allergens *via* transepidermal route. cADSCs and cASC-EVs regulate the immune and inflammatory response by regulating mast cell infiltration, decreasing serum levels of IgE, inflammatory cytokines and epidermal chemokines (IL-4, IL-13, and IL-31) that intervene in Th2. By decreasing IL-31, a decrease in pruritus was also observed by inhibiting the activation of JAK-STATs signaling [38].

The use of UC-MSCs secretome has been associated with the improvement of atopic dermatitis, due to the secretion of epidermal growth factor, which regulates the inflammatory response of mast cells, Th2 cells, and keratinocytes [44].

5.3 Application of MSCs in autoimmune skin diseases

Autoimmune skin diseases occur when the body itself causes self-destruction of its cells and tissues [45].

Pemphigus describes a group of cutaneous autoimmune diseases. Pemphigus vulgaris consists in the appearance of mucocutaneous blisters that are characterized by the presence of autoantibodies against desmogleins (1 and 3). It can be life threatening, and the treatment with systemic corticosteroids has improved the mortality rates [46].

PF is a common autoimmune skin disease characterized by acantholysis. This pathology is associated with the production of autoantibodies that target protein in the desmosomes of keratinocytes [47]. The desmoglein-1 and the desmocollin-1, which are epidermal adhesion proteins, are the main antigens implicated in PF [48]. It is characterized by the production of self-antibodies by B cells that attack desmoglein-1, causing cell apoptosis and disruption of the skin layers, resulting in vesicles, intra-epidermal pustules, and crust lesions [49]. The cause is usually unknown, but some situations are a sequel to a chronic inflammatory skin disease or probably drug-induced [47]. The treatment and control of PF is difficult and often requires lifelong therapy with immunosuppressive drugs (corticosteroids or cyclosporine), having severe side effects such as polyuria/polydipsia, diarrhea, weigh gain, and predisposition to recurrent infection [50]. Furthermore, it has been described that only 53% of treated cases of PF survive more than 1 year after the treatment initiation [47]. Due to their immunomodulatory, anti-inflammatory, and antiapoptotic abilities, MSCs are a promising therapeutic option, not showing the side effects of the conventional treatment.

In 2015, a 10-year-old neutered Shih-Tzu dog diagnosed with PF refractory to corticosteroid treatment was treated with cytotoxic T-lymphocyte antigen 4 (CTLA4)-overexpressing ADSCs. CTLA4-ADSCs and/or naive ADSCs were administered 21 times over a 20-month period (every 2 to 8 weeks) with a positive result. The prednisolone dose was progressively lowered with no relapse of the lesions. At the end of treatment, the lesions had improved considerably, and the disease was under control with a low dose of corticosteroids for 12 months [47].

Canine anal furunculosis is a chronic inflammatory disease that leads to perianal fistulas and that shares a large part of etiology and clinical manifestation with Crohn's disease in humans [51].

In 2015, six dogs with perianal fistulas were treated with human embryonic stem cell-derived mesenchymal stem cells (hESC-MSCs). One month after the injection, reduced serum levels of IL-2 and IL-6 and two inflammatory cytokines associated with Crohn's disease were observed, and after 3 months all animals were controlled and remained free of fistulas for 6 months [51].

Psoriasis is another chronic autoimmune disease, characterized by silvery white scaly patches projecting from the inflamed skin, mainly present in humans, but that can also appear in dogs and monkeys [52]. In patients with psoriasis, the histology of damaged skin demonstrates that epidermal keratinocytes are hyperproliferative and a huge number of immune cells infiltrate into the skin layers (dermis and epidermis). The first treatment used for this pathology was crude coal tar or a combination of the last with ultraviolet irradiation, both with the purpose to restrain keratinocyte proliferation and therefore restoring normal epidermopoiesis. With time, retinoids were also proved to be an efficient treatment for psoriasis since they were able to inhibit the keratinocytes proliferation. For that reason, in the beginning keratinocytes were considered as the main inducer of psoriasis. Later, cyclosporine was discovered to be efficient in psoriasis treatment by inhibiting cytokines produced by T cells [53]. Therefore, keratinocytes can trigger psoriasis and actively participate in a complex environment coordinated by cytokines [54]. The treatments depend on the severity of the disease, from topical agents and phototherapy to the usual immunosuppressant drugs [55]. However, these therapies are expensive and are related to adverse reactions, and therefore, there is a need to discover a more effective and safer treatment. For that reason, there are some expectations in the use of MSCs for psoriasis.

A study testing a treatment with umbilical cord-derived MSCs (UC-MSCs) resulted in comparison with the conventional treatments (betamethasone cream) on imiquimod-induced psoriasis-like skin lesion in adult male albino rat model. MSCs showed efficacy in reducing the severity of the disease, demonstrating that the cells had anti-inflammatory and immunomodulatory effects by inhibiting the clinical manifestation [55].

The use of the MSCs secretome in psoriasis is also able to inhibit the maturation and activation of DC and IL17, decreasing psoriasis score in a rat model [56].

Systemic lupus erythematosus (SLE) is a multisystemic autoimmune disease, with clinical manifestations on every organ. The production of antigen-antibodies complexes that settle in the basement membrane zone of the skin can make this disease manifest as cutaneous lupus erythematosus, with the appearance of rashes. It is a multifactorial disease that can be caused by genetic factors, B cell hyperactivity, T cell defects, virally induced antigen-antibody complex formation, and even hormonal alterations [57]. The cutaneous inflammation is due to Th1 cells, neutrophils, B cells, and even complex cascades of native skin cell types (keratinocytes and endothelial cells) [58]. The conventional treatment options consist in the use of corticosteroids and cyclophosphamide.

The use of allogenic MSCs administrated intravenously has improved multiorgan dysfunction in both MRL/lpr mice and NZB/W1 F1 mice, used as SLE animal models [59].

The use of human AD-MSCs also improved the survival rate and histological, serological, and immunological function of NZB × NZW mice, models for SLE, without adverse effects [57].

5.4 Application of MSCs in alopecia

Alopecia is a frequent dermatologic disorder, affecting both veterinary species and humans. The pathophysiology of this group of disorders is still unclear, but can be associated with trauma, stress, autoimmune disorders, hormones, and even genetics [60]. Alopecia can be caused by a several disorders, such as infections, allergenic reasons, nutritional deficits (mineral deficiency), parasites, bacteria or hot spots, and fungi. A complete physical examination and history are needed to an accurate diagnosis for the reason of hair loss [61]. Hair loss is usually accompanied by a section of thinned skin at the site with hair loss. Additionally, these clinical symptoms occur because of the functional loss of follicular stem cell activity. Nowadays, there are various treatments for alopecia, such as oral medications, that only improve the situation temporary and often with reduced effectiveness. For this reason, alternative strategies are fundamental for alopecia [62]. The use of BM-MSCs and UC-MSCs *in vitro* and in an athymic nude mouse model has been able to create dermal papilla-like structures, as well as hair follicles [12]. In a study, the use of UC-MSCs increased the regeneration of new follicles and improved onset of anagen phase [60]. To determine if UC-MSCs promote the hair cycle, these cells were injected intra-dermally at multiple sites in the dorsal skin field of depilated mouse. The control was the use of daily topical treatments with 3% minoxidil, and the hair cycle stage was determined with the measurement of skin hair regrowth. The results showed that the UC-MSCs emphasized hair follicle morphogenesis, but only without the ablation of the neonatal dermal cell, indicating that UC-MSCs facilitate hair growth and regeneration *via* a paracrine mechanism [62]. Several studies using ADSCs secretome had positive results when used to treat alopecia, as they were able to restore hair loss, due to the activation of hair regeneration pathways [63, 64].

5.5 Application of MSCs in scar tissue

Scar tissue is produced due to cutaneous wound healing, in which there is excessive deposition of extracellular matrix, allowing the skin to restore its integrity after a lesion. It occurs due to specific mechanisms that are modulated by local pro-inflammatory mediators, in the inflammatory phase of wound healing [65]. It has a different appearance, and the tissue does not function as normal skin, lacking some structures, such as hair follicles, sensory nerve receptors, and even sebaceous glands. Its tensile strength is also diminished in about 20%, which leads to re-injures, as the scar is considered a weak point [65].

The current treatments include sterile dressing and topical antibiotics to diminish infection risk and to advance into the proliferation and remodeling phases of the wound healing process, then allowing the regeneration of the tissue. It may also be necessary to debride the wound and irrigate it, to remove necrotic tissue [65].

The use of ADSCs has been reported to have the capacity to remodel scar tissue or block its formation, when used with a fat graft, in human plastic surgery [12].

A study has shown that the use of silk fibroin scaffolds containing human Wharton's jelly MSCs (Wj-MSCs-SF) in a murine model reduced the formation of fibrotic scar tissue, improving reepithelization and vascularized granulation tissue [66].

Gentile *et al* have demonstrated that the use of ADSCs contained in fat grafts has positive effects in scar signs and symptoms [67].

The use of ADSCs secretome in full skin defects demonstrated that it is capable of reducing scar formation, as well as accelerate wound closure and improve angiogenesis [68].

5.6 Application of MSCs in burns

Burns are very common lesions both in veterinary and human medicine and occur due to thermal, electrical, chemical, or radiation exposure. They are associated with the loss of normal tissue and cells, which complicates the wound healing process. Their severity is characterized by the depth and size of tissue damage, as first-, second-, third-, or fourth-degree burns. A first-degree burn is red or pink and sensitive, and can swell slightly. A second-degree burn is painful and often associated with the presence of blisters that reach the reticular dermal layer and have a high risk of chronic inflammation and keloid/hypertrophic scar formation. A third-degree burn presents necrosis of the skin and deep tissues, and is compact and immobile. Fourth-degree burns presents as dry, very compact, and wrinkled. There are alterations in blood composition associated with a burn that occupies 10% or more of the body, which leads to metabolic complications [69, 70].

Current treatments consist in antibiotics, fluids, and detoxification. First- and second-degree burns are treated with antibiotics and anti-inflammatory drugs. Third- and fourth-degree burns require regular dressing change and sometimes surgery [70]. In several studies, the use of local injections of UC-MSCs and ADSCs in rodent models has diminished burn wound progression, as well as burn-induced inflammation. They have also accelerated wound healing in burned lesions, increased re-epithelization, vascularization, and granulation tissue formation [71–73].

The use of a hydrogel containing unsaturated arginine-based poly(ester amide) and chitosan associated with BM-MSCs also demonstrated an increased re-epithelization, granulation tissue formation, and wound healing rate [73, 74]. Also, the use of systemically delivered BM-MSCs in rodent models has increased wound healing [73].

Hackers *et al.* demonstrated the effects of secretome from peripheral blood mononuclear cells on pig models of skin burns. The results showed a decrease in the amount of mast cells in the wound area, demonstrating a lower inflammation of the burn area when using MSCs secretome [75].

In the study by Kudinov et al. using secretome from UC-MSCs combined with a chitosan hydrogel in burned rats, the results showed that this combination cleared the wound of bacteria, promoted re-epithelization and the formation of vascularized granulation tissue, and decreased inflammation [76].

6. Conclusion

Dermatological pathologies are increasingly common and often have a chronic nature, resulting in a real challenge to owners and veterinaries. This leads to animals having to receive long-term or lifelong medications with its consequent systemic side effects. Veterinary regenerative medicine is an area field of research that is becoming more explored and active. Therefore, in the recent years, there have been significant advances in developing effective and safe stem cell therapies. Those studies reveal that MSCs have anti-inflammatory, anti-apoptotic, anti-fibrotic, and immunomodulatory potential, which ensures success in the treatment of degenerative, immunological, and inflammatory diseases in animals. In this review, some relevant cited studies in the field of veterinary dermatology demonstrated better results in the treatment of chronic wounds, especially with the use of UC-MSCs and ADSCs. These studies also showed accelerated wound healing in different clinical conditions. Although more studies are still necessary in this regard, the use of MSCs seems to be a very promising and safe therapeutic option.

Acknowledgements

All authors had made substantial contributions to the work, with well-established division of tasks. All authors reviewed the final work and approved its submission. All authors agreed to be personally accountable for the author's own contributions and for ensuring that questions related to the accuracy or integrity of any part of the work, even ones in which the author was not personally involved, are appropriately investigated, resolved, and documented in the literature. All authors have read and agreed to the published version of the manuscript.

This research was funded by Projects PEst-OE/AGR/UI0211/2011 and LA/P/0059/2020 funded by the Portuguese Foundation for Science and Technology (FCT), and COMPETE 2020, from ANI–Projetos ID&T Empresas em Copromoção, by the project "Print-on-Organs–Engineering bioinks and processes for direct printing on organs" with the reference POCI-01-0247-FEDER-033877, by the project "Bone2Move-Development of 'in vivo' experimental techniques and modelling methodologies for the evaluation of 4D scaffolds for bone defect in sheep model: an integrative research approach" with the reference POCI-01-0145-FEDER-031146 and by the PhD scholarships Mariana Vieira Branquinho (SFRH/BD/146172/2019), Ana Catarina Sousa (SFRH/BD/146689/2019), and Bruna Lopes (2021.05265.BD). The author Rui D. Alvites acknowledges Centro de Estudos de Ciência Animal (CECA), Instituto de Ciências, Tecnologias e Agroambiente (ICETA), Porto University (UP), and Fundação para a Ciência e Tecnologia (FCT) for the funding and availability of all technical, structural, and human resources necessary for the development of this work. The author Patrícia Sousa acknowledges Instituto Politécnico de Leiria—Center for Rapid and Sustainable Product Development (CDRSP), University of Porto (UP), Centro de Estudos de Ciência Animal (CECA), Instituto de Ciências, Tecnologias e Agroambiente (ICETA) for the funding (UIDB/04044/2020) and availability of all resources needed for this work. The work was supported through the projects UIDB/04044/2020 and UIDB/00211/2020 funded by FCT/MCTES through national funds.

Conflict of interest

The authors declare that there are no conflicts of interest regarding the publication of this chapter.

Abbreviations

ADSCs	Adipose-derived MSCs
ASC	Adult stem cells
BM-MSCs	Bone marrow-derived MSCs
CADLI	CAD lesion index
CAD	Canine atopic dermatitis
CADESI-4	Canine atopic dermatitis extent and severity lesion, version 4
CTLA4	Cytotoxic T-lymphocyte antigen 4
DCs	Dendritic cells
ESC	Embryonic stem cells
cASCs – EVs	Extracellular vesicles derived from cASCs
hESC-MSCs	Human embryonic stem cell-derived mesenchymal stem cells
hiPSC-SMCs	Human-induced pluripotent stem cell-derived smooth muscle cells
IDO	Indoleamine-2,3-dioxygenase
MCSs	Mesenchymal stem cells
mOMSCs	Mouse oral mucosa stem cells
NK	Natural killer
PF	Pemphigus foliaceus
PRGF	Plasma rich in growth factors

PGE2	Prostaglandin E2
PVAS	Pruritus visual analog scales
SLE	Systemic Lupus Erythematosus
Th1	T-helper 1
Th2	T-helper 2
THF-B	Transforming growth factors
TSG6	Tumor necrosis factor stimulated gene 6 protein
UC-MSCs	Umbilical cord-derived MSCs
Wj-MSCs-SF	Wharton's jelly MSCs

Author details

Carolina Mesquita[1,2,3†], Bruna Lopes[1,2,3†], Patrícia Sousa[1,2,3†], Mariana Branquinho[1,2,3], Ana Catarina Sousa[1,2,3], Ana Lúcia Luís[1,2,3], Rui Alvites[1,2,3,4] and Ana Colette Maurício[1,2,3*]

1 Departamento de Clínicas Veterinárias, Instituto de Ciências Biomédicas de Abel Salazar (ICBAS), Universidade do Porto (UP), Porto, Portugal

2 Centro de Estudos de Ciência Animal (CECA), Instituto de Ciências, Tecnologias e Agroambiente da Universidade do Porto (ICETA), Porto, Portugal

3 Associate Laboratory for Animal and Veterinary Sciences (AL4AnimalS), Lisboa, Portugal

4 Instituto Universitário de Ciências das Saúde – CESPU (IUCS-CESPU), Gandra, Portugal

*Address all correspondence to: acmauricio@icbas.up.pt

† The authors should be considered as first authors.

References

[1] Lopes B et al. The application of mesenchymal stem cells on wound repair and regeneration. Applied Sciences. 2021;**11**(7):3000

[2] Quinones-Vico MI et al. The role of exosomes derived from mesenchymal stromal cells in dermatology. Frontiers in Cell and Development Biology. 2021;**9**:647012

[3] Dias IE et al. Mesenchymal stem cells therapy in companion animals: Useful for immune-mediated diseases? BMC Veterinary Research. 2019;**15**(1):358

[4] Lopes B et al. Peripheral nerve injury treatments and advances: One health perspective. International Journal of Molecular Sciences. 2022;**23**(2):10-14

[5] Han Y et al. Mesenchymal stem cells for regenerative medicine. Cell. 2019;**8**(8):1-3

[6] Xing SJ et al. Isolation, characterization, and therapeutic application of extracellular vesicles from cultured human mesenchymal stem cells. Journal of Visualized Experiments. 2022;(187):1-2

[7] Ayala-Cuellar AP et al. Roles of mesenchymal stem cells in tissue regeneration and immunomodulation. Biomolecules and Therapeutics (Seoul). 2019;**27**(1):25-33

[8] Guillamat-Prats R. The role of MSC in wound healing, scarring and regeneration. Cell. 2021;**10**(7):1729

[9] Huang Y-Z et al. Mesenchymal stem cells for chronic wound healing: Current status of preclinical and clinical studies. Tissue Engineering Part B: Reviews. 2020;**26**(6):555-570

[10] Izzah N et al. Cell secretomes for wound healing and tissue regeneration: Next generation acellular based tissue engineered products. Journal of Tissue Engineering. 2022;**13**:1-21

[11] Rashid U et al. Characterization and differentiation potential of mesenchymal stem cells isolated from multiple canine adipose tissue sources. BMC Veterinary Research. 2021;**17**(1):388

[12] Harman RJ. Stem cell therapy in veterinary dermatology. Veterinary Dermatology. 2013;**24**(1):90-e24

[13] Voga M et al. Stem cells in veterinary medicine—Current state and treatment options. Frontiers in veterinary. Science. 2020;7:7

[14] Villatoro AJ et al. Allogeneic adipose-derived mesenchymal stem cell therapy in dogs with refractory atopic dermatitis: Clinical efficacy and safety. The Veterinary Record. 2018;**183**(21):654

[15] Alvites RD et al. Rat olfactory mucosa mesenchymal stem/stromal cells (OM-MSCs): A characterization study. International Journal of Cell Biology. 2020;**2020**:1-21

[16] Mao AS, Mooney DJ. Regenerative medicine: Current therapies and future directions. Proceedings of the National Academy of Sciences of the United States of America. 2015;**112**(47):14452-14459

[17] Peroni JF, Borjesson DL. Anti-inflammatory and immunomodulatory activities of stem cells. The Veterinary Clinics of North America. Equine Practice. 2011;**27**(2):351-362

[18] Strong AL, Neumeister MW, Levi B. Stem cells and tissue engineering:

Regeneration of the skin and its contents. Clinics in Plastic Surgery. 2017;**44**(3):635-650

[19] Glenn JD, Whartenby KA. Mesenchymal stem cells: Emerging mechanisms of immunomodulation and therapy. World Journal of Stem Cells. 2014;**6**(5):526-539

[20] Kim N, Cho SG. New strategies for overcoming limitations of mesenchymal stem cell-based immune modulation. International Journal of Stem Cells. 2015;**8**(1):54-68

[21] Li H, Dai H, Li J. Immunomodulatory properties of mesenchymal stromal/stem cells: The link with metabolism. Journal of Advanced Research. 2022;**45**:15-29

[22] Carrade DD, Borjesson DL. Immunomodulation by mesenchymal stem cells in veterinary species. Comparative Medicine. 2013;**63**(3): 207-217

[23] Shi Y et al. Immunoregulatory mechanisms of mesenchymal stem and stromal cells in inflammatory diseases. Nature Reviews. Nephrology. 2018;**14**(8):493-507

[24] Lanci A et al. Heterologous Wharton's jelly derived mesenchymal stem cells application on a large chronic skin wound in a 6-month-old filly. Frontiers in Veterinary Science. 2019;**6**:6

[25] Marfia G et al. Mesenchymal stem cells: Potential for therapy and treatment of chronic non-healing skin wounds. Organogenesis. 2015;**11**(4):183-206

[26] Arnhold S et al. Biological macromolecules and mesenchymal stem cells: Basic research for regenerative therapies in veterinary medicine. International Journal of Biological Macromolecules. 2019;**123**:889-899

[27] Suzdaltseva Y et al. Locally delivered umbilical cord mesenchymal stromal cells reduce chronic inflammation in long-term nonhealing wounds: A randomized study. Stem Cells International. 2020;**2020**:5308609

[28] Kuperman S et al. Examination of the therapeutic potential of mouse Oral mucosa stem cells in a wound-healing diabetic mice model. International Journal of Environmental Research and Public Health. 2020;**17**(13):8-9

[29] Gorecka J et al. Induced pluripotent stem cell-derived smooth muscle cells increase angiogenesis and accelerate diabetic wound healing. Regenerative Medicine. 2020;**15**(2):1277-1293

[30] Chicharro D et al. Combined plasma rich in growth factors and adipose-derived mesenchymal stem cells promotes the cutaneous wound healing in rabbits. BMC Veterinary Research. 2018;**14**(1):288

[31] Sasaki M et al. Mesenchymal stem cells are recruited into wounded skin and contribute to wound repair by transdifferentiation into multiple skin cell type. Journal of Immunology. 2008;**180**(4):2581-2587

[32] Javazon EH et al. Enhanced epithelial gap closure and increased angiogenesis in wounds of diabetic mice treated with adult murine bone marrow stromal progenitor cells. Wound Repair and Regeneration. 2007;**15**(3):350-359

[33] Chen L et al. Analysis of Allogenicity of mesenchymal stem cells in engraftment and wound healing in mice. PLoS One. 2009;**4**(9):e7119

[34] Su N et al. Fibrous scaffolds potentiate the paracrine function of mesenchymal stem cells: A new

dimension in cell-material interaction. Biomaterials. 2017;**141**:74-85

[35] Park SR et al. Stem cell Secretome and its effect on cellular mechanisms relevant to wound healing. Molecular Therapy. 2018;**26**(2):606-617

[36] Marsella R. Advances in our understanding of canine atopic dermatitis. Veterinary Dermatology. 2021;**32**(6):547-e151

[37] Hensel P et al. Canine atopic dermatitis: Detailed guidelines for diagnosis and allergen identification. BMC Veterinary Research. 2015;**11**(1):196

[38] Kim SY et al. Mesenchymal stem cells and extracellular vesicles derived from canine adipose tissue ameliorates inflammation, skin barrier function and pruritus by reducing JAK/STAT Signaling in atopic dermatitis. International Journal of Molecular Sciences. 2022;**23**(9):2-3

[39] Black L et al. The effect of uterine-derived mesenchymal stromal cells for the treatment of canine atopic dermatitis: A pilot study. Frontiers in Vetenary Science. 2022;**9**:1011174

[40] Klinger C. Mesenchymal stem cells: A potential therapy for canine atopic dermatitis? The Veterinary Record. 2018;**183**(21):651-653

[41] Enciso N et al. Multidose intramuscular allogeneic adipose stem cells decrease the severity of canine atopic dermatitis: A pilot study. Vetenary World. 2019;**12**(11):1747-1754

[42] de Oliveira Ramos F et al. Canine atopic dermatitis attenuated by mesenchymal stem cells. Journal of Advanced Veterinary and Animal Research. 2020;7(3):554-565

[43] Kaur G et al. A double-blinded placebo-controlled evaluation of adipose-derived mesenchymal stem cells in treatment of canine atopic dermatitis. Veterinary Research Communications. 2022;**46**(1):251-260

[44] Jung N et al. Immunomodulatory effect of epidermal growth factor secreted by human umbilical cord blood-derived mesenchymal stem cells on atopic dermatitis. International Journal of Stem Cells. 2022;**15**(3):311-323

[45] Chase K et al. Understanding the genetics of autoimmune disease: Two loci that regulate late onset Addison's disease in Portuguese water dogs. International Journal of Immunogenetics. 2006;**33**(3):179-184

[46] Agarwal A et al. Comparison of rituximab and conventional adjuvant therapy for pemphigus vulgaris: A retrospective analysis. PLoS One. 2018;**13**(9):e0198074

[47] Han SM et al. CTLA4 overexpressing adipose tissue-derived mesenchymal stem cell therapy in a dog with steroid-refractory pemphigus foliaceus. BMC Veterinary Research. 2015;**11**:49

[48] Chong E, Austel M, Banovic F. A retrospective evaluation of the steroid-sparing effect of Oral modified Ciclosporin for treatment of canine pemphigus Foliaceus. Veterinary Sciences. 2022;**9**(4):153

[49] Olivry T. A review of autoimmune skin diseases in domestic animals: I - superficial pemphigus. Veterinary Dermatology. 2006;**17**(5):291-305

[50] Putra A, Austel M, Banovic F. A retrospective evaluation of the steroid sparing effects of oral mycophenolate mofetil (MMF) as an adjunct immunosuppressant for the treatment of canine pemphigus foliaceus. Veterinary Dermatology. 2022;**33**(1):77-e24

[51] Ferrer L et al. Treatment of perianal fistulas with human embryonic stem cell-derived mesenchymal stem cells: A canine model of human fistulizing Crohn's disease. Regenerative Medicine. 2016;**11**(1):33-43

[52] Sandra, R.M., et al., Psoriatic animal models developed for the study of the disease, in Psoriasis, C. Anca, Editor. London, UKIntechOpen: Rijeka. 2017. p. Ch. 5

[53] Ni X, Lai Y. Keratinocyte: A trigger or an executor of psoriasis? Journal of Leukocyte Biology. 2020;**108**(2):485-491

[54] Bhopale MK et al. DAB(389) IL-2 recombinant fusion toxin effect on lymphocyte- and macrophage-producing cytokine subpopulation cells in experimentally induced demyelinating disease in mice. Immunopharmacology and Immunotoxicology. 2017;**39**(6):318-329

[55] Attia SS et al. A potential role of mesenchymal stem cells derived from human umbilical cord blood in ameliorating psoriasis-like skin lesion in the rats. Folia Morphologica. 2022;**81**(3):614-631

[56] Eaton LH et al. Impaired Langerhans cell migration in psoriasis is due to an altered keratinocyte phenotype induced by interleukin-17. British Journal of Dermatology. 2018;**178**(6):1364-1372

[57] Choi EW et al. Reversal of serologic, immunologic, and histologic dysfunction in mice with systemic lupus erythematosus by long-term serial adipose tissue–derived mesenchymal stem cell transplantation. Arthritis and Rheumatism. 2012;**64**(1):243-253

[58] Prieto MH, et al. New Approaches to Dermatological Conditions Employing Mesenchymal Stem Cell Therapies. Clinical Dermatology Open Access Journal. 2018;**3**(6)

[59] Shin T-H et al. Mesenchymal stem cell therapy for inflammatory skin diseases: Clinical potential and mode of action. International Journal of Molecular Sciences. 2017;**18**(2):244

[60] Anudeep TC et al. Advancing regenerative cellular therapies in non-scarring alopecia. Pharmaceutics. 2022;**14**(3):612

[61] Siam M, Elsheikh AK, Attia N. Alopecia in dogs causes, incidance and clinical signs with special reference to nutritional alopecia. Zagazig Veterinary Journal. 2022;**50**(2):136-147

[62] Bak DH et al. Human umbilical cord blood mesenchymal stem cells engineered to overexpress growth factors accelerate outcomes in hair growth. Korean Journal of Physiology and Pharmacology. 2018;**22**(5):555-566

[63] Salhab O, Khayat L, Alaaeddine N. Stem cell secretome as a mechanism for restoring hair loss due to stress, particularly alopecia areata: Narrative review. Journal of Biomedical Science. 2022;**29**(1):77

[64] Schmidt B, Horsley V. Unravelling hair follicle-adipocyte communication. Experimental Dermatology. 2012;**21**(11):827-830

[65] Jackson WM, Nesti LJ, Tuan RS. Mesenchymal stem cell therapy for attenuation of scar formation during wound healing. Stem Cell Research & Therapy. 2012;**3**(3):20

[66] Millán-Rivero JE et al. Silk fibroin scaffolds seeded with Wharton's jelly mesenchymal stem cells enhance re-epithelialization and reduce formation

of scar tissue after cutaneous wound healing. Stem Cell Research & Therapy. 2019;**10**(1):126

[67] Gentile P. New strategies in plastic surgery: Autologous adipose-derived mesenchymal stem cells contained in fat grafting improves symptomatic scars. FBL. 2021;**26**(8):255-257

[68] An Y-H et al. High-efficient production of adipose-derived stem cell (ADSC) Secretome through maturation process and its non-scarring wound healing applications. Frontiers in Bioengineering and Biotechnology. 2021;**9**:9

[69] Lukiswanto BS et al. Evaluation of wound healing potential of pomegranate (Punica granatum) whole fruit extract on skin burn wound in rats (Rattus norvegicus). Journal of Advanced Veterinary and Animal Research. 2019;**6**(2):202-207

[70] Efimova IO, et al. Treatment of burns All-Russian student scientific-practical conference with participation of pupils of 10-11 128 forms, in Student science - the first step and academic science. In: IOP Conference Series, Earth Environment Science. 2019;**346**:012057

[71] Zhang J et al. Immunosuppressive effects of mesenchymal stem cell transplantation in rat burn models. International Journal of Clinical and Experimental Pathology. 2015;**8**(5):5129-5136

[72] Chen Y-W et al. The effects of adipose-derived stem cell–differentiated adipocytes on skin burn wound healing in rats. Journal of Burn Care & Research. 2017;**38**(1):1-10

[73] Rangatchew F et al. Mesenchymal stem cell therapy of acute thermal burns: A systematic review of the effect on inflammation and wound healing. Burns. 2021;**47**(2):270-294

[74] Alapure BV et al. Accelerate healing of severe burn wounds by mouse bone marrow mesenchymal stem cell-seeded biodegradable hydrogel scaffold synthesized from arginine-based poly(ester amide) and chitosan. Stem Cells and Development. 2018;**27**(23):1605-1620

[75] Hacker S et al. Paracrine factors from irradiated peripheral blood mononuclear cells improve skin regeneration and angiogenesis in a porcine burn model. Scientific Reports. 2016;**6**:25168

[76] Kudinov VA et al. Antimicrobial and regenerative effects of placental multipotent mesenchymal stromal cell Secretome-based chitosan gel on infected burns in rats. Pharmaceuticals (Basel). 2021;**14**(12):17-18

Chapter 2

Scarless Wound Healing

Shalini Sanyal

Abstract

Wound healing is a complex, multiple-step mechanism and most lead to the development of scars, which may or may not affect the functional capability of the healed tissue. However, with the advanced healing techniques and our improved understanding of the wound-healing process, there has been some development towards limiting the scarification that develops as part of the process. This chapter will explore the major types of scar tissue as well as their development and complications arising from the same. With wound healing being a complex process, there have also been attempts towards modulating the wound environment to increase the rate of healing as well as limit the formation of scars. While there is no definitive procedure that can ascertain rapid, scar-free healing as yet, this chapter aims to explore both, the traditional and alternative techniques that are used (during or after the complete healing of the wound) to mitigate the development of scars.

Keywords: wound healing, keloid, hypertrophic scar, scarless healing, wound healing factors

1. Introduction

Scarless Wound healing is considered as the elusive *Holy Grail* of wound management [1]. While scars are considered as 'badges of honour' in some cultures and highly prized [2, 3]; in most scenarios, people prefer to avoid or minimise them as much as possible. And in some cases, formation of a 'scar' leads to functional impairment that hampers the quality of one's life—such as scars from abrasions on the ocular surface that lead to corneal opacity and hamper vision [4–8].

Wound healing is composed of three overlapping stages involving cellular and molecular processes that generally culminate into a fibrotic patch to 'repair' the wound with [3]. These 'scar tissues' have no hair follicles or sweat glands, and are inflexible and weaker than regular skin. They also limit movement and do not easily adapt to temperature changes [9].

Wound healing is a complex series of reactions primarily involving three distinct stages: *inflammation*, *proliferation* and *maturation* or remodelling of the tissue [10]. Each stage involves a complex series of interactions among the involved cells and their mediators (**Figure 1**).

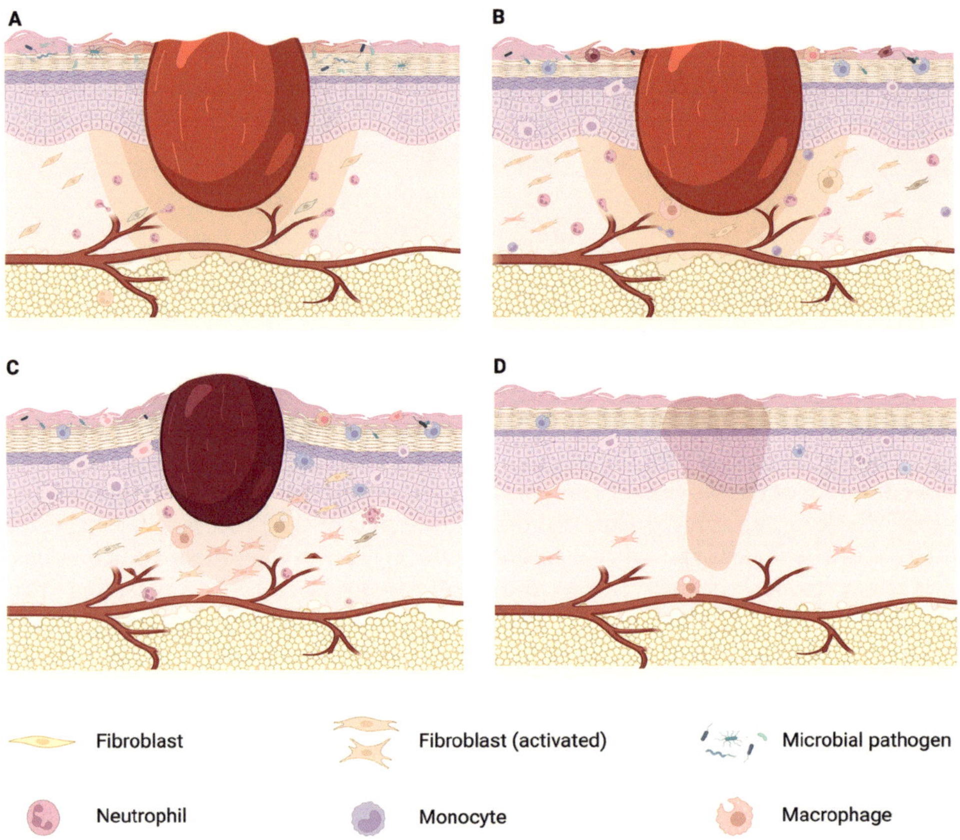

Figure 1.
Stages of wound healing- representative image indicating the four primary stages involved in wound healing since the inception of the injury (A), and the pathogens on the epidermal surface which may lead to opportunistic infections. The inflammation stage (B) when the scab is formed to staunch the bleeding and macrophages activated to combat pathogens. The injury leads to 'signals' that summon fibroblasts, macrophages, neutrophils and platelets to the site of the injury. The proliferation stage (C) when the arriving cells proliferate and re-structure the ECM. The maturation stage (D) when the wound contracts and leads to the development of a scar.

2. Steps involved in traditional wound healing

2.1 Inflammatory phase

The initial healing begins with the formation of a fibrin clot at the site of the wound that serves as a temporary extra-cellular matrix (ECM) and provides the necessary stimulus to summon inflammatory cells [11].

Characterised by haemostasis and inflammation, collagen exposure during injury leads to the activation of the intrinsic and extrinsic pathways of the clotting cascade, thereby initiating the inflammatory phase. Vasoconstrictors like thromboxane A2 and prostaglandin 2-α are immediately released, leading to the formation of a clot made of collagen, platelets, thrombin and fibronectin. The release of cytokines and growth factors initiates the inflammatory response and the fibrin clot serves as ECM for the arriving cascade of inflammatory cells (including neutrophils, monocytes, fibroblasts and endothelial cells) with the neutrophils being the first cells to arrive (**Figure 1A** and **B**). As these inflammatory regulators arrive, the signal released changes from vasoconstrictors (that aided in initial clot formation) to vasodilators to allow for the increased cellular traffic [10].

The presence of Interleukin (IL)-1, Tumour Necrosis factor (TNF)- α, Transforming Growth factor (TGF)-β, Platelet Factor-4 (PF-4) attract monocytes from nearby tissue and blood that convert into macrophages which in turn are essential for transitioning the wound from its initial inflammatory phase to the proliferative phase. Macrophage activation generally occurs between 2 and 4 days post injury and leads to angiogenesis (the formation of new blood vessels) and fibroplasia (growth of fibrous tissue). It also leads to the synthesis of nitric oxide that plays multiple roles including providing pain relief by serving as a partial agonist at opioid receptors, encouraging vasodilation and having anti-inflammatory effects [10]. Interestingly, nitric oxide is considered as a pro-inflammatory mediator that induces inflammation due to its overproduction in pathophysiological situations [10, 12].

2.2 Proliferation phase

The proliferation phase is another complex stage in wound healing that involve multiple simultaneous processes occurring at the site of the injury including (but not limited to) epithelialisation, angiogenesis, fibroplasia, granular tissue formation and collagen deposition (**Figure 1C**) [10, 11].

Epithelialisation, one of the early steps in wound repair occurs in one of two ways based on the severity of the wound:

Basement membrane intact—If the wound is shallow, leaving the basement membrane intact; epithelial cells migrate upwards in a normal pattern as epithelial progenitor cells remain undamaged. This type of injury allows the epidermis to be restored within 2–3 days.

Basement membrane damage—In case of deeper wounds where the basement membrane has been affected, the epithelial cells at the edges begin proliferation and sending out projections to aid in clot formation and re-establishment of protective barrier. This is followed by angiogenesis, which leads to endothelial cell migration and capillary formation, which allows granulation and tissue deposition due to the nutrient supply. The protective barrier formed by the epithelial cell projections from the edge of the wound plays crucial role in providing a protective role by preventing bacterial invasion and fluid loss.

Epithelialisation, while initially stimulated by inflammatory cytokines from the inflammatory phase of wound healing, leads to upregulation of keratinocyte growth factor (KGF) by the stimulation of IL-1 and TNF-α. KGF, in turn stimulates keratinocytes from wound-adjacent regions to migrate to the site of injury and proliferate as well as differentiate in the epidermis [10].

Granulation tissue formation is the final stage in the proliferation phase, characterised by activation of fibroblasts which in turn initialise collagen synthesis and turn into myofibroblasts that aid in wound contraction. Wound contraction, induced by the TGF-β1 that is secreted by macrophages, is primarily carried out by the fibroblasts present at the wound site (wound fibroblasts) that have less proliferative potential as compared to those at the periphery. Platelet-derived growth factor (PDGF) and epidermal growth factor (EGF) are the primary signals that drive the attraction of fibroblasts and their activation [10, 11].

This in turn leads to the synthesis of a provisional matrix that is made up of collagen type-III, glycosaminoglycans and fibronectin [9–11].

2.3 Maturation phase

The maturation phase is often deemed as the most important phase from a clinical perspective as it is characterised by collagen deposition (**Figure 1D**). Any issue with collagen deposition and deviation in the orderly networked fashion it is meant to take can lead to compromised wound strength. Conversely, excessive collagen deposition leads to the development of a hypertrophic or keloid scar [8, 9].

As the wound matures, the collagen that is initially thinner than that produced over uninjured skin changes to become thicker and organised along the wound such that they are organised around the regions that are under greater stress than their surroundings. It must be noted that the collagen in these granulation tissues that develop in wound regions has greater hydroxylation and glycosylation of lysine residues, making it different from those that are found in uninjured areas. While the tissue strength rarely returns to its pre-injury state, wound strength gradually increases over time with the region needing a minimum of 90 days to regain 80% of its original strength (this may be compared with its strength during the first week of wound healing which is only 3%) [10, 11].

3. Scarless wound healing

While scars are revered in some cultures, with elaborate rituals centred around developing aesthetically pleasing, elaborate scars, they are more commonly categorised as a cosmetic concern. Apart from aesthetic concerns, scars can also lead to reduced functionality and limit mobility. Furthermore, unsightly scars, particularly those on the face or other visible areas of the body; can often lead to crippling self-esteem issues and affect the quality of life of the effected individual. The United States of America alone has a $12 million industry targeted to reducing or limiting scars [8, 10].

Scarless wound healing as it occurs in nature is a rare phenomenon that is limited to specific scenarios.

3.1 Foetal wound healing

While wounds in the early mammalian gestational period heal without the formation of scars, wounds beyond that period form scars. It has been speculated that the early foetal wound healing occurs by a process resembling regeneration. While the exact mechanism is elusive, it is speculated that the characteristics that differentiate foetal skin at the tissue and cellular levels plays a role such as the decreased tensile strength [11].

A fascinating study by Wong et al. [13] has connected mechano-transduction with fibrosis through the focal adhesion kinase (FAK) pathway. It was observed that the extra cellular-related kinase (ERK) initiated the secretion of monocyte chemoattractant protein-1(MCP-1) in the FAK pathway is associated with multiple fibrotic disorders in humans. When components of the inflammatory FAK-ERK-MCP-1 pathways are inhibited, the development of scars is attenuated [13].

3.2 Oral mucosa

In the mammalian system, the oral mucosa demonstrates minimal scarring and is the closest model of regenerative healing. It is often described as a 'protected environment' for wound healing as the underlying mucosa in the oral cavity is protected from mechanical damage or infection from pathogens by hydrophilic viscoelastic gels that are formed by the salivary mucins [14]. Fascinatingly, they lose this property when transplanted [15].

Studies comparing the oral mucosa to the foetal wound healing environment have found similarities in the ECM with the mucosa revealing increased fibronectin, its splice variant ED-A and chondroitin sulphate as compared to the skin. Also, elastin levels were found to be higher in dermal cells, with those exhibiting greater differentiation property as opposed to the greater proliferative property demonstrated by the mucosa [16].

4. Difference between traditional and scarless wound healing

While not conclusive, studies have indicated that the mechanism of wound healing itself is different in the case of traditional wound healing and the scarless wound healing of early foetal cells (**Figure 2**). One of the primary differences being the niche and its composition itself. For instance, it has been observed that the early gestational cells modify their environmental, embryonic niche to promote regeneration during wound healing as a cell-intrinsic property [17]. However, late gestational cells are restricted to repetitive healing, in the sense that they are capable of modulating fibroblasts to increase proliferation and migration.

This is further confirmed by proteome analysis comparisons of foetal and adult fibroblasts which have revealed completely different patterns of protein expression such as the types of collagen that are more prevalent in scarless wound healing and wound healing with scar formation [11].

These findings were further supported by Siebert and his team [18], who had performed several histological and biochemical analyses on the healing of foetal wounds

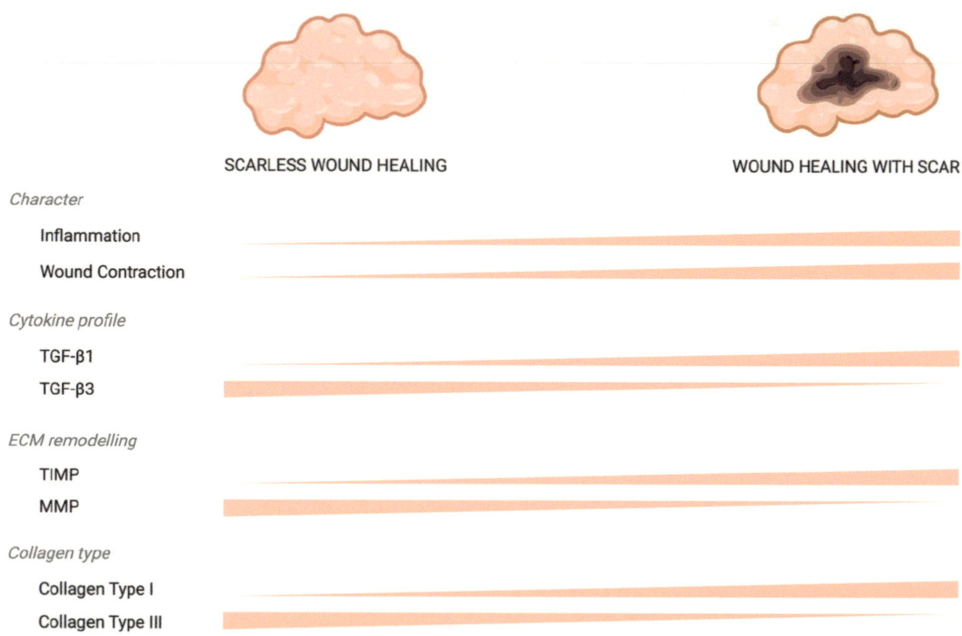

Figure 2.
Differences between scarless wound healing and traditional wound healing- representative image indicating the factors that influence traditional and scarless wound healing.

to determine how it differs from adult wound healing to lead to a scarless wound closure, and observed that the collagen (collagen type-I) that is identical to the one found in adult wound healing sites was minimal while it was abundant in a different type of collagen (collagen type-III). Additionally, the foetal wound matrix was also rich in hyaluronic acid that had earlier been associated with decreased scar-formation during post-natal wound closure [18]. This in turn, led to the development of a theory pertaining to a hyaluronic acid/collagen/protein complex with a highly efficient matrix reorganisation potential leading wound healing in the early foetal stage debunking the theory of 'true regeneration' wherein a completely new individual is formed from a small tissue/cell.

While the quantities of collagen deposited in foetal and in adult wounds are known to be different; it has been theorised that the collagen present in foetal wounds is more for 'structural' purposes than in the form of 'scar tissue' [18]. This is further supported by the deposition of glycosaminoglycans at the wound site which promotes the migration towards, differentiation and maturation of mesenchymal stem cells (MSCs) [18, 19].

Additionally, inflammation, that is the bedrock of adult wound healing, is absent in foetal wound healing. Thus, while epithelialisation occurs in foetal wound healing, the accompanying angiogenesis that is prevalent in adult injury repairing mechanisms is absent and, as already observed by Siebert and his team, has minimal, highly organised, deposition of (the same type of) collagen and is instead dominated by the presence of hyaluronic acid [18, 20–23].

It has been speculated that altering the levels of growth factors and their inhibitors might aide in replicating the scarless wound healing mechanisms in the adult system. To that end, Bone morphogenetic protein-2, hypoxia-inducible factor 1α (HIF-1α), decorin (a TGF-β modulator), α- and β-fibroblast growth factors, IL-6, and IL-8; as well as Tenascin, which is a large, extracellular matrix glycoprotein synthesised by fibroblasts during embryogenesis are currently being explored by various teams. It has been theorised that Tenascin, which is present in early foetal wounds might be the factor responsible for initiating the rapid cell-migration and re-epithelialisation that is characteristic of foetal wound healing [24, 25].

5. Factors involved in wound healing

Physiological responses as well as cellular functions influence wound healing, and interruptions at any stage enhance the chances of scar development.

5.1 Local factors

5.1.1 Ischemia

Inadequate supply of blood to any part of the body is termed as ischemia, and since wounds require multiple elements such as energy (in the form of adenosine triphosphate or ATP), glucose and oxygen; that are all borne by the blood to the site of the wound, ischemia affects wound healing dramatically. The rate of wound healing is significantly lower in cases of Hypoxia, which in turn may be triggered by ischemia [26].

Hypoxia leads to vasodilation and stimulates fibrin deposition which increases pro-inflammatory activity, capillary leak and neovascularisation. Pro-inflammatory property is stimulated by Tumour Necrosis Factor (TNF)-α, leading to apoptosis and affecting the collagen organisation of the injured tissue [26, 27].

Similarly, fibroblasts exposed to long periods of hypoxia may not involve in extra cellular matrix, thereby delaying wound healing/closure [27].

5.1.2 Oedema (edema)

Swelling that arises due to excess fluid trapped in the body's tissues is medically termed as an Oedema (/edema). This is most commonly associated with ischemia and severely delay wound healing as inflammatory response is delayed due to raised tissue pressure. This in turn compromises cellular function and lead to severe hypoxia or even cell death, thereby leading to necrosis and impairing wound healing [26].

5.1.3 Foreign bodies

Clinically, any object found in the wound, apart from its natural tissues is demarcated as a foreign body, the presence of which severely inhibits wound closure. This is primarily because foreign bodies prevent wound contraction and epithelialisation, thereby leading to the development of necrotic tissues. Unfortunately, necrotic tissues further prevent wound healing to the extent that *all* the necrotic tissue has to be removed before wound healing can commence [28].

'Foreign bodies', which may also indicate non-viable tissue; further complicate matters by serving as an asylum to bacteria and other pathogens.

5.1.4 Infection

Presence of bacteria or other pathogens at the site of the wound is termed as 'wound infection', and characterised by the one or more of the four cardinal signs of inflammation:

Rubor—the infected region might appear red,
Calor—the affected region might be warmer than the surrounding tissues,
Dolor—there might be increased pain and,
Tumour—or swelling.

A fascinating study by Robson and his team in 1997 [29] exhibited that bacterial counts exceeding 10^5 organisms per gram of tissue prevent wound closure to the extent that skin-graft replacement or even primary sutures failed to heal the wound. Similarly, presence of beta-haemolytic streptococcus will also inhibit wound healing. This is because endotoxins present in bacteria stimulate phagocytosis and the release of the enzyme collagenase that contributes to collagen degradation and destruction of the priory normal tissue that surrounds the site of injury [29, 30].

5.2 Systemic factors

Certain factors such as obesity, cardiovascular and respiratory disease etc. might affect an individuals' wound healing capacity and pre-dispose them to wound healing dysfunction [31, 32]. While wound healing is slower with age, it has been observed that those with co-morbidities also exhibit delayed healing which is indistinguishable from the delay caused due to the effects of age alone. This was confirmed with observations of improved healing ability in elderly female patients when they were prescribed/given topical oestrogen supplements [33, 34].

Although it is a prevalent belief that senior patients heal at a slower rate than their younger counterparts, it must also be acknowledged that older patients are more prone to co-morbidities which may interfere with wound healing. Fascinatingly, while longitudinal studies in animal models [35] support this theory, studies in humans have been inconclusive in the sense that dermal collagen deposition is equivalent in patients undergoing skin-grafting irrespective of age, however their re-epithelialisation rates are reduced [36]. While further research is needed to understand the consequences of age in wound repair, it has been speculated that it may be attributed to reduced availability of growth factors.

Some of the known chronic conditions that interfere with wound healing are listed below:

5.2.1 Diabetes mellitus

Increased serum glucose and hyperglycaemia related deleterious impact has been evidenced in cellular and molecular pathophysiology. For instance, sorbitol, a toxic by-product of glucose metabolism has been found to accumulate in tissues in case of hyperglycaemia and thereby involved in the renal, ocular as well as vascular complications commonly associated with diabetes. Additionally, collagen; which plays a vital role in wound healing mechanisms is more prevalent in its glycosylated form that is comparatively more resistant to enzymatic degradation and less soluble than normal protein product. These defects in collagen maturation led to decreased granulations and reduced collagen in granulation tissue, thereby hampering wound healing [37–39].

5.2.2 Hypothyroidism

Experimental studies have indicated that hypothyroidism leads to decreased collagen production and decreases tensile wound strength. These issues are further complicated by the co-morbidities that are often caused/present in hypothyroidism patients [40, 41].

5.3 Other factors influencing wound healing

5.3.1 Tissue perfusion

Tissue perfusion, which may be local due to external compression, or even systemic, when arising from alterations in circulatory volumes may lead to tissue hypoxia; which, as already noted earlier; interferes with wound healing [28].

5.3.2 Hypothermia

Hypothermia leads to peripheral vasoconstriction which in turn has an impact on cutaneous perfusion, thereby affecting wound healing [42, 43].

5.3.3 Debilitating pain

The pain stimuli may lead to the diffuse of an adrenergic discharge, which in turn is responsible for cutaneous vasoconstriction. Consequently, it has often been observed that proper pain control leads to improved wound healing [44, 45].

5.3.4 Major trauma

Severe trauma often results in hypo-volemic shock as a consequence of compromised cardiac functionality, thereby enhancing circulating cytokines as well as inflammatory mediators such as TNF- α and leading to anomalies in wound closure such as abnormalities in clotting [46, 47]. Thus, it is essential to maintain normo-volemic conditions as well as body temperature for proper wound management [31, 32, 46–48].

5.3.5 Septicaemia

Excessive secretion of pro-inflammatory mediators due to endotoxins is a critical part of systemic inflammation that leads to sepsis or septicaemia. Systemic inflammation has a hypo-inflammatory state characterised by monocyte deactivation and immunosuppression that compromises leukocytic activity and has inhibitory effect on wound healing.

Septicaemia also causes plasma and endothelial-related inflammatory modifications that impact coagulation and has been implicated in micro circulatory thrombosis that affects tissue perfusion and may even lead to fatalities due to associated multiple-organ failure [49, 50].

5.3.6 Nutrition

Wound healing is nutrition intensive as there is significant protein loss to maintain normoglycaemia, thus patients' bodies consume body stores of fats and protein during this process and it is essential to maintain proper nutrition to ensure proper wound remediation. While glucose is the main fuel for wound healing, protein malnutrition, especially deficiencies of specific amino acids such as arginine and methionine have been associated with compromised wound repair due to prolonged inflammation stage, disruption of matrix deposition, cellular proliferation, and angiogenesis. Decreased rates of collagen deposition during dermal wound healing have also been associated with malnutrition [51–53].

5.3.7 Smoking

The detrimental impact of smoking on wound healing has been elegantly demonstrated nearly four decades ago by Mosely and Finseth in 1977 and re-assessed by Goldminz and Bennet in 1991 [54, 55].

The impact of smoking is multi-factorial: Nicotine has vasoconstriction properties that additionally decrease the proliferation of erythrocytes, macrophages, and fibroblasts - different cells that play indispensable role in wound-closure. Additionally, carbon monoxide severely limits the oxygen-carrying capacity of haemoglobin (thereby inducing tissue hypoxia) while simultaneously increasing platelet aggression and viscosity of blood and interfering with collagen deposition and prostacyclin formation [56].

5.3.8 Corticosteroids

Anti-inflammatory steroids are known to inhibit cell development. Additionally, they are known to decrease inflammatory response. Macrophage response to chemotactic signals as well as phagocytosis by polymorphonuclear neutrophils and macrophages is negatively affected by the stabilising impact of steroids on lysosomes. Epithelialisation, which is a critical step in wound healing is inhibited by glucocorticoids such as hydrocorticosterone [57].

Things are further complicated by the low-secretory state induced by corticosteroids due to their effect on the endoplasmic reticulum. Thus, risk of wound dehiscence is consequently enhanced due to the reduced deposition of collagen [58].

5.4 Genetic syndromes associated with abnormal wound healing

5.4.1 Cutis laxa

Defective elastin fibres as evidenced in cutis laxa- an acquired or congenital disorder, impacts wound healing. Characterised by skin that is loose (lax), wrinkled, sagging, and lacking elasticity (inelastic). The inelastic skin returns to place abnormally slowly when stretched. The skin around the face, arms and legs etc. are the predominantly affected parts and give patients a prematurely-aged appearance [59].

5.4.2 Ehlers-Danlos Syndrome

Characterised by deficit in collagen metabolism, it is a group of connective tissue abnormalities that lead to defects in the inherent strength, elasticity, integrity, and healing properties of the tissues [60, 61]. Even mild injury in Ehlers-Danlos patients may lead to severe bruising and the development of wide, 'open' wounds due to the delayed healing [27, 60, 61].

5.4.3 Osteogenesis imperfecta

An inheritable disorder of connective tissue, clinical features of this condition include bone fragility, neonatal dwarfism, deformities of the long bones, scoliosis, ligamentous laxity, blue sclerae, defective dentinogenesis, and deafness. While there are four major forms, mutations in the genes that encode type I collagen is a common trait that result in the formation of wide scars [27, 62].

6. Adjuncts to wound healing

6.1 Bioengineered skin

One of the best examples of Bioengineered skin is the *Apligraf:* a bi-layered bioengineered skin substitute composed of 'bovine type I collagen matrix populated with human male neonatal fibroblasts and an epidermal sheet derived from male neonatal epidermal keratinocytes', that has been approved by the US Food and Drug Administration (FDA) for cases where standard wound care has failed to treat ulcers. The mechanism that initiates wound healing by the use of these bioengineered products is still being researched but it has been revealed that these cells grow and proliferate, and produce growth factors, collagens, and extracellular matrix proteins, all of which are known to positively stimulate re-epithelialisation, formation of granulation tissue, angiogenesis, and neutrophil and monocyte chemotaxis. Thus, these have the potential to provide a potent cellular remedy and adaptable response in acute and chronic wounds [63].

6.2 Electrostimulation

While the first exploration of electrical current in skin was described as early as 1860 by DuBois-Reymond; the fact that wounds treated with electrostimulation had a positive potential compared with the surrounding skin was only confirmed in 1945 [64]. It is believed that electro-stimulations aides in wound healing by accelerate the wound-healing process by tissue increasing the migration of vital cells to the site of injury i.e., neutrophils, macrophages [64–66] and fibroblasts [67–69] by imitating the natural electrical current that occurs in skin when it is injured and thereby accelerates the healing process [70–72].

6.3 Hydrotherapy

One of the oldest adjunct treatment modalities that is still practiced today is the Whirlpool therapy that accelerates wound healing by wound debridation, warming the wounded tissue, and providing buoyancy and gentle limb resistance for physical therapy [73]. However, despite their prevalence, Whirlpool treatments have been subject to disapprobation in recent years because of the enhanced risk of nosocomial contamination and transmission of virulent infections associated with them [74–78]. These days, modified forms of the whirlpool therapy, such as the pulsed lavage and the *VersaJet* are more popular as they provide the benefits of hydrotherapy without the associated collateral trauma of traditional methods [78, 79].

6.4 Hyperbaric oxygen

Although hyperbaric oxygen treatment for narcotising soft-tissue infections has not always been successful, the treatment has been found to be beneficial for a variety of conditions including amputations, [80] osteoradionecrosis, [81, 82] surgical flaps, and skin grafts [81, 83, 84]. However, studies have failed to statistically corroborate significant outcomes regarding differences with respect to mortality rates and length of hospitalisation [82, 85–88]. Benefits are suspected to primarily originate from the benefits of the increased nitric oxide levels that are developed by increasing oxygen pressure as nitric oxide is known to be vital for wound-healing [88].

Fascinatingly, in a study using an ischemic rabbit ear model, hyperbaric oxygen therapy was used in combination with PDGF or TGF-β1 and was found to have a synergistic effect that completely reversed the healing issues caused by ischemia [89].

7. Scars

A scar refers to a growth of tissue marking the spot where skin has healed after an injury. And while scars are used for body modification and 'body art' in some cultures, most take it to be a sign of someone surviving a catastrophic event or a debilitating disease [2, 3]. They are predominantly of two types:

Keloid scar: these are scars that have overgrown their boundaries with large collagen bundles in their midst and being limited in macrophage content but abundant in eosinophils, mast cells, plasma cells and lymphocytes [90–92].

Hypertrophic scar: Hypertrophic scars do not have collagen bundles, but nodules of α-smooth muscle actin–staining myofibroblasts that contain cells and collagen [93].

7.1 Treatment

While multiple treatments are promoted/suggested to minimise the development of scars, none have been proven to be completely effective. Keloid scars especially are difficult to treat because of their high recurrence rate.

Common scar-treatment modalities include:

Excision: While one of the more popular treatments, excision alone (especially in the case of keloid scars) has been proven to have a high recurrence rate ranging from 45 to 93 percent.

However, when coupled with other treatment practices, excision has been known to lower recurrence risk [90–92].

Laser excision: Lasers cause a range of specific thermal tissue reactions in a dry and bloodless environment and was initially utilised in the hopes of reducing scar formation, however they are not frequently used in the present date owing to their high recurrence levels [94, 95].

Radiation Therapy: Radiations have been used in the eradication of this benign lesion since the 1960s; however current concerns regarding the safety of patients - due to increased risks of developing skin cancer; have limited the perpetuity of this therapeutic modality [94].

Steroids: While steroids themselves are known to interfere with wound healing, they are used in initial treatment of scars as they suppress the inflammatory stage [95, 96].

Cryo-surgery: Traditionally, cryotherapy have been used for managing hypertrophic scars and keloids, with pre-treatment and post-treatment histological analyses indicating significant improvement in scar organisation after needle cryosurgery [93].

Interferon: IFN-α-2b normalises the collagen and glycosaminoglycan of the keloid, thereby interfering with the fibroblasts collagen synthesis [97]. Complications with IFN-α-2b include flu-like symptoms, headache, fever, and myalgias.

However, till date; prevention is the best keloid therapy.

8. Problems with current strategies to reduce scarring

Current strategies for non-surgical therapy for the treatment of keloids and hypertrophic scars include topical therapy and intra-lesional injections of corticosteroids. While literature has reported a success rate ranging between 50 to 100 percent; these methods have also been associated with hypopigmentation, dermal atrophy, telangiectasia, widening of the scar, and delayed wound healing [98].

8.1 Prospects being explored to promote scarless-wound healing

8.1.1 Dermal stem cells

While advances in genetic lineage-tracing technologies, cellular assays, and imaging techniques have revealed important stem and progenitor cell reservoirs in the inter- follicular epidermis, the eccrine sweat glands, and the hair follicle; given excisional wounds develop into areas lacking sweat and sebaceous glands as well as hair follicles, further understanding of stem and progenitor cells would aide in achieving the ultimate goal of scarless wound healing following injury [99].

8.1.2 Interfollicular epidermis

During wound healing of the interfollicular epidermis, a population of 'slow-cycling cells' is suspected to demonstrate autocrine regulation [100, 101] until mobilised by a wound healing signal. The cell division frequency of these slow-cycling cells increases following a wound, which provides excess daughter cells that help in repairing the damage. Further, injured epithelium has been known to demonstrate behavioural plasticity with progenitors capable of reverting to multipotent states and multipotent cells differentiating to fill unipotent roles, [102, 103]. Exploring these avenues may eventually allow us to discover the hitherto undiscovered processes that would allow regenerative wound healing with negligible scarring.

8.1.3 Sweat glands

Loss of sweat glands in burn patients remains an unsolved problem. However, recent studies of these epidermal appendages have identified gland-specific progenitors, [104] and indicated the role of these cells in development, homeostasis, and wound repair [104–107].

8.1.4 Hair follicles

Mammalian hair follicles are known to house numerous progenitor cell populations that might play indispensable role in the repair of injured dermal tissue and exploring them might give us ground breaking insight towards achieving scarless wound healing [106, 108, 109].

8.2 Future prospects for scarless wound healing

8.2.1 Gene targets

Genes involved in the scarring response that influence fibrosis by regulating collagen production and degradation have been identified. If they can be safely down-regulated by emerging medical techniques, they may provide the answer to the mechanisms involved in the minimisation of scars [110].

8.2.2 Dermal substitutes

Wound coverage as well as a matrix to encourage engraftment and proliferation of endogenous cells and the function of transplanted cells is provided by dermal substitutes. These are typically acellular in nature, but biocompatible and morphologically similar to natural tissue structure with mechanical properties similar to host dermal tissue [111].

8.2.3 Mechanical offloading

Another alternative to limiting fibrosis in cutaneous injuries is mechanical offloading since mechanical tension plays a significant role in the development of fibrosis, activating numerous mechano-responsive signalling pathways such as the focal adhesion kinase (FAK) [112, 113].

8.3 Cellular targets for scarless wound healing

Identification of populations of cells contributing to scar formation allows us to explore options that reduce these specific cell populations during wound healing, thereby minimising scarification.

For instance, Dulauroy and team (2012) successfully distinguished a pro- inflammatory subset of perivascular cells that are activated upon acute injury in muscle and dermis by transient expression of a disintegrin and metalloprotease (ADAM12) [114]. Knocking down ADAM12 expression or ablating these cells was shown to decrease fibrosis and resulting scar formation.

This has been concordant with the findings of Rinkevich et al. [115] who found that fibroblasts originating from En1-lineages were the main culprits in the cutaneous scarring. These cells majorly contribute to scar formation in connective tissue.

Selective abrogation of the En1-fibroblast lineage with diprotin A by accompanying CD26 (also known as dipeptidyl peptidase-4, DPP4) surface marker has also been found to reduce cutaneous scarring without compromising the integrity of the healed tissue [115].

The ability of DPP4 inhibitors to curb the fibrogenic phenotypes of keloid-derived fibroblasts and normal fibroblasts have been further verified through various *in vivo* experiments. Observed decrease in collagen production and TGF-β1 expression have also been found to be enabled by underlying mechanisms involving the pro-fibrotic pp38 and pERK1/2 pathways [116].

Further, Myofibroblasts have been identified as the key players in the standard wound healing response, as they contribute to wound contraction and ECM production [117], making them ideal targets for reducing scar formation [118]. However, during the maturation phase of normal wound healing, the majority of these cells undergo apoptosis [119]. Thus, reversal of the myofibroblast phenotype might also help in decreasing this cell population [120, 121].

Unfortunately, like fibroblasts, myofibroblasts (or myofibroblast-like cells) also form a functionally heterogeneous population with potential precursors including fibroblasts, mesenchymal stem cells (MSCs), smooth muscle cells, endothelial cells, and fibrocytes [122]. Although it is still being determined whether fibroblasts and adipocytes share a common progenitor, Schmidt and Horsley [123] have demonstrated that dermal adipocytes are essential for fibroblast recruitment during wound healing mechanisms. Experimental interventions with direct and indirect targeting at both populations have been demonstrated to be responsible for scar formation.

Interestingly, Desai and his team [120] have found indications that the myofibroblast differentiation process is not terminal with basic fibroblast growth factor (bFGF) functioning as a phenotypic reversing agent as it led to diminishing expression of α-Smooth Muscle Actin (SMA), collagen I, and fibronectin, and a loss of focal adhesions and stress fibres being inversely co-related with tenascin-C and vimentin upregulation, in agreement with a more fibroblast-like phenotype [120]. These findings are in tune Rinella et al. [124] work that indicate that extracorporeal shockwaves (ESW), which cause myofibroblast precursors to differentiate into more fibroblast-like cells with lower contractility and higher migration potential, simultaneously reducing α-SMA and type I collagen expression may play a significant role in scar reduction.

8.4 Stem cells

Stem cells are known to modulate the wound environment and improve healing by reducing inflammation [125–127]. A recent study by Li et al. [128] has demonstrated the potential benefits of conditioned media from umbilical cord (UC)-MSC cultures wherein, dermal fibroblasts under the paracrine influence exhibit characteristics similar to those of foetal fibroblasts: low myofibroblast forming capacity, decreased TGF-β1/TGF-β3 ratio, as well as increased expression of enzymes (matrix metalloproteinases or MMPs) involved in ECM remodelling [128]. Other *in vitro* studies have indicated that human amniotic-fluid-derived MSC-conditioned media also has the potential to inhibit the pro-fibrotic actions of TGF-β1 and even reverse the myofibroblast phenotype to a fibroblast-like state. Conditioned media from ASCs produced similar results, but to a lesser extent [129]. However, this enhanced healing mechanism may not always translate to reduced scar-formation as these experiments do not have similar results when performed *in vivo* [130, 131]. Additionally, ethical, legal as well as practical barriers associated with stem-cell- based therapies might restrict their use in the exploration of scarless wound healing [132].

8.5 Wnt and regeneration

Various signalling pathways, such as the canonical Wnt/β-catenin have been implicated in the expression of foetal mouse keratinocytes and fibroblasts at embryonic day (E)16 and E18 time points, straddling the transition from scarless to scar-forming repair [117, 133]. While Wnt signalling is a key component of embryological development, it is also involved in various wound healing mechanisms with the canonical Wnt pathway being the most relevant [134]. In this pathway, the Wnt-ligand binding at the cell surface leads to cytoplasmic β-catenin accumulation, which subsequently translocates to the nucleus to exert its effects as a transcriptional co-activator [135].

Additionally, a link between TGF-β and the canonical Wnt/β-catenin pathway has been observed in the case of fibrosis with analysis of pathological scars (hypertrophic scars and keloids) revealing upregulated Wnt signalling secondary to TGF-β [136]. β-catenin levels have been shown to double during the proliferative phase in normal wound healing (with scarring) as well [137]. Keloids in humans also display Wnt-3a over-expression by inducing fibroblasts of endothelial origin to transition to mesenchymal cells that leads to collagen accumulation [138].

8.6 MicroRNA

MicroRNA (miRNA) gene therapies are a more recent avenue for potential therapeutic interventions as these molecules exert an inhibitory role on mRNA transcription within eukaryotic cells, effectively silencing genes at a post- transcriptional level [139]. Comparison of genome-wide miRNA expression between mid-gestational (E16) and late-gestational (E19) mouse skin discovered global repression of these molecules at the earlier time point where scarless healing is the norm [140]. miR-34 family have been established as potential candidates for scarless wound healing in human foetal keratinocytes, however; expression of these miRNAs was found to be significantly lower as gestation progressed [103].

Regenerative wound healing using miRNAs has been explored to reduce scarification [141–143]. For instance, miR-145 has been found at three times its normal levels in hypertrophic scars and pro-fibrotic TGF-β1-induced myofibroblasts. However, with the help of a commercial inhibitor of miR-145, Gras et al. (2015) were able to significantly decrease type I collagen expression, TGF-β1 secretion, and contractility in skin myofibroblasts [144].

Similarly, miRNAs have been combined with biomimetic scaffolds to enhance wound healing, and furthering their clinical potential [145]. Future *in vivo* studies will hopefully enumerate the clinical potential for other miRNA-based therapies.

9. Conclusions

Our current understanding of wound healing and cell subpopulations within the skin has allowed us to develop scar-reducing therapies, however, they are not as effective as needed to make them the mainstay of available wound healing modalities. While research regarding this elusive therapeutic modality is underway, successful scarless wound healing would require not only an understanding of signalling molecules and growth factors but also a thorough understanding of lineage-specific cellular origin and function during both foetal and adult stages.

Acknowledgements

I would sincerely like to thank Priya Ashrit and Dr. Shweta Sharma for their assistance and encouragement during the preparation of this chapter. I also acknowledge the kind aid of Mr. Subhasis Bhattacharjee in the design of the images that have been used in this chapter.

Conflict of interest

The author declares that there is no conflict of interest.

List of abbreviations/acronyms

ADAM	a disintegrin and metalloprotease
ASC	acellular stem cell (bioengineered cells)
ATP	adenosine triphosphate
ECM	extra-cellular matrix
ERK	extra-cellular related kinase
ESW	extracorporeal shockwaves
FAK	focal adhesion kinase
FDA	Food and Drug Administration (of the USA)
HIF	hypoxia inducible factor
IFN	interferon
IL	interleukin
KGF	keratinocyte growth factor
MCP	monocyte chemo-attractant protein
MMPs	matrix metalloproteinases
MSCs	mesenchymal stem cells
PDGF	platelet derived growth factor

PF	platelet factor
SMA	smooth muscle actin
TGF	transforming growth factor
TNF	tumour necrosis factor
bFGF	basic fibroblast growth factor

Author details

Shalini Sanyal
Laboratory of Self-assembled Biomaterials and Translational Science, Institute for Stem Cell Science and Regenerative Medicine, Bengaluru, Karnataka, India

*Address all correspondence to: sanyal.shalini@gmail.com

References

[1] Rodrigues AD, editor. Scarless Wound Healing. Florida, United States: CRC Press; 2000

[2] Covino DC. Amending the Abject Body: Aesthetic Makeovers in Medicine and Culture. Illustrated. Research foundation for the State University of New York: SUNY Press; 2012

[3] Beswick C, Coombs K. More Than Skin Deep: Managing the Psychological Impact of Scars. Scar Prevention and Treatment; 2018

[4] Sanyal S, Law A, Law S. Chronic pesticide exposure and consequential keratectasia & corneal neovascularisation. Experimental Eye Research. 2017;**164**:1-7

[5] Sanyal S, Law S. Chronic pesticide exposure induced aberrant Notch signalling along the visual pathway in a murine model. Environmental Pollution. 2021;**282**:117077

[6] Sanyal S, Law S. Ocular surface and chronic pesticide exposure: Evaluating the alterations in corneal cellular turnover concerning cell cycle and apoptosis. Experimental Eye Research. 2019;**178**:122-132

[7] Sanyal S, Das P, Law S. Effect of chronic pesticide exposure on murine cornea: A histopathological, cytological and flow cytometric approach to study ocular damage by xenobiotics. Cell Biology and Toxicology. 2016;**32**(1):7-22

[8] El Ayadi A, Jay JW, Prasai A. Current approaches targeting the wound healing phases to attenuate fibrosis and scarring. International Journal of Molecular Science. 2020;**21**(3):1105

[9] Broek LJ, Limandjaja GC, Niessen FB, Gibbs S. Human hypertrophic and keloid scar models: Principles, limitations and future challenges from a tissue engineering perspective. Experiment in Dermatology. 2014;**23**(6):382-386

[10] Broughton G, Janis JE, Attinger CE. Wound healing: An overview. Plastic and Reconstructive Surgery. 2006;**117**:1-32

[11] Walmsley GG, Maan ZN, Wong VW, Duscher D, Hu MS, Zielins ER, et al. Scarless wound healing. Plastic and Reconstructive Surgery. 2015;**135**(3):907-917

[12] Witte MB, Barbul A. Role of nitric oxide in wound repair. American Journal of Surgery. Apr 2002;**183**(4):406-412

[13] Wong VW, Rustad KC, Akaishi S, Sorkin M, Glotzbach JP, Januszyk M, et al. Focal adhesion kinase links mechanical force to skin fibrosis via inflammatory signaling. Nature Medicine. 2012;**18**(1):148-152

[14] Hof W, Veerman ECI, Nieuw Amerongen A V., Ligtenberg AJM. Antimicrobial defense systems in saliva. 2014;**24**:40-51

[15] Longaker MT, Whitby DJ, Ferguson MWJ, Lorenz HP, Harrison MR, Adzick NS. Adult skin wounds in the fetal environment heal with scar formation. Annals of Surgery. 1994;**219**(1):65-72

[16] Glim JE, Everts V, Niessen FB, Ulrich MM, Beelen RHJ. Extracellular matrix components of oral mucosa differ from skin and resemble that of foetal skin. Archives of Oral Biology. 2014;**59**(10):1048-1055

[17] Ho S, Marçal H, John L, Foster R. Towards Scarless Wound Healing: A Comparison of Protein Expression between Human, Adult and Foetal Fibroblasts. 2014. Available from: http://dx.doi.org/10.1155/2014/676493

[18] Siebert JW, Burd AR, McCarthy JG, Weinzweig J, Ehrlich HP. Fetal wound healing: A biochemical study of scarless healing. Plastic and Reconstructive Surgery. 1990;**85**(4):495-504

[19] Whitby DJ, Ferguson MWJ. Immunohistochemical localization of growth factors in fetal wound healing. Developmental Biology. 1991;**147**(1):207-215

[20] Longaker MT, Scott Adzick N, Hall JL, Stair SE, Crombleholme TM, Duncan BW, et al. Studies in fetal wound healing, VII. Fetal wound healing may be modulated by hyaluronic acid stimulating activity in amniotic fluid. Journal of Pediatric Surgery. 1990;**25**(4):430-433

[21] Longaker MT, Harrison MR, Crombleholme TM, Langer JC, Decker M, Verrier ED, et al. Studies in fetal wound healing: I. A factor in fetal serum that stimulates deposition of hyaluronic acid. Journal of Pediatric Surgery. 1989;**24**(8):789-792

[22] Longaker MT, Whitby DJ, Adzick NS, Crombleholme TM, Langer JC, Duncan BW, et al. Studies in fetal wound healing VI. Second and early third trimester fetal wounds demonstrate rapid collagen deposition without scar formation. Journal of Pediatric Surgery. 1990;**25**(1):63-69

[23] Bruce A, Diegelmann RF, Krummel TM, Cohen K. scarless wound healing in the mammalian fetus. Surgery, Gynecology & Obstetrics. 1992;**174**:441-450

[24] Whitby DJ, Longaker MT, Harrison MR, Adzick NS, Ferguson MW. Rapid epithelialisation of fetal wounds is associated with the early deposition of tenascin. Journal of Cell Science. 1991;**99**(3):583-586

[25] Luomanen M, Virtanen I. Distribution of tenascin in healing incision, excision and laser wounds. Journal of Oral Pathology & Medicine. 1993;**22**(1):41-45

[26] Senel O, Cetinkale O, Ozbay G, Ahçioğlu F, Bulan R. Oxygen free radicals impair wound healing in ischemic rat skin. Annals of Plastic Surgery. 1997;**39**(5):516-523

[27] Steinbrech DS, Longaker MT, Mehrara BJ, Saadeh PB, Chin GS, Gerrets RP, et al. Fibroblast response to hypoxia: The relationship between angiogenesis and matrix regulation. The Journal of Surgical Research. 1999;**84**(2):127-133

[28] Kadota Y, Nishida K, Hashizume K, Nasu Y, Nakahara R, Kanazawa T, et al. Risk factors for surgical site infection and delayed wound healing after orthopedic surgery in rheumatoid arthritis patients. Modern Rheumatology. 2016;**26**(1):68-74

[29] Robson MC. Wound infection: A failure of wound healing caused by an imbalance of bacteria. The Surgical Clinics of North America. 1997;**77**(3):637-650

[30] Bang RL, Gang RK, Sanyal SC, Mokaddas EM, Lari AR. Beta-haemolytic Streptococcus infection in burns. Burns. 1999;**25**(3):242-246

[31] Riou J-PA, Cohen JR, Johnson H. Factors influencing wound dehiscence. American Journal of Surgery. 1992;**163**(3):324-330

[32] Lingen MW, M. Role of leukocytes and endothelial cells in the development

of angiogenesis in inflammation and wound healing. Archives of Pathology & Laboratory Medicine. 2001;**125**(67):67-71

[33] Al-Attar A, Mess S, Thomassen JM, Kauffman CL, Davison SP. Keloid pathogenesis and treatment. Plastic and Reconstructive Surgery. 2006;**117**(1):286-300

[34] Ashcroft GS, Greenwell-Wild T, Horan MA, Wahl SM, Ferguson MWJ. Topical estrogen accelerates cutaneous wound healing in aged humans associated with an altered inflammatory response. The American Journal of Pathology. 1999;**155**(4):1137-1146

[35] Bruce SA, Deamond SF. Longitudinal study of in vivo wound repair and in vitro cellular senescence of dermal fibroblasts. Experimental Gerontology. 1991;**26**(1):17-27

[36] Freedland M, Karmiol S, Rodriguez J, Normolle D, Smith D, Garner W. Fibroblast responses to cytokines are maintained during aging. Annals of Plastic Surgery. 1995;**35**(3):290-296

[37] Bucalo B, Eaglstein WH, Falanga V. Inhibition of cell proliferation by chronic wound fluid. Wound Repair and Regeneration. 1993;**1**(3):181-186

[38] He Z, King GL. Microvascular complications of diabetes. Endocrinology and Metabolism Clinics of North America. 2004;**33**(1):215-238

[39] Chow LWC, Loo WTY, Yuen K-Y, Cheng C. The study of cytokine dynamics at the operation site after mastectomy. Wound Repair and Regeneration. 2003;**11**(5):326-330

[40] Kowalewski K, Yong S. Hydroxyproline in healing dermal wounds of normal and hypothyroid rats. Acta Endocrinologica. 1967;**54**(1):1-7

[41] Lennox J, Johnston ID. The effect of thyroid status on nitrogen balance and the rate of wound healing after injury in rats. The British Journal of Surgery. 1973;**60**(4):309

[42] Armstrong SR, Roberts BK, Aronsohn M. Perioperative hypothermia. Journal of Veterinary Emergency and Critical Care. 2005;**15**(1):32-37

[43] Esclamado RM, Damiano GA, Cummings CW. Effect of local hypothermia on early wound repair. Archives of Otolaryngology–Head & Neck Surgery. 1990;**116**(7):803-808

[44] Woo KY. Exploring the effects of pain and stress on wound healing. Advances in Skin & Wound Care. 2012;**25**(1):38-44

[45] Widgerow AD, Kalaria S. Pain mediators and wound healing—establishing the connection. Burns. 2012;**38**(7):951-959

[46] Schmidt GH, Drucker WR. Effect of hemorrhagic shock on wound healing in rats and guinea pigs. The Journal of Surgical Research. 1967;7(11):513-519

[47] Jurkiewicz MJ, Garrett LP. Studies on the influence of anemia on wound healing. Plastic and Reconstructive Surgery. 1964;**34**(1):109

[48] Gando S, Nanzaki S, Kemmotsu O. Disseminated intravascular coagulation and sustained systemic inflammatory response syndrome predict organ dysfunctions after trauma. Annals of Surgery. 1999;**229**(1):121-127

[49] Rico RM, Ripamonti R, Burns AL, Gamelli RL, DiPietro LA. The effect of

sepsis on wound healing. The Journal of Surgical Research. 2002;**102**(2):193-197

[50] Hardaway RM. A review of septic shock. The American Surgeon. 2000;**66**(1):22-29

[51] Gore D, Wolf S, Herndon D, Wolfe R. Relative influence of glucose and insulin on peripheral amino acid metabolism in severely burned patients. Journal of Parenteral and Enteral Nutrition. 2002;**26**(5):271-277

[52] Ruberg RL. Role of nutrition in wound healing. The Surgical Clinics of North America. 1984;**64**(4):705-714

[53] Haydock DA, Hill GL. Impaired wound healing in surgical patients with varying degrees of malnutrition. Journal of Parenteral and Enteral Nutrition. 1986;**10**(6):550-554

[54] Mosely LH, Finseth F. Cigarette smoking: Impairment of digital blood flow and wound healing in the hand. Hand. 1977;**9**(2):97-101

[55] Goldminz D. Cigarette smoking and flap and full-thickness graft necrosis. Archieves in Dermatology. 1991;**127**:1012

[56] Goldman B. Caffeine may counter systemic inflammation. Stanford Medicine. 2017;**23**:1-6

[57] Brauchle M, Fässler R, Werner S. Suppression of keratinocyte growth factor expression by glucocorticoids in vitro and during wound healing. The Journal of Investigative Dermatology. 1995;**105**(4):579-584

[58] Beck E, Duckert F, Ernst M. The influence of fibrin stabilizing factor on the growth of fibroblats in vitro and wound healing. Thrombosis and Haemostasis. 1961;**06**(03):485-491

[59] Berk DR, Bentley DD, Bayliss SJ, Lind A, Urban Z. Cutis laxa: A review. Journal of the American Academy of Dermatology. 2012;**66**(5):842.e1-842.e17

[60] Kumar P, Sethi N, Friji MT, Poornima S. Wound healing and skin grafting in Ehlers-Danlos syndrome. Plastic and Reconstructive Surgery. 2010;**126**(4):214e-215e

[61] Freeman LJ, Hegreberg GA, Robinette JD. Cutaneous wound healing in Ehlers-Danlos syndrome. Veterinary Surgery. 1989;**18**(2):88-96

[62] Wong RS, Follis FM, Shively BK, Wernly JA. Osteogenesis imperfecta and cardiovascular diseases. The Annals of Thoracic Surgery. 1995;**60**(5):1439-1443

[63] Jimenez PA, Jimenez SE. Tissue and cellular approaches to wound repair. American Journal of Surgery. 2004;**187**(5):S56-S64

[64] Eberhardt A, Szczypiorski P, Korytowski G. Effect of transcutaneous electrostimulation on the cell composition of skin exudate. Acta Physiological Polish. 1986;**37**(1):41-46

[65] K. F. Studies of galvanotaxis of leukocytes. Medical Journal of Osaka University. 1953;**4**:195-208

[66] Orida N, Feldman JD. Directional protrusive pseudopodial activity and motility in macrophages induced by extracellular electric fields. Cell Motility. 1982;**2**(3):243-255

[67] Cruz NI, Bayrón FE, Suárez AJ. Accelerated healing of full-thickness burns by the use of high-voltage pulsed galvanic stimulation in the pig. Annals of Plastic Surgery. 1989;**23**(1):49-55

[68] Alvarez OM, Mertz PM, Smerbeck RV, Eaglstein WH. The healing

of superficial skin wounds is stimulated by external electrical current. The Journal of Investigative Dermatology. 1983;**81**(2):144-148

[69] Bourguignon GJ, Bourguignon LYW. Electric stimulation of protein and DNA synthesis in human fibroblasts. The FASEB Journal. 1987;**1**(5):398-402

[70] Barker AT, Jaffe LF, Vanable JW. The glabrous epidermis of cavies contains a powerful battery. American Journal of Physiological Integrated Composite Physiology. 1982;**242**(3):R358-R366

[71] Foulds IS, Barker AT. Human skin battery potentials and their possible role in wound healing. The British Journal of Dermatology. 1983;**109**(5):515-522

[72] Barnes TC. Healing rate of human skin determined by measurement of the electrical potential of experimental abrasions. American Journal of Surgery. 1945;**69**(1):82-88

[73] Hess CL, Howard MA, Attinger CE. A review of mechanical adjuncts in wound healing: Hydrotherapy, ultrasound, negative pressure therapy, hyperbaric oxygen, and Electrostimulation. Annals of Plastic Surgery. 2003;**51**(2):210-218

[74] Meldrum R. Survey of Staphylococcus aureus contamination in a hospital's spa and hydrotherapy pools. Communicative Diseases in Public Health. 2001;**4**(3):205-208

[75] Chinn RYW, Sehulster L. Guidelines for environmental infection control in health-care facilities : Recommendations of CDC and Healthcare Infection Control Practices Advisory Committee (HICPAC) [Internet]. (U.S.) HICPAC, Engineering AS for H, (U.S.) C for DC and P, Promotion. NC for ID (U. S). D of HQ, editors. U.S. Department of Health and Human Services, Centers for Disease Control and Prevention; printed by the American Society for Healthcare Engineering of the American Hospital Association; 2003. Available from: https://stacks.cdc.gov/view/cdc/11303

[76] Simor AE, Lee M, Vearncombe M, Jones-Paul L, Barry C, Gomez M, et al. An outbreak due to multiresistant *Acinetobacter baumannii* in a burn unit: Risk factors for acquisition and management. Infection Control Hospital. 2002;**23**(5):261-267

[77] Berrouane YF, McNutt L, Buschelman BJ, Rhomberg PR, Sanford MD, Hollis RJ, et al. Outbreak of severe *Pseudomonas aeruginosa* infections caused by a contaminated drain in a Whirlpool Bathtub. Clinical Infectious Diseases. 2000;**31**(6):1331-1337

[78] Haynes LJ, Brown MH, Handley BC. Comparison of Pulsavac and sterile whirlpool regarding the promotion of tissue granulation. Physical Theraphy. 1994;**74**(suppl):S4

[79] Klein MB, Hunter S, Heimbach DM, Engrav LH, Honari S, Gallery E, et al. The Versajet??? Water Dissector: A new tool for tangential excision. The Journal of Burn Care & Rehabilitation. 2005;**26**(6):483-487

[80] Nichter LS, Morwood DT, Williams GS, Spence RJ. Expanding the limits of composite grafting: A case report of successful nose replantation assisted by hyperbaric oxygen therapy. Plastic Reconstruction Surgery. 1991;**87**(2):337-340

[81] Bowersox JC, Strauss MB, Hart GB. Clinical experience with hyperbaric oxygen therapy in the salvage of ischemic skin flaps and grafts. Journal of Hyperbaric Medicine. 1986;**1**(3):141-149

[82] Mounsey RA, Brown DH, O'Dwyer TP, Gullane PJ, Koch GH. Role of hyperbaric oxygen therapy in the management of mandibular osteoradionecrosis. Laryngoscope. 1993;**103**(6):605-608

[83] Bill TJ, Hoard MA, Gampper TJ. Applications of hyperbaric oxygen in otolaryngology head and neck surgery. Otolaryngologic Clinics of North America. 2001;**34**(4):753-766

[84] Perrins D. Influence of hyperbaric oxygen on the survival of split skin grafts. Lancet. 1967;**289**(7495):868-871

[85] Shupak A, Oren S, Goldenberg I, Barzilai A, Moskuna R, Bursztein S. Necrotizing fasciitis: An indication for hyperbaric oxygenation therapy? Surgery. 1995;**118**(5):873-878

[86] Brown DR, Davis NL, Lepawsky M, Cunningham J, Kortbeek J. A multicenter review of the treatment of major truncal necrotizing infections with and without hyperbaric oxygen therapy. American Journal of Surgery. 1994;**167**(5):485-489

[87] Kuncir EJ, Tillou A, Hill CR, Petrone P, Kimbrell B, Asensio JA. Necrotizing soft-tissue infections. Emergency Medicine Clinics of North America. 2003;**21**(4):1075-1087

[88] Boykin JVJ. The nitric oxide connection: Hyperbaric oxygen therapy, becaplermin, and diabetic ulcer management. Advanced Skin Wound Care. 2000;**13**(4):169

[89] Xia Y-P, Zhao Y, Marcus J, Jimenez PA, Ruben SM, Moore PA, et al. Effects of keratinocyte growth factor-2 (KGF-2) on wound healing in an ischaemia-impaired rabbit ear model and on scar formation. The Journal of Pathology. 1999;**188**(4):431-438

[90] Lawrence WT. In search of the optimal treatment of keloids: Report of a series and a review of the literature. Annals of Plastic Surgery. 1991;**27**(2):164-178

[91] Apfelberg DB, Maser MR, Lash H. The use of epidermis over a keloid as an autograft after resection of the keloid. The Journal of Dermatologic Surgery and Oncology. 1976;**2**(5):409

[92] Weimar VM, Ceilley RI. Surgical gems: Treatment of keloids on earlobes. The Journal of Dermatologic Surgery and Oncology. 1979;**5**(7):522-523

[93] Zouboulis CC. Outcomes of cryosurgery in keloids and hypertrophic scars. Archives in Dermatology. 1993;**129**(9):1146

[94] Akita S, Akino K, Yakabe A, Imaizumi T, Tanaka K, Anraku K, et al. Combined surgical excision and radiation therapy for keloid treatment. The Journal of Craniofacial Surgery. 2007;**18**(5):1164-1169

[95] Connell PG, Harland CC. Treatment of keloid scars with pulsed dye laser and intralesional steroid. Journal of Cutaneous Laser Therapy. 2000;**2**(3):147-150

[96] Tang YW. Intra-and postoperative steroid injections for keloids and hypertrophic scars. British Journal of Plastic Surgery. 1992;**45**(5):371-373

[97] Fitzpatrick FA, Soberman R. Regulated formation of eicosanoids. The Journal of Clinical Investigation. 2001;**107**(11):1347-1351

[98] Rabello FB, Souza CD, Farina Júnior JA. Update on hypertrophic scar treatment. Clinics. 2014;**69**:565-573

[99] Alcolea MP, Jones PH. Lineage analysis of epidermal stem cells. Cold

Spring Harbor Perspectives in Medicine. 2014;**4**(1):a015206-a015206

[100] Çankirili NK, Altundag O, Çelebi-Saltik B. Skin stem cells, their niche and tissue engineering approach for skin regeneration. 2019;**6**: 107-126

[101] Frede J, Jones PH. Permission to proliferate. Science. 2013;**342**(6163):1184-1183

[102] Buczacki SJA, Zecchini HI, Nicholson AM, Russell R, Vermeulen L, Kemp R, et al. Intestinal label-retaining cells are secretory precursors expressing Lgr5. Nature. 2013;**495**(7439):65-69

[103] Tata PR, Mou H, Pardo-Saganta A, Zhao R, Prabhu M, Law BM, et al. Dedifferentiation of committed epithelial cells into stem cells in vivo. Nature. 2013;**503**(7475):218-223

[104] Lu CP, Polak L, Rocha AS, Pasolli HA, Chen S-C, Sharma N, et al. Identification of stem cell populations in sweat glands and ducts reveals roles in homeostasis and wound repair. Cell. 2012;**150**(1):136-150

[105] Rittié L, Sachs DL, Orringer JS, Voorhees JJ, Fisher GJ. Eccrine sweat glands are major contributors to reepithelialization of human wounds. The American Journal of Pathology. 2013;**182**(1):163-171

[106] Nowak JA, Polak L, Pasolli HA, Fuchs E. Hair follicle stem cells are specified and function in early skin morphogenesis. Cell Stem Cell. 2008;**3**(1):33-43

[107] Biedermann T, Pontiggia L, Böttcher-Haberzeth S, Tharakan S, Braziulis E, Schiestl C, et al. Human eccrine sweat gland cells can reconstitute a stratified epidermis. The Journal of Investigative Dermatology. 2010;**130**(8):1996-2009

[108] Ito M, Liu Y, Yang Z, Nguyen J, Liang F, Morris RJ, et al. Stem cells in the hair follicle bulge contribute to wound repair but not to homeostasis of the epidermis. Nature Medicine. 2005;**11**(12):1351-1354

[109] Levy V, Lindon C, Zheng Y, Harfe BD, Morgan BA. Epidermal stem cells arise from the hair follicle after wounding. The FASEB Journal. 2007;**21**(7):1358-1366

[110] Branski LK, Pereira CT, Herndon DN, Jeschke MG. Gene therapy in wound healing: Present status and future directions. Gene Therapy. 2007;**14**(1):1

[111] Shridharani SM, Tufaro AP. A systematic review of acelluar dermal matrices in head and neck reconstruction. Plastic and Reconstructive Surgery. 2012;**130**:35S-43S

[112] Silver FH, Siperko LM, Seehra GP. Mechanobiology of force transduction in dermal tissue. Skin Research and Technology. 2003;**9**(1):3-23

[113] Stephens DJ. Collagen secretion explained. Nature. 2012;**482**(7386): 474-475

[114] Lo DD, Zimmermann AS, Nauta A, Longaker MT, Lorenz HP. Scarless fetal skin wound healing update. Birth Defects in Research Part C. 2012;**96**(3): 237-247

[115] Rinkevich Y, Walmsley GG, Hu MS, Maan ZN, Newman AM, Drukker M, et al. Identification and isolation of a dermal lineage with intrinsic fibrogenic potential. Science. 2015;**348**:6232

[116] Thielitz A, Vetter RW, Schultze B, Wrenger S, Simeoni L, Ansorge S, et al. Inhibitors of dipeptidyl peptidase IV-like activity mediate antifibrotic effects in normal and keloid-derived skin fibroblasts. The Journal of Investigative Dermatology. 2008;**128**(4):855-866

[117] Hu MS, Januszyk M, Hong WX, Walmsley GG, Zielins ER, Atashroo DA, et al. Gene expression in fetal murine keratinocytes and fibroblasts. The Journal of Surgical Research. 2014;**190**(1):344-357

[118] Powell DW, Mifflin RC, Valentich JD, Crowe SE, Saada JI, West AB. Myofibroblasts. I. Paracrine cells important in health and disease. American Journal of Physiology. 1999;**277**(1):C1-C19

[119] Desmoulière A, Redard M, Darby I, Gabbiani G. Apoptosis mediates the decrease in cellularity during the transition between granulation tissue and scar. American Journal of Pathology. 1995;**146**(1):56-66

[120] Desai VD, Hsia HC, Schwarzbauer JE. Reversible modulation of myofibroblast differentiation in adipose-derived mesenchymal stem cells. PLoS One. 2014;**9**(1):e86865

[121] Maltseva O, Folger P, Zekaria D, Petridou S, Masur SK. Fibroblast growth factor reversal of the corneal myofibroblast phenotype. Investigative Ophthalmology & Visual Science. 2001;**42**(11):2490-2495

[122] Hinz B, Phan SH, Thannickal VJ, Galli A, Bochaton-Piallat M-L, Gabbiani G. The myofibroblast. The American Journal of Pathology. 2007;**170**(6):1807-1816

[123] Schmidt BA, Horsley V. Intradermal adipocytes mediate fibroblast recruitment during skin wound healing. Development. 2013;**140**(7):1517-1527

[124] Rinella L, Marano F, Berta L, Bosco O, Fraccalvieri M, Fortunati N, et al. Extracorporeal shock waves modulate myofibroblast differentiation of adipose-derived stem cells. Wound Repair and Regeneration. 2016;**24**(2):275-286

[125] Corcione A, Benvenuto F, Ferretti E, Giunti D, Cappiello V, Cazzanti F, et al. Human mesenchymal stem cells modulate B-cell functions. Blood. 2006;**107**(1):367-372

[126] Di Nicola M, Carlo-Stella C, Magni M, Milanesi M, Longoni PD, Matteucci P, et al. Human bone marrow stromal cells suppress T-lymphocyte proliferation induced by cellular or nonspecific mitogenic stimuli. Blood. 2002;**99**(10):3838-3843

[127] Loots MAM, Lamme EN, Zeegelaar J, Mekkes JR, Bos JD, Middelkoop E. Differences in cellular infiltrate and extracellular matrix of chronic diabetic and venous ulcers versus acute wounds. The Journal of Investigative Dermatology. 1998;**111**(5):850-857

[128] Li T, Xia M, Gao Y, Chen Y, Xu Y. Human umbilical cord mesenchymal stem cells: An overview of their potential in cell-based therapy. Expert Opinion on Biological Therapy. 2015;**15**(9):1293-1306

[129] Ruud A, Bank MMM. Paracrine factors of human amniotic fluid-derived mesenchymal stem cells show strong anti-fibrotic properties by inhibiting myofibroblast differentiation and collagen synthesis. Journal of Stem Cell and Research Theraphy. 2015;**5**(5):2-16

[130] Doi H, Kitajima Y, Luo L, Yan C, Tateishi S, Ono Y, et al. Potency of umbilical cord blood- and Wharton's

jelly-derived mesenchymal stem cells for scarless wound healing. Scientific Reports. 2016;**6**(1):18844

[131] Sabapathy V, Sundaram B, Mankuzhy P, Kumar S. Human Wharton's Jelly mesenchymal stem cells plasticity augments scar-free skin wound healing with hair growth. PLoS One. 2014;**9**(4):e93726

[132] Nuschke A. Activity of mesenchymal stem cells in therapies for chronic skin wound healing. Organogenesis. 2014;**10**(1):29-37

[133] Leavitt T, Hu MS, Marshall CD, Barnes LA, Lorenz HP, Longaker MT. Scarless wound healing: Finding the right cells and signals. Cell and Tissue Research. 2016;**365**(3):483-493

[134] Clevers H, Loh KM, Nusse R. An integral program for tissue renewal and regeneration: Wnt signaling and stem cell control. Science. 2014;**346**:6205

[135] Houschyar KS, Momeni A, Pyles MN, Maan ZN, Whittam AJ, Siemers F. Wnt signaling induces epithelial differentiation during cutaneous wound healing. Organogenesis. 2015;**11**(3):95-104

[136] Sato M. Upregulation of the Wnt/?-catenin pathway induced by transforming growth factor-? in Hypertrophic Scars and Keloids. Acta Dermato-Venereologica. 2006;**86**(4):300-307

[137] Cheon SS, Cheah AYL, Turley S, Nadesan P, Poon R, Clevers H, et al. β-Catenin stabilization dysregulates mesenchymal cell proliferation, motility, and invasiveness and causes aggressive fibromatosis and hyperplastic cutaneous wounds. Proceedings of the National Academy of Sciences. 2002;**99**(10):6973-6978

[138] Lee WJ, Park JH, Shin JU, Noh H, Lew DH, Yang WI, et al. Endothelial-to-mesenchymal transition induced by Wnt 3a in keloid pathogenesis. Wound Repair and Regeneration. 2015;**23**(3):435-442

[139] Sen CK, Ghatak S. miRNA control of tissue repair and regeneration. The American Journal of Pathology. 2015;**185**(10):2629-2640

[140] Cheng J, Yu H, Deng S, Shen G. MicroRNA profiling in mid- and late-gestational fetal skin: Implication for scarless wound healing. Tohoku Journal of Experimental Medicine. 2010;**221**(3):203-209

[141] Shilo S, Roy S, Khanna S, Sen CK. MicroRNA in cutaneous wound healing: A new paradigm. DNA and Cell Biology. 2007;**26**(4):227-237

[142] Soliman AM, Das S, Abd Ghafar N, Teoh SL. Role of microRNA in proliferation phase of wound healing. Frontiers in Genetics. 2018;**9**:38

[143] Banerjee J, Sen CK. microRNA and wound healing. In: MicroRNA: Medical Evidence. Champions: Springer; 2015. pp. 291-305

[144] Gras C, Ratuszny D, Hadamitzky C, Zhang H, Blasczyk R, Figueiredo C. miR-145 contributes to hypertrophic scarring of the skin by inducing myofibroblast activity. Molecular Medicine. 2015;**21**(1):296-304

[145] Monaghan M, Browne S, Schenke-Layland K, Pandit A. A collagen-based scaffold delivering exogenous MicroRNA-29B to modulate extracellular matrix remodeling. Molecular Therapy. 2014;**22**(4):786-796

Chapter 3

Surgical Wound Closure and Healing

Liza G. Ovington

Abstract

This chapter will review the most recent advances in surgical wound closure devices and how they impact and support surgical wound healing. An overview of surgical wound healing and its potential complications will be provided. Wound closure technologies will be described with a focus on how they may also minimize complications of surgical wound healing such as infection, dehiscence, and incisional hernia. Evidence will be summarized to support these effects along with an explanation of mechanisms of action. Broad categories of wound closure technologies to be discussed will include absorbable suture materials, antibacterial sutures, surgical staples, and topical skin adhesives.

Keywords: surgical wound, wound closure techniques, postoperative complications, incisional hernia, surgical wound infection, surgical wound dehiscence, sutures, antibacterial sutures, absorbable sutures, topical skin adhesives

1. Introduction

Surgical wounds are unique in the spectrum of acute and chronic wounds. They are technically acute wounds that progress through the phases of normal healing, resulting in wound closure within an expected timeframe of about 4 weeks [1]. They differ however from all other acute wounds in three important ways. First, they are planned and executed under the best of conditions, second, they present as incisions or excisions with clean edges and minimal tissue damage or loss, and third, their edges are precisely approximated with the mechanical support of a wound closure device to facilitate healing [2]. Wound closure devices are essential tools in surgery but can entail both benefits and risks to successful wound healing. The major categories of surgical wound closure devices will be described and discussed from the standpoint of their potential impact on both surgical wound healing and surgical wound complications.

2. Classifications and healing of surgical wounds

The global volume of surgery was estimated to be 312.9 million procedures in 2012, which represented an increase of 38.2% from a prior estimate in 2004 [3]. Almost all of these surgical procedures begin with the creation of an incisional wound to provide access to the organ or anatomy of interest and end with the closure of the incision. Surgical incisions can be made at any location on the body, be of any length, variable depths, and different shapes. With over fourteen surgical specialties creating multiple types of incisions, classifying these wounds can be complex [4]. There are however, two classification systems for surgical wounds that are widely used [5, 6].

In the first, surgical wounds are classified preoperatively into one of four categories according to the likelihood and degree of wound contamination at the time of operation [5]. The Centers for Disease Control and Prevention (CDC), using an adaptation of the American College of Surgeons' wound classification schema, divides surgical wounds into four classes [5]. Class I or clean wounds are defined as uninfected operative wounds in which no inflammation is encountered and the respiratory, alimentary, genital, or uninfected urinary tracts are not entered [5]. Class II or clean-contaminated wounds are defined as operative wounds in which the respiratory, alimentary, genital, or urinary tracts are entered under controlled conditions and without unusual contamination [5]. Operations involving the biliary tract, appendix, vagina, and oropharynx are included in this category provided no evidence of infection or major break in sterile technique is encountered [5]. Class III or contaminated wounds are defined as open, fresh, accidental wounds. In addition, operations with major breaks in sterile technique (e.g., open cardiac massage) or gross spillage from the gastrointestinal tract, and incisions in which acute, nonpurulent inflammation is encountered [5]. Class IV or dirty-infected wounds are defined as old traumatic wounds with retained devitalized tissue and those that involve existing clinical infection or perforated viscera [5]. This definition suggests that the organisms causing postoperative infection were present in the operative field before the operation [5].

The second classification system for surgical wounds is determined postoperatively and refers to when and how they are closed and will heal. Primary wound closure refers to the immediate closure of a surgical incision (usually within 4–8 h) and is also known as healing by primary intention [6]. Wounds that heal by primary intention are those with little or no tissue loss in which the wound edges can be easily approximated or brought together [6]. Primary intention healing occurs via epithelization and connective tissue deposition [7]. Most incised surgical wounds will heal by primary intention [6]. Secondary wound closure, also known as healing by secondary intention, applies to wounds with significant tissue loss in which the wound edges cannot be approximated. Secondary intention healing requires a granulation tissue matrix to form and fill the defect prior to epithelialization of the surface [7]. Less frequently, surgical wounds are managed by tertiary or delayed primary closure, also known as healing by tertiary intention [6]. This approach is usually taken in wounds where there is not significant tissue loss but an elevated risk or presence of infection [7]. Examples include traumatic injuries such as animal bites or lacerations involving foreign bodies. These wounds can usually be surgically closed, or skin grafted after thorough cleansing, debridement of any necrotic tissue, and observation for up to 7 days to ensure adequate tissue viability and perfusion [8].

Wound healing, whether in chronic wounds or acute wounds like closed surgical incisions involves a complex series of molecular and cellular events that culminate in fibrotic repair or a scar [9]. These wound healing events can be described as four overlapping phases of hemostasis, inflammation, proliferation (collagen formation) and maturation (collagen remodeling) [9]. Hemostasis begins at the moment of incision with a complex series of enzymatic events that result in the formation of a fibrin clot [9]. The clot establishes a temporary extracellular matrix and subsequent platelet mediated stimuli recruit neutrophils to the wound environment to initiate the inflammatory phase with the initial function of defending against bacterial infection [9]. Within 2–3 days, monocytes from the bloodstream enter the tissues and transition into macrophages [9]. Early wound macrophages phagocytize dead neutrophils, bacteria, and tissue debris [9]. Later these macrophages take on an anti-inflammatory role in preparation for tissue repair and begin to secrete a variety of growth factors to stimulate fibroblast migration and activation [9]. The acute inflammatory phase can last 3–7 days dependent on tissue type [7]. During this phase of healing, a surgical incision does not gain appreciable tensile strength, and is dependent upon the wound closure material to hold it in approximation [7]. The arrival of fibroblasts signals the beginning of the proliferative phase [9]. The fibroblasts and endothelial cells begin to produce a highly vascularized extracellular matrix composed of glycosaminoglycans, proteoglycans, and collagen called granulation tissue [9]. The ratio of type III to type I collagen in granulation tissue is higher than in unwounded tissue or mature/remodeled scar and it accounts for the weaker tissue strength in a healing wound [9]. Although collagen deposition by fibroblasts is at its maximal level around 3 weeks after injury, wound strength is still at a minimum [9]. Surgical incisional wounds have minimal to no tissue loss, so the proliferative phase may be attenuated with lower volume of granulation tissue relative to wounds with significant tissue loss. Epithelial cells resurface the wound only after granulation in wounds with tissue loss, however in incisional wounds with close wound edge approximation, epithelization is complete within about 48–72 h [10]. The maturation phase begins after proliferation subsides and involves remodeling of the newly deposited matrix with changes in collagen fibril orientation and a shift toward a higher proportion of type I to type III collagen [9]. This remodeling process results in a mature scar that can regain up to 80% of the strength of normal skin after 3–4 months [9]. Remodeling involves reorganization of extracellular matrix by matrix metalloproteinases and collagenases and is accompanied by decreased cellularity and vascularity of scar tissue [7]. Epithelial appendages such as hair follicles, sweat glands, and sebaceous glands are not reformed, so a healed scar is an acellular arrangement of epithelialized extracellular matrix composed primarily of collagen [9].

There are many elements of an operative procedure that can impact the surgical wound healing process [7]. The patient's overall health status will affect the duration of healing with many factors to be considered, including but not limited to age, BMI, nutrition, hydration, diabetes, tobacco use, blood supply, polypharmacy, and immunodeficiencies [7]. Likewise, there are factors related to the surgical procedure itself, such as the length and orientation of the incision, dissection technique, tissue handling, elimination of dead space, closing tension, and the choice of wound closure materials [7].

3. Surgical wound healing complications

Several of the most common surgical wound healing complications which can be impacted by wound closure materials or technique will now be briefly discussed.

3.1 Surgical site infection

Surgical incisions are made under sterile conditions, however multiple infection prevention measures must be observed pre-, post-, and intraoperatively to minimize risks of post-operative infections. Surgical site infection (SSI) is the most common surgical wound complication, affecting up to one-third of patients who have undergone a surgical procedure [11]. SSIs are commonly classified as one of three types: superficial incisional (involving only the skin or subcutaneous tissue of the incision), deep incisional (involving the deep soft tissues of the incision, such as fascia and muscle layers) or organ/space (involving any part of the anatomy which was opened or manipulated during an operation other than the incision) [5]. It has been estimated that two-thirds of SSI are confined to the incision [5].

Infection occurs when microorganisms in a wound proliferate to a level that produces a local and/or systemic response [12]. Many of the factors that impact surgical wound healing also affect the potential for infection. Risk factors for SSI include patient-specific and process/procedural-specific variables. Some variables are not modifiable, such as patient age and gender, however, others can be improved to reduce the risk of infection such as nutritional status, tobacco use, correct timing and dosing of antibiotics and aspects of intraoperative technique [11]. A particular risk factor for SSI is the presence of foreign bodies in the wound which can provide a surface for bacteria colonization and biofilm formation [13]. While such foreign bodies are often thought to be exemplified by larger, permanent implantable medical devices such as joint protheses or heart valves, devices for wound closure such as surgical sutures can present similar risks for surgical wound infection [13]. Clinical data as early as the 1950s has shown that the presence of suture in an incision can reduce the infective dose of bacteria by 10,000-fold; from a dose of millions down to hundreds [14]. The rationale for this is that within hours, small numbers of bacteria released into the wound from lower layers of the stratum corneum and dermal appendages during creation of the surgical incision can colonize the suture surface and develop into a biofilm which is resistant to phagocytic immune cells as well as to antibiotics [15].

Surgical site infections are the most common of all healthcare associated infections (HAI) [16]. A 2022 retrospective analysis of the largest all-payer US inpatient databases—the Agency for Healthcare Cost and Utilization Project's 2016 National Inpatient Sample, provides some of the most up-to-date information on the incidence of HAI [16]. This database covers more than 97% of the US population and contains data from more than 35 million inpatient admissions [16]. The analysis considered all inpatient encounters with primary or secondary ICD-10 diagnosis codes corresponding to infection with catheter-associated urinary tract infections (CAUTI), catheter- and line-associated bloodstream infections (CLABSI), SSI, ventilator-associated pneumonia (VAP), and infection with *Clostridioides difficile* (CDI) to determine incidence [16]. For the 280,575 admissions with HAI as a primary diagnosis, SSI was the most frequent at 47%, followed by CDI as 37.4%, CLABSI at 10.2%, CAUTI at 5% and VAP at 0.4% [16]. The additional costs associated with these SSI were 3.7 billion USD [16].

3.2 Surgical wound dehiscence

Surgical wound dehiscence (SWD) is a wound healing complication that has a wide range of definitions [17]. It can refer broadly to any separation of a surgical incision ranging from a superficial separation of part of the incision to complete separation of the full thickness of the incision with exposure of organs or surgical implants [17]. Conversely, the term can be used specifically to describe the failure of an abdominal incision and evisceration of the abdominal contents [17]. Further, literature reports may use a variety of alternative descriptors for SWD such as wound disruption, wound opening, wound breakdown, fascial dehiscence, or surgical site failure, among others [17]. A standardized definition of SWD for all closed surgical incision types was proposed in 2018 by the World Union of Wound Healing Societies to facilitate accurate identification and reporting as well as management [17]. The definition is as follows: "Surgical wound dehiscence (SWD) is the separation of the margins of a closed surgical incision that has been made in the skin, with or without exposure or protrusion of underlying tissue, organs, or implants. Separation may occur at single or multiple regions, or involve the full length of the incision, and may affect some or all tissue layers. A dehisced incision may, or may not, display clinical signs and symptoms of infection" [17].

Dehiscence can be caused by technical issues with incision closure such as failure of the closure material or technique, postoperative mechanical stresses placed on the incision by local edema or patient activity levels, endogenous healing issues or any combination of these [17]. There is also a correlation between SWD and other surgical wound complications, such as seroma, hematoma, incisional hernia, and SSI [17].

Determination of SWD incidence is hampered by the lack of a uniform definition and rates in the literature vary widely by surgical procedure type and surgical wound classification [17]. SWD rates have been reported to range from 0.65% in cardiothoracic surgery up to 41.8% in pilonidal sinus surgery [17].

3.3 Incisional hernia

Incisional hernias (IH) are a common surgical wound complication after abdominal surgical procedures (especially midline incisions) and are defined as "abdominal wall gaps around postoperative scars, perceptible or palpable by clinical examination or imaging" [18]. Incisional hernias develop because of the failure of the abdominal wall to close properly due to patient related factors, disease related factors and or technical factors related to surgical technique or wound closure materials [19]. Wound infection, obesity, and suture closure technique (in particular a suture length/wound length ratio > 4/1) are thought to be the most important risk factors for the development of IH [19].

The incidence of IH after midline laparotomy ranges from 0 to 44% in the literature; however, a pooled rate of 12.8% has been reported at two years postoperatively from a systematic review and meta-analysis of 56 papers involving 14,618 patients [18].

4. Surgical wound closure options and impact on healing

While there are different approaches to the closure of surgical incisions, the goals of all are to (1) facilitate the natural healing process leading to restoration of tissue function, (2) supply exogenous strength until tissue strength is restored by the endogenous healing process, and (3) avoid potential complications through appropriate closure technique and choice of closure approach [7]. Hence, clinicians closing wounds are concerned about the wound closure strength provided by the device they select, with not interfering with endogenous wound healing and ideally avoiding or minimizing complications [7]. Apposition of tissue edges by a wound closure device is maintained until the endogenous healing process restores enough wound tensile strength such that the wound becomes self-supporting [7]. The duration of time that a wound is completely dependent on the closure device for its initial holding strength is often referred to as the "critical wound healing period" [20]. The critical wound healing period is longer or shorter depending on the tissue type as well as on an individual patient's healing ability based on their health status as described earlier [20].

Surgeons have several types of wound closure devices/materials to choose from when closing a surgical incision. There is no single wound closure choice that is ideal for all situations, the physician must decide which material is best suited to a particular wound and situation based on their knowledge and experience [21]. Surgeons may choose to close the tissue layers that have been separated by the incision in two general ways; en masse (e.g., using a single closure material and technique to close multiple tissue layers at once) or layer by layer (e.g., making specific wound closure choices of material and technique for different tissue layers) [21]. There are differing opinions on closing specific tissue layers separately versus en masse. For example, some surgeons question the need of separately closing the subcutaneous fat layer because it has little tensile strength due to its composition, which is mostly water, whereas others believe it is necessary to place at least a few sutures in a thick layer of subcutaneous fat to prevent dead space, where tissue fluids can accumulate to create seromas or hematomas which can delay healing and potentiate infection [7].

Regarding the tissue layers, there are multiple types of devices for skin (epidermal) closure including sutures, staples, and topical skin adhesives. For the tissue layers below the epidermis—dermis, subcutaneous fat, fascia, muscle—sutures are still the only option for wound closure [7].

4.1 Sutures for wound closure

4.1.1 Suture technique and impact on healing

A suture is any strand of material attached to a surgical needle designed to carry that material through tissue with minimal trauma to approximate two opposing tissue edges [7]. Regardless of the type of suture material selected, an important aspect of their use is how they are deployed by the surgeon. Suturing techniques require considerable skill by surgeons and affect wound closure outcomes. The method of where the suture enters and exits the tissue, the distance between throws, the distance from the wound edges, the suture length to wound length ratio, the way knots are performed, etc. are all aspects of suture technique [22]. Frequently used suturing techniques for tissue approximation include, but are not limited to simple interrupted, continuous (also referred as a running), mattress (horizontal or vertical), and subcuticular (interrupted or continuous) [22].

Suturing technique alone can have an impact on wound closure success [22]. For example, the European Hernia Society undertook a systematic review of the literature to establish guidelines for the optimal wound closure technique for elective midline incisions of the abdominal wall with the goal of decreasing the occurrence of the surgical wound complications of both burst abdomen and incisional hernia [23]. These guidelines were intended for all surgeons performing abdominal incisions in any type of surgery including visceral, gynecological, aortic vascular, urological, or orthopedic, and for both open and laparoscopic approaches [23]. Their final recommendations regarding the optimal suture technique included using a continuous suturing in a single layer aponeurotic closure technique without separate closure of the peritoneum [23]. Further, a small bites technique (stitches placed 5 mm apart and 5–8 mm from the wound edges) with a suture to wound length (SL/WL) ratio of at least 4/1 was recommended [23]. They went on to make specific recommendations also regarding the optimal suture material and suggested the use of slowly absorbable monofilament suture when using this closure technique [23].

4.1.2 Suture materials

Most sutures used today are composed of either natural materials such as gut or silk or an increasing variety of manmade synthetic polymers [23]. Their physical formats can be either monofilament, multifilament (braids) or barbed monofilaments [23]. They can be nonabsorbable (permanent) or absorbable (temporary) [7]. Desirable characteristics of sutures include pliability for ease of handling, adequate tensile strength, knot security, minimal tissue reactivity, infection resistance, and good elasticity and plasticity to accommodate wound swelling or tissue growth [7]. The choice of a suture material depends on factors such as the number of tissue layers involved in wound closure, the critical wound healing period for the tissue involved, tension across the wound, depth of suture placement, presence of edema, and expected time of suture removal among others [24].

4.1.3 Absorbable versus nonabsorbable sutures

While sutures can be made of many different natural and synthetic materials, the most significant categorization is that of their status as nonabsorbable versus absorbable sutures [21]. Nonabsorbable sutures which cannot be removed (e.g., those used below the skin surface) persist in the body even after tissue has regained enough tensile strength to be self-supporting and may elicit a foreign body response as they become encapsulated by fibrous connective tissue [7]. They may also be palpable and perceived as painful by the patient. Ideally, a suture material will remain strong enough to support the wound through the critical healing period and then gradually be absorbed [20]. With the advent of synthetic absorbable polymers for suture in the late 1960s, it became possible to design suture material that maintained its wound holding strength for specific durations of time (also called breaking strength retention or BSR) and were then absorbed by the body via hydrolysis and required no return visit for suture removal if used for skin closure [24]. The breaking strength retention times can be specifically controlled through the molecular composition of the polymers [21]. Among the various types of synthetic absorbable sutures, there are polymers that retain their breaking strength for one, two, four or six weeks before the absorption process significantly reduces it (**Table 1**).

The surgeon will choose the type of absorbable suture with the breaking strength retention period appropriate for the tissue being approximated and the specific clinical scenario [21]. For example, in a rapidly healing tissue such a mucosa, a short-term absorbable suture such as low molecular weight polyglactin with a BSR of one week may be the optimal choice but for a longer healing tissue subject to mechanical stresses such as abdominal fascia, a slowly absorbable polydioxanone monofilament may be the best choice [7]. In fact, the EHS Guidelines just discussed have made that specific recommendation for fascial closure in elective midline incisions [23].

An initial concern with the advent of synthetic absorbable suture materials was their ability to maintain effective wound closure in different tissue types as compared to nonabsorbable suture materials [25]. There have been multiple meta-analyses performed to compare the performance of absorbable and nonabsorbable sutures for wound closure in various tissue types including skin, dermis, fascia, and muscle and comparing rates of wound healing complications [18, 25–28]. The largest such comparison across multiple procedure types reviewed outcomes post absorbable and nonabsorbable suture use in 25 randomized controlled trials and 5781 patients and

Approximate % of original strength remaining[a] at:						
	1 week	2 weeks	3 weeks	4 weeks	5 weeks	6 weeks
LMW Polyglactin (Vicryl Rapide)	50%	0				
Poliglecaprone (Monocryl)	60%	30%		0		
Polyglactin 910 (Vicryl)		75%	40–50%	25%	0	
Polyglycolic acid (Dexon II)		65%	35%			
Polyglyconate (Maxon)	80%	75%	65%	50%		25%
Polydioxanone (PDS II)		80%		70%		60%

[a]*Data taken from respective suture instructions for use.*

Table 1.
Breaking strength retention times of different absorbable polymers.

found no significant differences in surgical site infection, dehiscence, or other post-operative complications [25]. A 2016 meta-analysis compared outcomes for absorbable versus nonabsorbable sutures in skin closure (1748 patients in 19 RCTs) and confirmed that an absorbable suture for skin closure was an acceptable alternative for traditional nonabsorbable sutures with no significant differences between the two suture types in the incidence of wound infections, cosmetic outcomes, wound dehiscence, or patients' or caregivers' satisfaction [26]. In three large meta-analyses (56 RCT/14618 patients, 55 RCT/19174 patients, 8 RCT/426 patients) comparing the use of absorbable versus nonabsorbable sutures in fascial closure of laparotomy incisions, none demonstrated any significant differences in the surgical healing complication outcomes of incisional hernia, surgical wound dehiscence, or surgical site infection [18, 27, 28]. It should be noted that these comparisons focused on absorbable versus nonabsorbable sutures in general and not on specifically on slowly absorbable sutures which have been recommended by the European Hernia Society as the optimal fascial closure choice for elective midline incisions based on reduced risks of incisional hernia and dehiscence as previously discussed [23].

4.1.4 Antibacterial sutures versus non-antibacterial sutures

Sutures with antibacterial coatings were developed to address an underappreciated yet known risk factor for surgical site infection– bacterial colonization and biofilm formation on the suture [24]. Currently, the only globally available antibacterial sutures are those coated with triclosan (Plus Antibacterial Sutures, Ethicon, Inc., Somerville NJ). There have been multiple randomized controlled trials (RCT) of triclosan coated sutures compared to non-triclosan sutures with the primary outcome of SSI within 30 days [29]. These studies have been performed in various procedure types encompassing all surgical wound classifications (clean, clean-contaminated, contaminated, and dirty) [30]. Subsequently, there have been serial meta-analyses of these randomized trials published over time. **Table 2** presents the most recent meta-analyses of triclosan coated sutures versus non-triclosan-coated sutures [29–33]. While each of these meta-analyses incorporates largely the same RCT data, none of the listed analyses completely replicates the data in another, either due to timing or to included surgical procedure types. Each meta-analysis, whether including all types of surgical procedures or limited to specific types of surgical procedures, found a

Procedure type	Author Yr. (#RCT, #pts)	Relative risk of surgical site infection
Multiple	Ahmed 2019 (25 RCT, 11,957 pts)	RR 0.73 (0.65–0.82) P = < 0.00001
Gastrointestinal surgery	Uchino 2018 (10 RCT, 3488 pts)	RR 0.67 (0.48–0.94) P = 0.02
Colorectal surgery	Uchino 2018 (9 RCT, 2433 pts)	RR 0.69 (0.49–0.98) P = 0.04
Abdominal fascial closure	Henriksen 2017 (8 RCT, 3641 pts)	OR 0.67 (0.46–0.98) P = 0.04
Multiple	de Jonge 2017 (21 RCT, 6462 pts)	RR 0.72 (0.60, 0.86) P < 0.001
Multiple	Leaper 2017 (34 studies, mean #pts./study 493)	OR 0.61 (0.52, 0.73) P = 0.001

Table 2.
Recent meta analyses of triclosan coated antibacterial sutures versus non-antibacterial sutures.

significant difference in the performance outcome of reduced risk of SSI with the use of triclosan coated sutures. The average reduction in risk of SSI ranged from 27 to 33% [29, 31]. A large meta-analysis focused primarily on economic outcomes included observational studies as well as RCT and found a risk reduction of 39% [32].

Two meta-analyses also employed trial sequential analysis (TSA) to quantify the statistical reliability of data in the cumulative meta-analysis adjusting significance levels for sparse data and repetitive testing on accumulating data [30, 32]. TSA is increasingly used as a tool to quantify the reliability of a meta-analytic outcome [30]. The TSA outcome of the meta-analysis of abdominal fascial closure was that triclosan coated sutures decrease the risk of SSI significantly and that further RCTs will not change that outcome [33]. The TSA outcome in the meta-analysis of triclosan coated sutures for any tissue closure was similar, concluding that the effect of the sutures was robust, and that additional data are unlikely to alter the summary effect [30]. No meta-analysis of triclosan-coated sutures reported any significant differences in any safety outcomes. These data collectively support the conclusion that triclosan-coated sutures are a valuable technology for wound closure in a wide variety of tissue types and procedures encompassing all surgical wound classifications with the intention of reducing the risk of SSI.

Furthermore, given that systematic reviews and meta-analysis cannot directly calculate the pooled SSI-attributable excess costs to healthcare, one investigator conducted an economic study to estimate the potential clinical and economic impact for NHS of using these sutures compared with conventional non-antimicrobial-coated absorbable sutures for wound closure [32]. Results showed that antimicrobial sutures may result in significant savings across various surgical wound types [32].

In 2021 the National Institute for Health and Care Excellence (NICE) commissioned an external assessment center to analyze the evidence base for Ethicon's Plus triclosan coated sutures as an innovative technology which consisted of 31 RCT involving over 14,000 patients [34]. Their analysis consisted of six de novo meta-analyses to establish the overall pooled effect size associated with Plus Sutures on the incidence of surgical site infections [34]. The primary outcome was the relative risk of developing a surgical site infection between Plus Sutures and control groups [34]. The six separate meta-analyses were done using: (1) all studies that provided enough

Meta analysis	#RCT	#Pts	Fixed effects RR	Random effects RR
All	28	13,667	**0.72** [0.64; 0.80] p < 0.001	**0.71** [0.59; 0.85] p < 0.001
Adults	25	9757	**0.73** [0.65; 0.82] p < 0.001	**0.74** [0.62; 0.88] p < 0.002
Children	2	1692	**0.52** [0.32; 0.87] p < 0.012	—
Clean wounds	15	6035	**0.75** [0.62; 0.90] p < 0.003	**0.71** [0.53; 0.96] p < 0.029
Non-clean wounds	12	2841	**0.66** [0.54; 0.80] p < 0.001	**0.67** [0.48; 0.92] p < 0.019
Sensitivity	31	13,821	**0.71** [0.64; 0.79] p < 0.001	**0.70** [0.58; 0.84] p < 0.001

Table 3.
NICE meta-analyses of triclosan coated suture evidence.

data; (2) a subset of studies in adults; (3) a subset of studies in children; (4) a subset of studies in patients with clean wounds; (5) a subset of studies in patients with non-clean wounds; and (6) all studies of Plus Sutures including STRATAFIX Plus that provided enough data, as a sensitivity analysis. The details and results of these meta-analyses are shown in **Table 3** and led to NICE making the following recommendations to the United Kingdom's National Health Service:

Recommendation 1.1: Evidence supports the case for adopting Plus Sutures as part of a bundle of care for preventing surgical site infection in the NHS for people who need wound closure after a surgical procedure when absorbable sutures are an appropriate option [34].

Recommendation 1.2: Cost modeling shows that Plus Sutures is cost saving compared with non-triclosan absorbable sutures by an average of £13.62 per patient. These savings are from reduced surgical site infections. Cost savings will vary by surgery type and baseline risk of surgical site infection [34].

4.2 Suture alternatives for skin closure

4.2.1 Staples

Skin staplers are medical devices that can be used to place "metallic sutures" or staples for closure of skin incisions. Skin staples provide a fast method for wound closure which allows for good eversion of skin edges without strangulation of tissue and minimal scarring [35]. Most modern skin staples are made from stainless steel. Skin staplers may be designed with a fixed head, a multi-directional release head or a 360° rotating head to improve visibility and facilitate access to wound areas, and with ergonomic handles (pistol-grip). The staples may have a dry film coating to facilitate removal which is accomplished with a special instrument called a staple extractor. The jaws of the device are used to grab the crossbar of the staple and bend the points out of the skin for removal. Both nonabsorbable/metallic and absorbable polymer-based skin staples are available [35].

Staples are often used for skin closure due to the rapidity of deployment compared to sutures [35]. A 2020 systematic review and meta-analysis of 42 RCT involving 11,067 patients comparing staples to sutures for skin closure in adults undergoing any type of surgery in a hospital setting examined primary outcomes of any SSI and severe SSI (defined as deep incisional or organ/space) and secondary outcomes of post-operative hospital stay, rates of readmission for wound complication, adverse events within 30 days and patient satisfaction with cosmetic results [36]. It was noted that overall, the body of evidence was low to very low quality and that many of the studies did not report on all desired outcomes [36]. The authors concluded that sutures may reduce pain and provide better satisfaction with the cosmetic results than staples; however, it was uncertain whether using sutures decreased the risk of overall and severe SSI, readmission rates, adverse events and postoperative pain compared to wound closure with staples [36]. A more recent meta-analysis compared staples to sutures for skin closure elective knee and hip arthroplasties with primary outcomes of SSI [37]. Eight RCT involving 1120 patients were included. The studies were classified using the Cochrane risk of bias tool: two were low risk, four had some concerns and two were high risk. Five of the studies involved knees only, two involved hips only, and one involved both knees and hips. When all eight studies were combined for meta-analysis, no significant differences in the risk of SSI were found between sutures and staples; but when limited to only the studies with low risk of bias, there was a significantly higher risk of SSI with staples versus sutures [37]. After additional subgroup analysis, the authors concluded that "stapling might carry a higher risk of surgical site infection than suturing in elective knee and hip arthroplasties, especially in hip arthroplasty" [37].

4.2.2 Topical skin adhesives

Tissue adhesives are a newer and potential alternative method of skin closure in surgical wounds (deeper tissue layers must still be closed with suture) [7]. Topical skin adhesives are commonly used in the emergency room setting for closure of acute traumatic lacerations and offer the advantage of reduced application time and reduced pain with no need for anesthesia as compared with standard wound-closure methods, which can be especially useful in pediatric patients [7]. Additionally, patients also avoid the need to return for removal of stitches or staples.

Topical skin adhesives come in a liquid monomer formulation and undergo a polymerization reaction when encountering moisture or a chemical initiator, leading to a slightly exothermic reaction and bonding to skin [38]. A chemical initiator can ensure consistent, dependable, and predictable polymerization times and is often located in the tip of the liquid adhesive applicator [38]. Monomers used in topical skin adhesives are cyanoacrylate-based (including n-butyl or 2-octyl side chains) and may contain other formulation additives to enhance strength, flexibility, or modulate viscosity and adherence to the skin [38]. Some topical skin adhesives incorporate a mesh patch. The purpose of combining a mesh patch with a topical adhesive as a system is to allow for temporary approximation of wound edges, (as opposed to digital approximation) prior to deployment of the liquid adhesive component which provides the definitive wound closure strength [39]. This temporary approximation can be especially useful in longer incisions where digital approximation along the length of the incision can be time-consuming [39]. In addition, the mesh component can provide added strength to the closure.

Topical skin adhesives can be used alone or in conjunction with other skin closure methods (sutures, staples). They provide sufficient strength to maintain skin edges approximation and distribute tension along the entire incision, preventing skin gaps from forming when the skin is stressed [38]. They can also create a strong, flexible barrier to prevent exogenous bacteria from entering the incision until the epidermis has fully resurfaced to re-establish the skin barrier [38]. Although initially widely used in the emergency room, surgeons are increasingly using topical skin adhesives for closure of surgical incisions in the operating room.

The most recent Cochrane systematic review of topical skin adhesives for closure of surgical incisions identified 33 RCT with 2793 patients [40]. Adhesives were compared to other methods of skin wound closure for outcomes of surgical wound dehiscence and infection and cosmesis. Meta-analysis found that sutures performed significantly better than adhesives for reducing the risk of wound dehiscence, but there were no significant differences between sutures and adhesives for wound infection or cosmesis [40].

5. Evidence based guidelines with wound closure recommendations

In addition to the 2015 European Hernia Society guidelines on the closure of abdominal wall incisions, there are two other evidence-based guidelines with specific recommendations for choice of wound closure materials [11, 41]. Both focus on reducing the risk of SSI. The 1999 CDC Guidelines for Prevention of Surgical Site Infection were finally updated in 2017 [41]. The update did not reevaluate a number of strong recommendations from the 1999 version as they were deemed to be accepted practice for the prevention of SSI. The 2017 update does however include a new recommendation for the choice of wound closure material—there is a specific Category II recommendation to "Consider the use of triclosan-coated sutures for the prevention of SSI" [41].

In addition to the CDC 2017 guideline, the WHO Global Guidelines for the Prevention of Surgical Site Infection 2018), also included a recommendation for wound closure: "The panel suggests the use of triclosan-coated sutures for the purpose of reducing the risk of SSI, independent of the type of surgery" [11]. This recommendation was categorized as Conditional Strength based on Moderate Quality of Evidence [11].

6. Conclusion

As acute wounds created under sterile conditions, the healing of surgical incisions is typically expected to occur without incident within an expected timeframe [1]. However, surgical wounds are atypical in that they depend on a wound closure device to facilitate their progress during a critical wound healing period [20]. The most common surgical wound healing complications of infection, dehiscence, and incisional hernia can all be impacted by the choice and method of wound closure [11, 17, 23, 41]. Sutures are a ubiquitous tool in surgical wound closure however, not all sutures are created equally. Absorbable and nonabsorbable sutures vary in terms of their initial and duration of tissue holding strengths, and some may be better choices than others for specific tissues [7]. Absorbable sutures are available with a range of different breaking strength retention times enabling surgeons to select the one that is strong enough long enough to support the healing timeframe dictated by the specific tissues and patient conditions and then resorb to reduce the potential for foreign body sensation and pain [24]. Absorbable antibacterial sutures are now available which have been shown to reduce the risk of surgical site infection in a wide variety of procedures and all surgical wound classes [30]. As the SSI is not only the most common surgical wound healing complication [16], but a risk factor for other complications such as wound dehiscence and incisional hernia [17], antibacterial sutures technology may have an impact on these healing complications as well. For example, while it is accepted that slowly absorbing sutures decrease the risk of incisional hernia after midline closure relative to faster absorbing sutures [23], a fast-absorbing antibacterial suture did not increase the incisional hernia rate compared to non-antibacterial slowly absorbing suture in a 3-year follow-up study of over one thousand patients [42]. Understanding the features and clinical benefits of different wound closure choices can be an important contribution to optimal surgical wound healing.

Acknowledgements

Ethicon, Inc. has provided publication support.

Conflict of interest

L. Ovington is a consultant for Ethicon, Inc. a part of Johnson and Johnson MedTech.

Author details

Liza G. Ovington
Ovington and Associates, Walnutport Pennsylvania, USA

*Address all correspondence to: lizao@msn.com

References

[1] Velnar T, Bailey T, Smrkolj V. The wound healing process: An overview of the cellular and molecular mechanisms. The Journal of International Medical Research. 2009;**37**(5):1528-1542. DOI: 10.1177/147323000903700531

[2] Leaper DJ. Traumatic and surgical wounds. British Medical Journal. 2006;**332**(7540):532-535. DOI: 10.1136/bmj.332.7540.532

[3] Weiser TG, Haynes AB, Molina G, et al. Estimate of the global volume of surgery in 2012: An assessment supporting improved health outcomes. Lancet. 2015;**385**(Global Surgery special issue):S11

[4] Available from: https://www.facs.org/for-medical-professionals/education/online-guide-to-choosing-a-surgical-residency/guide-to-choosing-a-surgical-residency-for-medical-students/faqs/specialties/#:~:text=The%20American%20College%20of%20Surgeons%20recognizes%2014%20surgical%20specialties%3A%20cardiothoracic,surgery%2C%20otorhin-olaryngology%2C%20pediatric%20surgery%2C. [Accessed: May 01, 2022]

[5] Mangram AJ, Horan TC, Pearson ML, Silver LC, Jarvis WR. Hospital infection control practices advisory committee. Guideline for prevention of surgical site infection, 1999. Infection Control and Hospital Epidemiology. 1999;**20**(4):250-278

[6] Salcido R. Healing by intention. Advances in Skin and Wound Care. 2017;**30**(6):246-247. DOI: 10.1097/01.ASW.0000516787.46060.b2

[7] Dunn DL, editor. Wound Closure Manual. 1st ed. New York: Ethicon Inc. Available from: <https://usermanual.wiki/Document/Ethicon WoundClosure Manual 101702.454226757/html; [Accessed: May 04, 2022]

[8] Azmat CE, Council M. Wound closure techniques. [Updated 2021 Nov 11]. In: StatPearls [Internet]. Treasure Island (FL): StatPearls Publishing; 2022. Available from: https://www.ncbi.nlm.nih.gov/books/NBK470598/

[9] Ovington L, Schultz G. The physiology of wound healing. In: Morison M, Ovington L, Wilkie K, editors. Chronic Wound Care: A Problem Based Learning Approach. London: Mosby; 2004. pp. 83-100

[10] Harris DR. Healing of the surgical wound. II. Factors influencing repair and regeneration. Journal of the American Academy of Dermatology. 1979;**1**(3):208-215. DOI: 10.1016/s0190-9622(79)80003-1

[11] Solomkin JS, Egger M, Balkhy HH, Balda JF, Berenholtz S, Boermeester MA, et al. Global Guidelines for the Prevention of Surgical Site Infection. second ed. Geneva: World Health Organization; 2018. License: CC BY-NC-SA 3.0 IGO

[12] International Wound Infection Institute (IWII). Wound infection in clinical practice. Wounds International. 2016. Available from: <https://www.woundchek.com/uploads/downloads/consensus_documents/iwii-consensus_wound%20infection%20in%20clinical%20practice.pdf>. [Accessed: May 01, 2022]

[13] Edmiston CE, Krepel CJ, Marks RM, et al. Microbiology of explanted suture

segments from infected and noninfected surgical cases. Journal of Clinical Microbiology. 2013;**51**:417-421

[14] Elek SD, Conen PE. The virulence of staphylococcus pyogenes for man; A study of the problems of wound infection. British Journal of Experimental Pathology. 1957;**38**(6):573-586

[15] Kathju S, Nistico L, Tower I, Lasko LA, Stoodley P. Bacterial biofilms on implanted suture material are a cause of surgical site infection. Surgical Infections (Larchmt). 2014;**15**(5):592-600. DOI: 10.1089/sur.2013.016

[16] Forrester JD, Maggio PM, Tennakoon l. Cost of health care-associated infections in the United States. Journal of Patient Safety. 2022;**18**(2):e477-e479

[17] World Union of Wound Healing Societies (WUWHS) Consensus Document. Surgical Wound Dehiscence: Improving Prevention and Outcomes. London: Wounds International; 2018. Available from: https://www.woundsinternational.com/resources/details/consensus-document-surgical-wound-dehiscence-improving-prevention-and-outcomes. [Accessed: May 05, 2022]

[18] Bosanquet DC, Ansell J, Abdelrahman T, Cornish J, Harries R, Stimpson A, et al. Systematic review and meta-regression of factors affecting midline incisional hernia rates: Analysis of 14 618 patients. PLoS One. 2015;**10**(9):e0138745. DOI: 10.1371/journal.pone.0138745

[19] Yahchouchy-Chouillard E, Aura T, Picone O, Etienne JC, Fingerhut A. Incisional hernias I. Related risk factors. Digestive Surgery. 2003;**20**(1):3-9. DOI: 10.1159/000068850

[20] Chintamani. Editorial. Ten commandments of safe and optimum abdominal wall closure. Indian Journal of Surgery. 2018;**80**(2):105-108. DOI: 10.1007/s12262-018-1776-6

[21] Pillai CK, Sharma CP. Review paper: Absorbable polymeric surgical sutures: Chemistry, production, properties, biodegradability, and performance. Journal of Biomaterials Applications. 2010;**25**(4):291-366. DOI: 10.1177/0885328210384890. Epub 2010 Oct 22

[22] Semer N. Suturing: The basics. In: Practical Plastic Surgery for Nonsurgeons. 1st ed. Philadelphia: Hanley and Belfus; 2001. pp. 1-20

[23] Muysoms FE, Antoniou SA, Bury K, Campanelli G, Conze J, Cuccurullo D, et al. European hernia society guidelines on the closure of abdominal wall incisions. Hernia. 2015;**19**(1):1-24. DOI: 10.1007/s10029-014-1342-5. Epub 2015 Jan 25

[24] Dennis C, Sethu S, Nayak S, Mohan L, Morsi YY, Manivasagam G. Suture materials - current and emerging trends. Journal of Biomedical Materials Research. Part A. 2016;**104**(6):1544-1559. DOI: 10.1002/jbm.a.35683. Epub 2016 Apr 4

[25] Sheik-Ali S, Guets W. Absorbable vs non absorbable sutures for wound closure. Systematic review of systematic reviews. Wound Medicine. 2018;**23**:35-37. DOI: doi.org/10.1016/j.wndm.2018.09.004

[26] Xu B, Xu B, Wang L, Chen C, Yilmaz TU, Zheng W, et al. Absorbable versus nonabsorbable sutures for skin closure: A meta-analysis of randomized controlled trials. Annals of Plastic Surgery. 2016;**76**(5):598-606. DOI: 10.1097/SAP.0000000000000418

[27] Patel SV, Paskar DD, Nelson RL, Vedula SS, Steele SR. Closure methods

for laparotomy incisions for preventing incisional hernias and other wound complications. Cochrane Database Systematic Reviews. 2017;**11**(11):CD005661. DOI: 10.1002/14651858.CD005661.pub2

[28] Sajid MS, Parampalli U, Baig MK, McFall MR. A systematic review on the effectiveness of slowly-absorbable versus non-absorbable sutures for abdominal fascial closure following laparotomy. International Journal of Surgery. 2011;**9**(8):615-625. DOI: 10.1016/j.ijsu.2011.09.006. Epub 2011 Oct 30

[29] Ahmed I, Boulton AJ, Rizvi S, Carlos W, Dickenson E, Smith NA, et al. The use of triclosan-coated sutures to prevent surgical site infections: A systematic review and meta-analysis of the literature. BMJ Open. 2019;**9**(9):e029727. DOI: 10.1136/bmjopen-2019-029727

[30] de Jonge SW, Atema JJ, Solomkin JS, Boermeester MA. Meta-analysis and trial sequential analysis of triclosan-coated sutures for the prevention of surgical-site infection. The British Journal of Surgery. 2017;**104**(2):e118-e133. DOI: 10.1002/bjs.10445. Epub 2017 Jan 17

[31] Uchino M, Mizuguchi T, Ohge H, Haji S, Shimizu J, Mohri Y, et al. SSI prevention guideline committee of the Japan society for surgical infection. The efficacy of antimicrobial-coated sutures for preventing incisional surgical site infections in digestive surgery: A systematic review and meta-analysis. Journal of Gastrointestinal Surgery. 2018;**22**(10):1832-1841. DOI: 10.1007/s11605-018-3832-8. Epub 2018 Jun 20

[32] Leaper DJ, Edmiston CE Jr, Holy CE. Meta-analysis of the potential economic impact following introduction of absorbable antimicrobial sutures. The British Journal of Surgery. 2017;**104**(2):e134-e144. DOI: 10.1002/bjs.10443. Epub 2017 Jan 17

[33] Henriksen NA, Deerenberg EB, Venclauskas L, Fortelny RH, Garcia-Alamino JM, Miserez M, et al. Triclosan-coated sutures and surgical site infection in abdominal surgery: The TRISTAN review, meta-analysis and trial sequential analysis. Hernia. 2017;**21**(6):833-841. DOI: 10.1007/s10029-017-1681-0. Epub 2017 Oct 17

[34] National Institute for Health and Care Excellence. Plus Sutures for preventing surgical site infection. Medical technologies guidance No. 59. Published 28 June 2021. Available from: www.nice.org.uk/guidance/mtg59

[35] Al-Mubarak L, Al-Haddab M. Cutaneous wound closure materials: An overview and update. Journal of Cutaneous and Aesthetic Surgery. 2013;**6**(4):178-188. DOI: 10.4103/0974-2077.123395

[36] Cochetti G, Abraha I, Randolph J, Montedori A, Boni A, Arezzo A, et al. Surgical wound closure by staples or sutures?: Systematic review. Medicine (Baltimore). 2020;**99**:25-e20573. DOI: 10.1097/MD.0000000000020573

[37] van de Kuit A, Krishnan RJ, Mallee WH, Goedhart LM, Lambert B, Doornberg JN, et al. Surgical site infection after wound closure with staples versus sutures in elective knee and hip arthroplasty: A systematic review and meta-analysis. Arthroplasty. 2022;**4**(1):12. DOI: 10.1186/s42836-021-00110-7

[38] Singer AJ, Quinn JV, Hollander JE. The cyanoacrylate topical skin adhesives. The American Journal of Emergency Medicine. 2008;**26**(4):490-496. DOI: 10.1016/j.ajem.2007.05.015

[39] Singer AJ, Chale S, Giardano P, Hocker M, Cairns C, Hamilton R, et al. Evaluation of a novel wound closure device: A multicenter randomized controlled trial. Academic Emergency Medicine. 2011;**18**(10):1060-1064. DOI: 10.1111/j.1553-2712.2011.01177.x

[40] Dumville JC, Coulthard P, Worthington HV, Riley P, Patel N, Darcey J, et al. Tissue adhesives for closure of surgical incisions. Cochrane Database of Systematic Reviews. 2014;(11):CD004287. DOI: 10.1002/14651858.CD004287.pub4

[41] Berríos-Torres SI, Umscheid CA, Bratzler DW, Leas B, Stone EC, Kelz RR, et al. Healthcare infection control practices advisory committee. Centers for disease control and prevention guideline for the prevention of surgical site infection, 2017. JAMA Surgery. 2017;**152**(8):784, 791. DOI: 10.1001/jamasurg.2017.0904. Erratum in: JAMA Surgery. 1 Aug 2017;**152**(8):803

[42] Justinger C, Slotta JE, Schilling MK. Incisional hernia after abdominal closure with slowly absorbable versus fast absorbable, antibacterial-coated sutures. Surgery. 2012;**151**(3):398-403. DOI: 10.1016/j.surg.2011.08.004. Epub 2011 Nov 16

Chapter 4

Skin Blister Formation and Subepidermal Bullous Disorders

Gamze Taş Aygar and Müzeyyen Gönül

Abstract

Blistering diseases comprise a large group of clinically polymorphic and sometimes devastating diseases. Blistering diseases are evaluated according to the level of the blister, the mechanism of blister formation and the type of inflammation. There are many connections in the normal structure of the skin that hold the cells together. These connections both hold the cells in the epidermis together and ensure that these cells attach to the basement membrane. As a result of damage to these connections by genetic, immune, infectious or physical reasons, intercellular connections are broken and blistering developments due to the accumulation of extracellular fluid in the intercellular spaces. Autoimmune bullous diseases are classified according to the decomposition site of the epidermis. While the pemphigus group is used to classify diseases with intraepidermal separation, the pemphigoid group diseases are used to classify diseases with subepidermal separation. In this section, pemphigoid group diseases, such as bullous pemphigoid, mucous membrane pemphigoid, acquired epidermolysis bullosa, linear IgA bullous dermatosis, and anti-p200 pemphigoid, will be explained with a brief introduction to blistering diseases of the skin.

Keywords: blistering diseases, subepidermal bullous disorders, pemphigoid, linear IgA bullous dermatosis, mucous membrane pemphigoid, anti-p200 pemphigoid

1. Introduction

Skin blistering diseases are clinically polymorphic large-group disorders and they sometimes may be devastating. These disorders may be classified according to [1] the level of the blister: subcorneal, mid epidermis, suprabasal, subepidermal; [2] the mechanism of blister formation (spongiosis, acantholysis, blistering degeneration, or epidermolysis); and [3] the type of inflammation (neutrophilic, lymphocytic, eosinophilic, mixed) [1]. In this section, pemphigoid group diseases such as bullous pemphigoid, mucous membrane pemphigoid, acquired epidermolysis bullosa, linear IgA bullous dermatosis, and anti p-200 pemphigoid will be explained with a brief introduction to blistering diseases of the skin. The features of subepidermal bullous disorders were summarized in **Table 1**.

	Bullous pemphigoid	Mucous membrane pemphigoid	Acquired epidermolysis bullosa	Linear IgA bullous dermatosis	Anti-p200 pemphigoid
Clinical symptoms Pathology Differential diagnosis Treatments	Tight bullae located on erythematous or normal ground in the lower abdomen, flexor surfaces of the limbs, groin, and axilla. It may also present with only pruritus or urticarial plaques. Subepidermal blisters with moderate to dense inflammatory infiltrate, especially eosinophils. DIF: The linear IgG and/or C3 deposition along the BMZ epidermolysis bullosa acquisita, mucous membrane pemphigoid, anti-p200 pemphigoid, pemphigus vulgaris, Oral/topical corticosteroids Azathioprine Mycophenolate mofetil Oxytetracycline/doxycyclin Methotrexate Dapsone Chlorambucil Cyclophosphamide Omalizumab Intravenous immunoglobulin(IVIG), Plasmaphereses	Mucosal blistering, ulceration, and subsequent scarring in the mucous membranes(oral mucosa, ocular conjunctiva, nasopharynx, larynx, anogenital region, and esophagus) and vesiculobullous lesions, ulceration, erosions, and scars in the head and the upper body. Subepithelial blisters with or without significant mixed inflammatory infiltrates and lamellar fibrosis in the upper dermis. DIF: The linear deposition of IgG, IgA, or C3 along the BMZ Bullous pemphigoid, epidermolysis bullosa acquisita, anti-p200 pemphigoid, pemphigus vulgaris Low-risk patients: Topical or intralesional corticosteroids, topical tacrolimus High-risk patients: Dapsone and/or prednisone, tetracycline, doxycycline pulsed steroid therapy, cyclophosphamide, IVIG, rituximab, azathioprine, mycophenolate mofetil, methotrexate, cyclophosphamide	Skin fragility, tense bullae, erosions, milium, and scar formation in trauma areas, especially the extensor surfaces of the acral regions In inflammatory type, the lesions can be seen on all skin and mucous membranes Subepidermal blister with eosinophilic-rich infiltrate, DIF: linear deposition of C3 and IgG along the BMZ Bullous pemphigoid Mucous membrane pemphigoid Linear IgA bullous dermatosis Anti-p200 pemphigoid Protecting from local traumas and infections. topical corticosteroids colchicine dapsone oral prednisone IVIG Pulse steroidsmycophenolate mofetil cyclosporine azathioprine rituximab Methotrexate cyclophosphamide plasma exchange	Vesicles and tense bullae are located on erythematous or normal ground in the trunk, extensor surfaces, buttocks, and face. Annular erythematous lesions with a ring of vesicles skin lesions heal without scarring, mucosal lesions may result in significant scarring. The mucosal involvement is more often in children than in adults Subepidermal blisters are associated with a dermal infiltrate of neutrophils, eosinophils, and mononuclear cells. Neutrophil microabscesses at the tip of the dermal papillae DIF: The linear accumulation of IgA along the BMZ. IgG, IgM, and C3 accumulation may be seen Bullous pemphigoid, Mucous membrane pemphigoid epidermolysis bullosa acquisita, anti-p200 pemphigoid, toxic epidermal necrolysis Dapsone sulfonamides oral corticosteroids, tetracycline and nicotinamide colchicine trimethoprim-sulfamethoxazole	Tense blisters with urticarial papules and plaque Acral and cephalic distribution and mucosal involvement subepidermal separation and a moderate to dense inflammatory infiltrate in the upper dermis, with a predominance of neutrophils DIF: Linear deposits of immunoglobulin IgG and C3 along the BMZ Bullous pemphigoid Mucous membrane pemphigoid Acquired epidermolysis bullosa Linear IgA bullous dermatosis Responds well to bullous pemphigoid treatment

DIF: direct immunofluorescence microscopy, Ig: Immunoglobulin, C3: complement 3, BMZ: basement membrane zone.

Table 1.
Features of subepidermal bullous disorders.

2. Blistering formation mechanisms

There are different mechanisms underlying vesicle and bulla formations, these are spongiosis, achantholysis, ballooning degeneration, and cytolysis (epidermolysis) [1, 2].

2.1 Loss of intercellular cohesion

Acantholysis is the loss of intercellular cohesion for various reasons. There may be many causes of primary acantholysis, the most known being pemphigus group diseases caused by autoantibodies against desmosome proteins. This condition can be caused by bacterial toxins, as in staphylococcal scalded skin syndrome, or by a genetic defect in the kertinocyte cell membrane, as in Hailey–Hailey disease [3–5].

Spongiosis, which describes intercellular edema causes secondary loss of intercellular cohesion although the intercellular connections are structurally normal. Loss of cohesion appears as small cavities in the epidermis in histopathology. It is called spongiosis because of its sponge-like appearance. As the severity of inflammation increases, the small spaces formed coalesce to form vesicle-bulla formation. The best example of this situation is allergic contact dermatitis [6].

Ballooning degeneration is the appearance of affected spinous cells with pale cytoplasm swollen due to intracellular edema. Necrosis of these cells and loss of attachment to neighboring cells is the cause of secondary acantholysis. It is characteristically seen in infections caused by some viruses, such as herpes, smallpox, and Coxsakie [7].

Cytolysis of basal layer cells of the epidermis causes loss of epidermal cohesion. In the epidermolytic form epidermolysis bullosa, bullae form due to post-traumatic damage to genetically defective basal layer cells [8].

2.1.1 Desmosomes, hemidesmosomes, and basal membrane

Preservation of the integrity of the epidermis depends on secure adhesion between adjacent keratinocytes, and between basal keratinocytes and the underlying epidermal basement membrane (BM). The major adhesion units are hemidesmosomes and desmosomes. As a result of damage to these connections by genetic, immune, infectious, or physical reasons, intercellular connections are broken and extracellular fluid accumulates in the intercellular spaces. This fluid accumulation appears as vesicles, intact or opened bullae, and erosions [2].

Desmosomes are structures that connect the intracellular skeleton to the cell membrane and other cells. Proteins, such as desmogleins, desmocollins, plakoglobins, plakophilins, and desmoplakins form the structure of the desmosome. The genetic absence of these proteins or the autoantibodies developed against these proteins cause genetic and autoimmune bullous diseases [9–11].

Basal keratinocytes adhere to connective tissue via extracellular matrix proteins that constitute BM [12]. Epidermal BM between the epidermis and dermis contains four principal basement membrane components; laminins, type IV collagens, perlecan, and nidogens [13].

Laminin-332, the most abundant laminin, distribute both throughout the epidermal BM and condenses in hemidesmosomes. Laminin-511 supports keratinocyte adhesion too and both laminins are important in maintaining the structural integrity of the BM and interact with integrin a3b1 and a6b4. In addition to integrin receptors, laminin-332 interacts with multiple proteins such as collagen XVII, syndecan 1 and 4, perlecan, nidogen 1, fibulin 2, and collagen VII [13, 14].

Collagen IV is the second major component of BM and is vital for maintaining epidermal BM integrity. The laminin and collagen IV networks need to be connected for BM stability. This task in the epidermal BM is performed by nidogens. Perlecan is an additional possible linker. Another BM component, fibrillin 1, interacts with perlecan and forms microfibrils participating in the anchorage of the epidermal BM to the papillary matrix [13, 15].

Collagen VII (anchoring fibrils) expressed by both epidermal keratinocytes and dermal fibroblasts has evolved as a specialized non-redundant component of the DEJ ensuring the firm attachment of the epidermal BM to the papillary matrix [13, 16]. As opposed to anchoring filaments, anchoring fibrils are much larger and have a characteristic structure anti-parallel alignment of type VII collagen molecules [16].

Epidermal BM has evolved to contain additional supportive structures that ensure firm adhesion of the epidermis to the dermis. This zone known as the dermal-epidermal junction (DEJ) is a functional unit composed of the plasma membrane of the basal keratinocyte with its hemidesmosomes, a lamina lucida, lamina densa, and a sublamina densa fibrous zone or reticular layer. DEJ plays a vital role in regulating communication between the epidermis and dermis and tissue reconstruction and repair [13–15].

Hemidesmosomes are cell-matrix junctions that connect epidermal keratinocytes to the BM. The core of each hemidesmosome consists of 180 kDa-bullous pemphigoid antigen (BP180, type XVII collagen, BPAG2), the two subunits of the α6β4 integrin, and a tetraspanin protein termed CD151. In BM, BP180 and α6β4 integrin interact with laminin–332. The cytoplasmic tail of the β4 integrin subunit binds both BP180 and two members of the plakin family, the 230 kDa bullous pemphigoid antigen (BP230 or BPAG1e) and plectin [12].

Subepidermal autoimmune bullous diseases (SABDs) are diseases characterized by subepidermal blisters that develop as a result of antibodies against DEJ components that are important structural proteins for the maintenance of dermo-epidermal integrity [17]. Bullous pemphigoid, mucous membrane pemphigoid, acquired epidermolysis bullosa, and linear IgA bullous dermatosis will be explained in these group disorders in this chapter.

3. Bullous phemphigoid

Bullous phemphigoid is the most common autoimmune blistering disease which affects the elderly, particularly in patients older than 70 years. The median age for bullous pemphigoid is 80 years. The incidence of the disease has increased significantly in last years due to the increased life expectancy of the aging population [18, 19]. BP has a significantly increased fatality, with 1-year mortality rates ranging from 6 to 41% in literature [17]. Infections are most important cause of death. Risk factors for mortality are advanced age, non-white ancestry, low health insurance accessibility, and the presence of neurological comorbidity and functional impairment at presentation [17, 20].

In the previous decades, neurological conditions including Parkinson's disease, dementia, stroke, epilepsy, and multiple sclerosis have been identified to be highly associated with BP patients. This association may be explained by the cross-reactivity between the neuronal (BP230) and epithelial isoforms of BP Ag1 which are both encoded by dystonin gene. Recently, psychiatric comorbidities, such as schizophrenia and bipolar disorder, as well as personality disorders have been reported in BP patients [17, 21]. A significant association with hematological malignancies between BP was revealed in the pooled analysis of cross-sectional studies while no association between BP and overall cancer was found in any of the study designs in the results of a meta-analysis [17]. Additionally, in BP risk of developing a thromboembolic disease is 15-fold higher [22].

A geographic or ethnic predilection of the disease is defined recently. Certain HLA class II alleles are more prevalent in patients with BP than in the general population. In Caucasians, a significant association with DQB1*0301 and in the Japanese population DRB1*04, DRB1*1101, and DQB1*0302 alleles have been found [17, 23].

It is associated with a humoral and cellular immune response directed against the components of the skin BM zone (BMZ). There are two self-antigens that are components of the hemidesmosomes: BP230 and BP180 [24]. *In vitro* studies have shown that human BP180 antibodies play a key role in the pathogenesis of the disease and are responsible for dermal-epidermal separation and subsequent subepidermal blister formation in patients with BP [18, 25]. In DIF, IgG-type antibodies are observed in 90–95% of cases and C3 accumulation is observed in 100% of cases, and this is a critical test for diagnosis. In a smaller group of patients, accumulation of IgE, IgA, and IgM can also be detected [26]. Those that are associated with pathogenesis are IgG and IgE-type antibodies. In particular, IgG1-type antibodies through complement activation, and IgE-type antibodies through mast cell degradation; cause neutrophil and eosinophil chemotaxis. Proteolytic enzymes released from these cells also cause separation at the dermo-epidermal junction. IgG4-type antibodies can also cause degradation by complement-independent antibody-dependent pathways. IgE-type antibodies are responsible for pruritic urticarial plaques, especially in the prebullous stage [27, 28].

The disease usually first presents with pruritus accompanied by localized or generalized excoriated lesions, eczematous, papular, and or urticarial lesions [29]. Blisters may accompany the first lesions or occur a few weeks up to months after the development of the first cutaneous signs [22]. Tense bullae can arise on an erythematous base or normal skin [29]. Blisters most commonly disperse symmetrically and predilection sites are the lower abdomen, flexor surfaces of the limbs, groin, and axilla [30]. The disease heals without scarring, but postinflammatory hypo-hyperpigmentation and milia can be seen [18]. Oral mucosal involvement is seen in 10–20% of affected patients [31–33].

The disease has a non-bullous phase in which typical clinical signs have not yet appeared. Classical bullous lesions are not seen in 20% of patients diagnosed with BP at the time of diagnosis [22, 30]. In this prodromal phase, patients may have only mild to severe pruritus. In an elderly patient who had especially neurological disorders, excoriations accompanied by severe pruritus should cause BP suspect. While eczematous patches can persist for months to years before the development of bullae progression from urticarial pemphigoid to bullous form is seen more quickly in approximately 6 weeks [22]. Another presentation form of BP are Prurigo nodularis-like lesions. Most Pemphigoid nodularis patients develop bullae within years but it is not necessary [22].

There is currently no standardized classification of BP. However, it is possible to recognize distinct variants of the disease according to the age of onset, clinical presentation, location of the lesions, and triggering factors [34]. The presence of concomitant lichen planus with BP is defined as lichen planus pemphigoid. Bullae that demonstrate classic immunopathologic findings of BP develop both on lichen planus lesions and on normal skin [22]. Pemphigoid vegetans is a form of BP in which clinical findings are similar to pemphigus vegetans but histopathology and immunofluorescence findings are identic with BP. BP rarely may manifest as exfoliative erythroderma characterized by generalized erythema and desquamation [34]. Another type is seborrheic pemphigoid involved seborrheic area and resembles pemphigus erythematosus. Also, BP may show ecthyma gangrenosum-like, erosive, toxic epidermal necrolysis-like presentations, and several localized forms. These localized forms that have better prognosis are dyshidrosiform pemphigoid characterized by pompholyx-like palmoplantar lesions, stomal pemphigoid sited stomal region, radiation aggravated pemphigoid limited to the site of radiation therapy, hemiplegic pemphigoid limited to the area of neurologic deficit, stump pemphigoid arised in a stump, pretibial umbilical and vulvar pemphigoid [22].

Pediatric BP is rare and has a more favorable prognosis than adults. Two peaks of incidence, one with an average age of 4 months in infantile BP and another with an age of 8 years in childhood BP were characterized [34]. Infantile BP significantly presents with face and acral involvement [22, 34]. Childhood BP may present localized lesions with genital involvement. Pediatric BP may be related to vaccination [34].

Drug-induced BP has been defined in the literature and several drugs, such as inhibitors of dipeptidyl peptidase-IV (especially vildagliptin and linagliptin, sitagliptin, anagliptin, alogliptin, teneligliptin, and saxagliptin) diuretics (furosemide and spironolactone), ACE inhibitors (captopril, enalopril, and lisinopril), β-blockers, NSAID's, TNF-a inhibitors, antipsychotics, calcium channel blockers and checkpoint inhibitors (Pembrolizumab, Nivolumab, and Durvalumab) are blamed for BP [21, 29, 34, 35].

Histopathology demonstrates subepidermal blister with a moderate to dense inflammatory infiltrate. Inflammatory cell infiltrates usually contain eosinophils and which are often seen in the blister cavity and basement membrane [18, 30]. These infiltrates may also contain neutrophils and lymphocytes [26, 36]. Direct immunofluorescence (DIF) examination shows linear immunoglobulin G (IgG) and/or C3 deposition along the basement membrane [25, 30]. The diagnosis is based on the combination of clinical features, histopathological and immunofluorescence findings.

Salt split DIF is useful in differentiating BP from other pemphigoid group diseases, such as epidermolysis bullosa acquisita, mucous membrane pemphigoid, and anti-p200 pemphigoid. The immune deposits are detected with salt-split DIF on the epidermal side of the skin in BP [18, 29].

Topical and systemic treatments can be used in the treatment of BP, depending on the severity of the disease, age, general health, medical history, and any contra-indications of the use of systemic medications for each patient. Topical clobetasol propionate should be the first choice in patients with < 5–10 new blisters per day. Clobetasol propionate cream can be applied only to the affected areas or to the whole body, sparing the face. If > 10 new blisters are present, systemic treatments can be used together with topical treatments. Oral corticosteroids are preferred first in systemic treatment to get the disease under control quickly. Azathioprine 1–3 mg/day, mycophenolate mofetil 2 g/day, oxytetracycline 2 g/day or doxycycline 200 mg/day with or without nicotinamide 2 g/day, methotrexate 15 mg/week, dapsone 1–5 mg/kg/day, chlorambucil 2–4 mg/day, cyclophosphamide 50 mg/day, anti-CD20 and anti-IgE monoclonal antibodies, intravenous immunoglobulin (IVIG), plasmaphereses and can be used to keep the disease under control and avoid steroid side effects in long-term treatment [37–39].

4. Mucous membrane pemphigoid

Mucous membrane pemphigoid (MMP) also known as cicatricial pemphigoid, is a rare subepidermal blistering disease with highly variable clinical heterogeneity and potential diagnostic delays. It predominantly affects the mucous membranes and, up to 30% of patients may also have skin involvement [37, 40, 41]. The disease most frequently involves the oral mucosa (85% of patients), followed by ocular conjunctiva (65%), nasopharynx, larynx, anogenital region, and esophagus involvement can be seen and results in mucosal blistering, ulceration, and subsequent scarring [41, 42]. The disorder if not recognized and treated early and aggressively in some cases, often may cause blindness, esophageal strictures, and even difficulty speaking and breathing [17, 22]. MMP mainly occurs in the elderly population, commonly observed between 60 and 80 years of age and seen in women more often than men [37, 42].

Certain HLA types like HLA DRB1*1503 have been associated with an increased risk of developing MMP [17, 22]. Autoantibodies against different antigens of the basement membrane zone, such as BP180, BP230, integrin subunits α6/β4, laminin-332 (also called epiligrin and laminin-5), laminin-6, and type VII collagen has been blamed for dermo-epidermal separation and blister formation in MMP [40, 42]. Generally, MMP has been classified into three types based on the antigenic target classic MMP (BP180); ocular MMP (α6β4 integrin); and anti-laminin 332 MMP (laminin 332) [18].

In the clinic, there are vesiculobullous lesions in all cases, but in contrast to BP oral involvement is in up to 85% of cases. The most commonly involved sites are the head and upper body and clinical evidence of scarring can clue in the diagnosis of MMP [18]. Healing of the lesions of the disease with scarring is an important cause of morbidity. Clinically, irreversible damage specific to the location of the lesions can be seen. Therefore, early diagnosis and effective treatment of the disease are important. Complications related to the eyes are very important as the eyes are the most frequently involved area. There may be non-specific conjunctivitis, as well as complications such as lagophthalmos, entropion, trichiasis, keratitis, glaucoma, and even blindness [43]. The most common finding of oral mucosal MMP is desquamative gingivitis. Ulcers and erosions due to the opening of bullae may also be seen. Patients complain of bleeding, pain, and dysphagia. As a result of oral mucosal involvement, speech and feeding difficulties may occur. Organ-specific complications can also be seen due to the involvement of other mucosal tissues [40, 44].

Diagnosis is made by clinical correlation with histopathologic, immunopathologic, and serologic findings [18]. Histology typically demonstrates the subepithelial split with or without significant mixed inflammatory infiltrates (predominantly neutrophilic and lymphocytic and variable eosinophilic) and lamellar fibrosis in the upper dermis [18, 45]. Lamellar fibrosis that can be seen underneath the subepidermal bullae is characteristic but is not always present. If it is, it can help distinguish MMP from other subepidermal blistering dermatoses [18]. In DIF examination, the linear deposition of IgG, IgA, or C3 along the BMZ is seen [45, 46]. As in BP, salt-split skin DIF shows epidermal staining in MMP except in anti-laminin 332 type [18, 41]. ELISA for the C-terminal domain of BP180, and laminin 332 MMP is not widely available so the benefit of serologic testing is limited for MMP diagnosis [18].

The choice of treatment depends on the severity of the disease and the patient's response to previous treatments. As in other chronic diseases, the patient's age, comorbid conditions, drug use, and severity of the disease are effective in the choice of treatment. In addition, a multidisciplinary approach and careful clinical examination are important in treatment because of irreversible tissue damage due to the disease [42].

In the choice of treatment, patients are evaluated as low and high risk. The "low-risk" patients are those with involvement of oral mucosa and/or skin. Patients with involvement of the ocular, nasopharyngeal, esophageal, laryngeal, and genital mucosa are considered "high-risk" patients [37].

Topical agents are the first line of treatment in low-risk patients. Topical or intralesional corticosteroids can be used. Topical tacrolimus can also be used for treatment, but topical steroids are more effective. When patients do not respond to topical treatments or in case of partial response to these treatments, systemic treatments should be started. Dapsone 50–200 mg/day and/or prednisone 0.5–1.0 mg/kg/day, tetracycline 1–2 g/day, and doxycycline 100 mg/day are the preferred agents in systemic therapy. In high-risk patients and low-risk patients who have a partial response to treatment, treatment should be more aggressive, and systemic therapy should be preferred primarily. Prednisone 1–2 mg/kg/day treatment can be used as the first choice for these patients. With or without prednisone treatment, depending on the patient's response to treatment; methylprednisolone 500 mg–1 g/day - 3 days (pulsed steroid therapy) or cyclophosphamide 1 g + dexamethasone 100 mg/day every 28/28 days or IV Immunoglobulin 2 g/kg/cycle and/or rituximab 375 mg/m2/week can be preferred. Also, azathioprine 1–3 mg/kg/day, mycophenolate mofetil 2–3 g/day, methotrexate 10–17.5 mg/week, and cyclophosphamide 1–2 mg/kg/day are also agents that can be used in the treatment [18, 37, 38, 42].

5. Epidermolysis bullosa acquisita (EBA)

Epidermolysis bullosa acquisita (EBA) is a rare, acquired subepidermal blistering disease of skin and mucous membranes, which is characterized by autoantibodies to collagen VII [47]. The disease occurs at similar rates in males and females and is common in the fourth and fifth decades, but 4.6% of patients are younger than 17 years of age [48].

The disease is divided into two types mechanobullous (non-inflammatory) and inflammatory type. Mechanobullous EBA is the most common type of EBA [49]. Skin fragility, tense bullae, erosions, milium, and scar formation can be observed in areas exposed to trauma, especially the extensor surfaces of the acral regions, in the mechanobullous type [50, 51]. Although mucosal involvement is less common than the inflammatory type, esophageal stenosis may develop. Milia, atrophic scars, hyper and hypopigmentation, nail dystrophy and loss, cicatricial alopecia, and digital contractures can be seen due to scar formation during healing [47]. This type should be distinguished from porphyria cutanea tarda in particular. While bullous lesions and erosions in acral areas seen in both are similar; In porphyria, hirsutism, photosensitivity, scleroderma-like skin changes, and high porphyrin in the urine are expected [52].

In the inflammatory type, the lesions can be seen in not only trauma-prone areas but also all skin, involving the trunk, central body, extremities and skin folds, and mucous membranes, so it is different from the mechanobullous type. It shows clinical findings similar to other subepidermal bullous diseases and is divided into subtypes named according to the diseases they resemble; BP-like EBA, cicatricial pemphigoid-like EBA, linear IgA bullous dermatosis (LABD)-like EBA and Brunsting-Perry pemphigoid-like EBA [47, 48].

Among inflammatory subtypes, BP-like EBA is the most common [47, 49]. Significant itching is observed in patients with BP-like EBA. It is usually present with tense bullae and erosions on urticarial or erythematous skin, which can occur in any part of the skin, including the face, and may affect the oral mucosa. In addition, lesions surrounded by intact skin can also be seen at trauma sites. Formation of cicatrice or millium is rare during healing [49]. Histopathology reveals a subepidermal blister with eosinophilic-rich infiltrate, and u-serrated pattern linear deposition of C3 and IgG in the basement membrane zone is detected in DIF examination [18, 47].

LABD-like EBA (IgA-EBA) patients present with tense bullae with annular or polycyclic array are seen on urticarial plaques with or without oral mucosal involvement. Milia and scar development are not expected. Subepidermal blisters are characterized by linear IgA deposits in the BMZ on direct immunofluorescence (DIF) [47, 53, 54].

MMP-like EBA mainly affects mucous membranes such as mouth, pharynx, esophagus, conjunctiva, anus, genital area, and respiratory tract and heals with scarring. As in MMP, organ-specific complications may occur due to scar formation in the mucous membranes [54, 55].

Brunsting-Perry pemphigoid-like EBA; subepidermal blisters located on the head and neck with atrophic scars with minimal or no mucosal involvement [56].

It is not clinically and histopathologically possible to distinguish all these inflammatory and non-inflammatory EBA forms from other subepidermal bullous diseases. As with most other subepidermal bullous dermatoses; linear deposits of IgG and C3 in BMZ can be demonstrated in perilesional skin. Diagnosis requires a demonstration of the presence of in situ and/or circulating IgG autoantibodies against collagen VII. At this point, the salt-split skin immunofluorescence test is can be used. EBA sera react on the dermal side of the salt-split skin, while BP sera react on the epidermal side [47, 55].

EBA may be associated with cancer as well as infectious, cardiovascular, metabolic, neurological, and chronic inflammatory diseases, such as inflammatory bowel disease, thyroiditis, rheumatoid arthritis, and psoriasis [48].

The choice of treatment for EBA depends on the severity of the disease. Although there are various methods to determine the severity of the disease, in recent research, patients with body surface area < 10%, without functional loss and severe mucosal involvement, are classified as non-severe. Patients with body surface area involvement > 10%, functional loss, and severe mucosal involvement are classified as severe [37, 47].

First of all, it is important to be protected from local traumas and infections. Topical corticosteroids are the first choice in mild and localized diseases. Depending on the condition of the disease, firstly colchicine(0.5–2 mg/day) or dapsone(50–100 mg/day) should be added to the treatment as an adjuvant in non-severe disease. If there is a partial response, oral prednisone (0.5–1 mg/kg/day) can be added to the treatment. In severe disease or resistance to other treatments, first-line treatment is intravenous immunoglobulin(IVIG) (2 g/kg over 5 days) and oral prednisone (1–1.5 mg/kg/day) or pulse therapy with methylprednisolone (1 g IV for 3 days). In case of partial response or unresponsiveness to previous treatments, mycophenolate mofetil (2–3 g/day) or cyclosporine (5 mg/kg/day), or azathioprine (100–200 mg/day) can be added to the treatment. If there is still no response to treatment, rituximab (1 g IV on D0 and D14 or 375 mg/m2 weekly for 4 weeks) is used every 6 months. Methotrexate, cyclosporine, cyclophosphamide, and plasma exchange are other treatment methods that can be used [37, 38, 47].

6. Linear IgA bullous dermatosis

Linear IgA bullous dermatosis (LABD) is a rare autoimmune subepidermal vesiculobullous disease, characterized by linear deposition of IgA along the basement membrane zone [57]. The disease is caused by IgA autoantibodies directed against different antigens of the basement membrane zone (BMZ) which are extracellular polypeptides of BP180 or collagen VII [58]. LABD may be idiopathic or due to different triggering factors including drugs and systemic autoimmune diseases (rheumatoid arthritis, psoriasis, systemic lupus erythematosus, Crohn's disease, and ulcerative colitis), infections (upper respiratory tract, gynecological infections, typhoid, brucellosis, varicella zoster, and tetanus), malignancies(bladder cancer) or less frequently, traumatic events such as burns and exposure to ultraviolet light [59–61].

The relationship between disease with drugs is well known. Vancomycin is the drug that most commonly causes LABD, followed by phenytoin and trimethoprim/sulfamethoxazole. The other commonly responsible drugs are antibiotics, non-steroidal anti-inflammatory agents, antiepileptic agents, or antihypertensives [60, 62].

The disease can occur in both adults and children. In children, the disease is known as "chronic bullous disease of childhood", that occurs in prepubertal children and has a self-healing course until adulthood [63].

LABD lesions, as in other subepidermal bullous diseases present as vesicles and tense bullae located on erythematous or normal skin and usually involve the trunk, extensor surfaces, buttocks, and face [61]. The typical clinical manifestation of LABD is an annular erythematous lesion with a ring of vesicles, a so-called "string of pearl, cluster of jewels, or rosette pattern" configuration [63, 64]. This configuration is more common in children and common locations are the trunk, the limbs, the perineum, and the perioral areas [65].

Mucous membrane involvement is common in both adults and children. The mucosa is involved more often in children than in adults [63]. While skin lesions heal without scarring, mucosal lesions may result in significant scarring. The disease is most commonly seen in the oral mucosa and conjunctiva. Mucosal strictures and corneal and conjunctival scars are the most important causes of morbidity [53, 66].

LABD clinical findings may be similar to toxic epidermal necrolysis (TEN), and even Nikolsky positivity may be seen. This situation should be kept in mind when making a differential diagnosis and a direct immunofluorescence examination should be performed [60].

Histopathological examination reveals the presence of subepidermal blisters associated with a dermal infiltrate of neutrophils and eventually eosinophils and mononuclear cells [64]. Neutrophil microabscesses at the tip of the dermal papillae may be seen [61]. In DIF examination, there is a linear accumulation of IgA along the basement membrane. IgG, IgM, and C3 accumulation may also be observed [67].

When the diagnosis of LABD is made, first of all, the patient's drug history should be well questioned. In drug-related diseases, first of all, the responsible drug should be discontinued [59]. Because drug-induced LABD has a good prognosis and most cases resolve within 2–6 weeks after discontinuation of the causative drug [66].

Topical potent corticosteroids can be used as the first choice in mild and localized diseases. In severe diseases, they are preferred in addition to systemic treatment [61].

Dapsone is considered the first-line therapy for LABD. The disease shows improvement within 2–3 days after dapsone therapy is started [66]. The dosage is 0.5–3 mg/kg/day for children and 25–150 mg/day for adults. The treatment should be started with a low dose, and the dose should be increased at intervals of 1–2 weeks until the disease is under control. Before starting treatment, the patient's glucose 6 phosphate dehydrogenase (G6PD) enzyme levels should be checked. This treatment should not be started for those with low enzyme levels. Due to the side effects of dapsone such as hemolytic anemia, agranulocytosis, dapsone hypersensitivity syndrome, leukopenia, methemoglobinemia, peripheral neuropathy, nephrotic syndrome, and abnormalities of liver function tests, patients should be followed closely during treatment and laboratory tests should be repeated at regular intervals. Hemogram and liver tests should be checked weekly for the first 1 month, then monthly for 6 months. In long-term treatment, controls can be made every 6 months [61, 66, 67].

Sulfonamides, including sulfapyridine and sulfamethoxy-pyridazine, oral corticosteroids, tetracycline and nicotinamide, colchicine, and trimethoprim-sulfamethoxazole can be used in the treatment of cases that do not response or partial response to dapsone [59, 61, 66].

7. Anti-p200 pemphigoid

Anti-p200 pemphigoid is a rare, recently described subepidermal autoimmune blistering disease characterized by autoantibodies against a 200 kDa glycoprotein localized within the lower lamina lucida in the basement membrane zone [68].

The disease presents as tense blisters with urticarial papules and plaque, as in bullous pemphigoid, and develops in the younger population, along with significant acral and cephalic distribution and mucosal involvement. Cases with similar findings with other subepidermal bullous diseases have also been reported. An association with psoriasis has been reported in 28.3% of patients mostly in Asian patients. In addition to the rarity of the disease, its exact incidence is unknown because it is clinically similar to other bullous diseases and unavailable detective technology in most countries.

Histopathological examination reveals subepidermal separation and a moderate to dense inflammatory infiltrate in the upper dermis, usually with a predominance of neutrophils but sometimes with significant numbers of eosinophils. Linear deposits of immunoglobulin (Ig)G and C3 are detected along the dermal-epidermal junction by direct immunofluorescence microscopy of perilesional skin [68]. In indirect immunofluorescence examination of salt-split skin, the serum sample is bound to the dermal side of the skin. Diagnosis of anti-p200 pemphigoid should be confirmed by the detection of antibodies directed against a 200 kDa dermal protein by enzyme immunoassay(ELISA). In addition, autoantibodies against the 200 kDa protein in the dermal extract can also be demonstrated by immunoblot [68].

Since the disease has been described recently, a standard treatment algorithm has not been defined. The disease usually responds well to bullous pemphigoid treatment [68]. As in other bullous diseases, topical corticosteroids are primarily used in the treatment of localized diseases. A combination of systemic corticosteroids and adjuvant immunomodulatory agents is preferred for systemic treatment. Unlike bullous pemphigoid, dapsone is the most preferred adjuvant agent in this disease [69].

8. Conclusion

Subepidermal bullous diseases are a group of diseases with skin and mucosal findings. To distinguish these diseases, which have many clinical similarities with each other, it is necessary to use tests such as histopathology, immunofluorescence, and ELISA. Complications due to these diseases themselves and the treatments applied are the cause of serious morbidity and mortality. Therefore, close follow-up of these patients and a multidisciplinary approach to treatment management are very important.

Author details

Gamze Taş Aygar and Müzeyyen Gönül*
University of Health Science, Dışkapı Yıldırım Beyazıt Education and Research Hospital, Dermatology Clinic, Ankara, Turkey

*Address all correspondence to: muzeyyengonul@gmail.com

References

[1] Kandemir NO, Barut F, Gün BD, Tekin NS, Keser SH, Özdamar ŞO. Histopathological analysis of vesicular and bullous lesions in Kaposi sarcoma. Diagnostic Pathology. 2012;**2012**:7. DOI: 10.1186/1746-1596-7-101

[2] Tintle SJ, Cruse AR, Brodell RT, Duong B. Classic findings, mimickers, and distinguishing features in primary blistering skin disease. Archives of Pathology and Laboratory Medicine. 2020;**144**:136-147. DOI: 10.5858/arpa.2019-0175-RA

[3] Egu DT, Schmitt T, Waschke J. Mechanisms causing acantholysis in pemphigus-lessons from human skin. Frontiers in Immunology. 2022;**13**:1-16. DOI: 10.3389/fimmu.2022.884067

[4] Prévost G, Couppié P, Monteil H. Staphylococcal epidermolysins. Current Opinion in Infectious Diseases. 2003;**16**:71-76. DOI: 10.1097/00001432-200304000-00002

[5] Ben Lagha I, Ashack K, Khachemoune A. Hailey–Hailey Disease: An update review with a focus on treatment data. American Journal of Clinical Dermatology. 2020;**21**:49-68. DOI: 10.1007/s40257-019-00477-z

[6] Streit M, Braathen LR. Contact dermatitis: Clinics and pathology. Acta Odontologica Scandinavica. 2001;**59**:309-314. DOI: 10.1080/000163501750541183

[7] Hookerman B. Dermatopathology: An abridged compendium of words. A discussion of them and opinions about them. Part 9 (T-Z). Dermatology Practical & Conceptual. 2015;**5**:3-5. DOI: 10.5826/dpc.0503a01

[8] Evtushenko NA, Beilin AK, Kosykh AV, Vorotelyak EA, Gurskaya NG. Keratins as an inflammation trigger point in epidermolysis bullosa simplex. International Journal of Molecular Sciences. 2021;**2021**:22. DOI: 10.3390/ijms222212446

[9] Delva E, Tucker DK, Kowalczyk AP. The desmoso

[10] sition. European Journal of Cell Biology. 2016;**95**:427-440

[11] Fine J-D. Structure and antigenicity of the skin basement membrane zone. Journal of Cutaneous Pathology. 1991;**18**:401-409. DOI: 10.1111/j.1600-0560.1991.tb01375.x

[12] Kridin K. Subepidermal autoimmune bullous diseases: Overview, epidemiology, and associations. Immunologic Research. 2018;**66**:6-17. DOI: 10.1007/s12026-017-8975-2

[13] Pratasava V, Sahni VN, Suresh A, Huang S, Are A, Hsu S, et al. Bullous pemphigoid and other pemphigoid dermatoses. Medicina (Kaunas, Lithuania). 2021;**57**:1061

[14] Joo JS, Yun SJ, Lee S, Lee J. Incidence of bullous pemphigoid and pemphigus in Korea. Annals of Dermatology. 2021;**33**:193-195

[15] Rozenblat M, Halaj A, Rozenblat T, Fisher S, Sah M, Dodiuk-Gad RP, et al. Mortality and risk factors among Israeli bullous pemphigoid patients. Archives of Dermatological Research. 2019;**311**:19-27. DOI: 10.1007/s00403-018-1875-z

[16] Moro F, Fania L, Linda J, Sinagra M, Salemme A, Di ZG. Bullous pemphigoid : Trigger and predisposing factors. Biomolecules. 2020;**10**:1432

[17] Amber KT, Murrell DF, Schmidt E, Joly P, Borradori L.

Autoimmune subepidermal bullous diseases of the skin and mucosae: Clinical features, diagnosis, and management. Clinical Reviews in Allergy and Immunology. 2018;**54**:26-51. DOI: https://doi.org/10.1007/s12016-017-8633-4

[18] Di ZG, Torre R, Zambruno G, Borradori L. Bullous pemphigoid : From the clinic to the bench. Clinics in Dermatology. 2012;**30**:3-16

[19] Bernard P, Antonicelli F, Bernard P. Bullous Pemphigoid: A review of its diagnosis , associations and treatment. American Journal of Clinical Dermatology. 2017;**18**:513-528. DOI: 10.1007/s40257-017-0264-2

[20] Sitaru C, Schmidt E, Petermann S, Munteanu LS, Bröcker EB, Zillikens D. Autoantibodies to bullous pemphigoid antigen 180 induce dermal-epidermal separation in cryosections of human skin. Journal of Investigative Dermatology. 2002;**118**:664-671. DOI: 10.1046/j.1523-1747.2002.01720.x

[21] Sadik CD, Schmidt E. Resolution in bullous pemphigoid. Seminars in Immunopathology. 2019;**2019**:645-654

[22] Genovese G, Di ZG, Cozzani E, Berti E, Cugno M, Marzano AV. New insights into the pathogenesis of bullous pemphigoid: 2019 update. Frontiers in Immunology. 2019;**10**:1-8. DOI: 10.3389/fimmu.2019.01506

[23] Ujiie H, Nishie W. Pa thogenesis of bullous pemphigoid. Dermatologic Clinics. 2011;**29**:439-446

[24] Bağcı IS, Horváth ON, Ruzicka T, Sárdy M. Bullous Pemphigoid. Autoimmunity Reviews. 2017;**16**:445-455

[25] Moar A, Azzolini A, Tessari G, Schena D, Girolomoni G. Non-bullous pemphigoid: A single-Center retrospective study. Dermatology. 2021;**237**:1039-1045. DOI: 10.1159/000515954

[26] Chen X, Zhao W, Jin H, Li L. Risk factors for mucosal involvement in bullous pemphigoid and the possible mechanism: A review. Frontiers in Medicine. 2021;**8**:1-8. DOI: 10.3389/fmed.2021.680871

[27] Kridin K, Bergman R. Assessment of the prevalence of mucosal involvement in bullous pemphigoid. JAMA Dermatology. 2019;**155**:166-171. DOI: 10.1001/jamadermatol.2018.5049

[28] Clapé A, Muller C, Gatouillat G, Le Jan S, Barbe C, Pham BN, et al. Mucosal involvement in bullous pemphigoid is mostly associated with disease severity and to absence of anti-BP230 autoantibody. Frontiers in Immunology. 2018;**9**:1-9. DOI: 10.3389/fimmu.2018.00479

[29] Miyamoto D, Santi CG, Maruta CW. Bullous pemphigoid. Anais Brasileiros de Dermatologia. 2019;**94**:133-146

[30] Tasanen K. Dipeptidyl Peptidase-4 inhibitor-associated bullous pemphigoid. Frontiers in Immunology. 2019;**10**:1-10. DOI: 10.3389/fimmu.2019.01238

[31] Schmidt E, Zillikens D. Pemphigoid diseases. The Lancet. 2013;**381**:320-332

[32] Santi CG, Gripp AC, Roselino AM, Mello DS, Gordilho JO, De MPF, et al. Bullous pemphigoid , mucous membrane pemphigoid and epidermolysis bullosa acquisita. Brazilian Society of Dermatology. 2019;**94**:33-47

[33] Patel PM, Jones VA, Murray TN, Amber KT. A review comparing international guidelines for the management of bullous pemphigoid, pemphigoid gestationis , mucous

membrane pemphigoid , and epidermolysis bullosa Acquisita. American Journal of Clinical Dermatology. 2020;**20**:557-565

[34] Feliciani C, Joly P, Jonkman MF, Zambruno G, Zillikens D, Ioannides D, et al. Management of bullous pemphigoid : The European dermatology forum consensus in collaboration. European Academy of Dermatology and Venereology. 2015:867-877. DOI: 10.1111/bjd.13717

[35] Carey B, Setterfield J. Mucous membrane pemphigoid and oral blistering diseases. Clinical and Experimental Dermatology. 2019;**44**:1-8. DOI: 10.1111/ced.13996

[36] Sollecito TP, Parisi E. Mucous membrane pemphigoid. The Dental Clinics of North America. 2005;**49**:91-106. DOI: 10.1016/j.cden.2004.07.004

[37] Xu HH, Werth VP, Parisi E, Sollecito TP. Mucous Membrane Pemphigoid. Dental Clinics of North America. 2013;**57**:611-630. DOI: 10.1016/j.cden.2013.07.003

[38] Srikumaran D, Akpek EK. Mucous membrane pemphigoid : recent advances. Current Opinion Ophthalmology. 2012;**23**:523-527

[39] Petruzzi M et al. Immunopharmacology and Immunotoxicology. 2012;**34**:363-367. DOI: 10.3109/08923973.2011.608684

[40] Yancey KB. Pemphigoid: Clinical histologic, immunopathologic, and therapeutic considerations. Journal of the American Medical Association. 2015;**284**:350-356

[41] Kourosh AS, Yancey KB. Pa thogenesis of mucous membrane pemphigoid. Dermatologic Clinics. 2011;**29**:479-484

[42] Miyamoto D, Gordilho JO, Santi CG, Porro AM. Epidermolysis bullosa acquisita. Anais Brasileiros de Dermatologia. 2022;**97**:409-423

[43] Iwata H, Vorobyev A, Koga H, Recke A, Zillikens D, Prost-Squarcioni C, et al. Meta-analysis of the clinical and immunopathological characteristics and treatment outcomes in epidermolysis bullosa acquisita patients. Orphanet Journal of Rare Diseases. 2018;**13**:1-9. DOI: 10.1186/s13023-018-0896-1

[44] Koga H, Prost-Squarcioni C, Iwata H, Jonkman MF, Ludwig RJ, Bieber K. Epidermolysis bullosa acquisita: The 2019 update. Frontiers in Medicine. 2019;**10**:362

[45] Kasperkiewicz M, Sadik CD, Bieber K, Ibrahim SM, Manz RA, Schmidt E, et al. Epidermolysis bullosa acquisita: From pathophysiology to novel therapeutic options. Journal of Investigative Dermatology. 2016;**136**:24-33

[46] Ishii N, Hamada T, Dainichi T, Karashima T, Nakama T, Yasumoto S, et al. Epidermolysis bullosa acquisita: What's new? Journal of Dermatology. 2010;**37**:220-230. DOI: 10.1111/j.1346-8138.2009.00799.x

[47] De Groot HJ, Jonkman MF, Pas HH, Diercks GFH. Direct immunofluorescence of mechanobullous epidermolysis bullosa acquisita, porphyria cutanea tarda and pseudoporphyria. Acta Dermato-Venereologica. 2018;**99**:26-32. DOI: 10.2340/00015555-3021

[48] Utsunomiya N, Chino T, Oyama N, Utsunomiya A, Yamaguchi Y, Takashima W, et al. Sublamina densa-type linear IgA bullous dermatosis

with IgA autoantibodies specific for type VII collagen: A case report and clinicopathological review of 32 cases. Dermatology Online Journal. 2017;**23**:1-6. DOI: 10.5070/d32311037250

[49] Kridin K, Kneiber D, Kowalski EH, Valdebran M, Amber KT. Epidermolysis bullosa acquisita: A comprehensive review. Autoimmunity Reviews. 2019;**18**:786-795

[50] Kim JH, Kim SC. Epidermolysis bullosa acquisita. Journal of the European Academy of Dermatology and Venereology. 2013;**27**:1204-1213. DOI: 10.1111/jdv.12096

[51] Asfour L, Chong H, Mee J, Groves R, Singh M. Epidermolysis bullosa Acquisita (Brunsting-Perry pemphigoid variant) localized to the face and diagnosed with antigen identification using skin deficient in type VII collagen. American Journal of Dermatopathology. 2017;**39**:e90-e96. DOI: 10.1097/DAD.0000000000000829

[52] Sarikaya Solak S, Ficicioglu S. Cephalosporin-induced linear IgA dermatosis in a child: Case report and literature review. Dermatologic Therapy. 2019;**2019**:32. DOI: 10.1111/dth.12927

[53] Inamura E, Nishie W, Yamaguchi Y, Fujimura Y, Ujiie H, Natsuga K, et al. Linear IgA/IgG bullous dermatosis with autoantibodies directing the native and processed forms of BP180. British Journal of Dermatology. 2020;**182**:1061-1062. DOI: 10.1111/bjd.18642

[54] Phyu H, Kobayashi T, Rastogi P, Cho C. Vancomycin- induced linear immunoglobulin a bullous dermatosis. BML Case Reports. 2019;**12**:1-2. DOI: 10.1136/bcr-2019-233281

[55] Lammer J, Hein R, Roenneberg S, Biedermann T, Volz T. Drug-induced linear IgA bullous dermatosis: A case report and review of the literature. Acta Dermato-Venereologica. 2019;**99**:508-515. DOI: 10.2340/00015555-3154

[56] Fortuna G, Marinkovich MP. Linear immunoglobulin A bullous dermatosis. Clinics in Dermatology. 2012;**30**:38-50

[57] Garel B, Ingen-housz-oro S, Afriat D, Prost-Squarcioni C, Tétart F, Bensaid B, et al. Drug-induced linear immunoglobulin a bullous dermatosis : A French retrospective pharmacovigilance study of 69 cases. British Journal of Clinical Pharmacology. 2019;**85**:570-579. DOI: 10.1111/bcp.13827

[58] Genovese G, Venegoni L, Fanoni D, Muratori S, Berti E, Marzano AV. Linear IgA bullous dermatosis in adults and children: A clinical and immunopathological study of 38 patients. Orphanet Journal of Rare Diseases. 2019;**14**:1-7. DOI: 10.1186/s13023-019-1089-2

[59] Mintz EM, Morel KD. Clinical features, diagnosis, and pathogenesis of chronic bullous disease of childhood. Dermatologic Clinics. 2011;**29**:459-462. DOI: 10.1016/j.det.2011.03.022

[60] Giraud L, Welfringer-Morin A, Boccara O, Frassati-Biaggi A, Leclerc-Mercier S, Grootenboer-Mignot S, et al. Neonatal and self-healing linear immunoglobulin a dermatosis. Journal of the European Academy of Dermatology and Venereology. 2020;**34**:86-87. DOI: 10.1111/jdv.15989

[61] Bernett C, Fong M. Linear IGA Dermatosis. Treasure Island, FL: StatPearls Publishing; 2022

[62] Carlos E, Dimatos OC, Porro AM, Santi CG. Consensus on the treatment of autoimmune bullous dermatoses: Dermatitis herpetiformis and linear IgA

bullous dermatosis. Brazilian Society of Dermatology. 2019;**94**:48-55

[63] Meijer JM, Diercks GFH, Schmidt E, Pas HH, Jonkman MF. Laboratory diagnosis and clinical profile of anti-p200 pemphigoid. JAMA Dermatology. 2016;**152**:897-904. DOI: 10.1001/jamadermatol.2016.1099

[64] Kridin K, Ahmed AR. Anti-p200 pemphigoid: A systematic review. Frontiers in Immunology. 2019;**10**:1-7. DOI: 10.3389/fimmu.2019.02466

[65] Goletz S, Hashimoto T, Zillikens D, Schmidt E. Anti-p200 pemphigoid. Journal of American Dermatology. 2014;**71**:185-191

[66] Xie Y, Wang S, Li S, Zuo Y. Coexistence of anti-p200 pemphigoid and psoriasis : A systematic review. Frontiers in Immunology. 2022;**13**:1-10. DOI: 10.3389/fimmu.2022.839094

[67] Rose C, Weyers W, Denisjuk N, Hillen U, Zillikens D, Shimanovich I. Histopathology of anti-p200 pemphigoid. American Journal of Dermatopathology. 2007;**29**:119-124

[68] Commin M-H, Schmidt E, Duvert-Lehembre S, Lasek A, Morice C, Estival J-L, et al. Clinical and immunological features and outcome of anti-p200 pemphigoid. British Journal of Dermatology. 2016;**175**:776-781. DOI: 10.1111/bjd.14629

[69] Laufer Britva R, Amber KT, Cohen AD, Kridin K. Treatment and clinical outcomes in anti-p200 pemphigoid: A systematic review. Journal of the European Academy of Dermatology and Venereology. 2020;**34**:465-472. DOI: 10.1111/jdv.15961

Section 2

Treatment and Management of Specific Skin Conditions

Chapter 5

Current Concepts: Pediatric Dog Bite Injuries

Katlin VanDerhoef and Jeffrey P. Louie

Abstract

Dog bite wounds are an increasingly common occurrence, particularly in children. Providers must be able to manage bite injuries, as well as identify wound infections and how to treat them. This chapter discusses common dog bite injuries, immediate and delayed sequelae of a bite wound, wound closure, and antibiotic treatment regimens. Facial injuries are common in pediatrics and may require surgical consultation. Knowledge of the immunization status of the patient and dog is essential in the prevention and sequala of tetanus and rabies. The subsequent information is essential for any physician working with children and their families, particularly in the emergency setting.

Keywords: dog bites, wound infection, bite management, antibiotics, trauma, rabies and tetanus vaccinations

1. Introduction

According to the American Veterinary Medical Association, over 48 million households in the United States own a pet dog. This equates to 38.4% of all Americans owning a dog. The estimated total number of dogs in the United States is approximately 76.8 million [1]. With these statistics in mind, it is not surprising that an estimated 4.5 million dog bites occur each year [1, 2]. Of these, approximately 800,000 seek medical attention and 386,000 require treatment in the Emergency Department [3].

Over the past 16 years, canines killed 568 Americans [2]. Pit bulls constitute 6.2% of the total US dog population but accounted for 380 (67%) of these fatalities [2]. Rottweilers had the second-largest contribution with 51 (9%) fatalities [2]. The other breeds implemented included American bulldogs, German shepherds, Mastiffs, Bull Terriers, Cane Corso, Belgian Malinois, Labrador retriever, and mixed-breeds [2].

In 2020, there were 46 fatalities from dog bites [2]. Pit bulls accounted for 33 (72%) of these deaths [2]. Of the dogs whose gender was known, 82% were male [2]. Fatal dog attacks involving multiple dogs accounted for 43% (20) of the victims [2]. Of these 20 attacks, 14 (70%) involved two or more pit bulls [2]. The data also showed that 20% (9) of dog bite fatalities involved dogs with a known history of human aggression and 13% (6) had a history of animal aggression [2].

In addition, the majority of dog bite victims were over 19 years of age (61%) [2]. Among the pediatric cohort of children 18 years or younger, 53% were infants less than 12 months of age [2]. Unfortunately, family dogs resulted in 59% (27) of the fatalities over the past year [2]. Of the 33 deaths inflicted specifically by pit bulls, 55% (18) were family members while 45% (15) were non-family members [2].

Location of dog bite injuries, laceration, or puncture wounds, is an important discussion point among children. Recent studies have reported that the average age of children who receive a dog bite is about 5 years of age [4, 5]. The most severe injuries requiring repair in an operating room involve children less than 3 years of age and tend to be above the clavicle [5, 6]. Rupture globes, avulsed ears, lips, nose, and eyelids have all been reported. The location of dog bite injuries appears to correlate with the child's age. As mentioned, younger children have a higher risk of sustaining injuries to their facial structures, scalp, and neck [5, 6]. Older children, because they are taller, are more likely to have injuries to their hands, feet, and extremities [5, 6]. One study reported that up to 92% of all dog bites in children are located in the head and neck region, followed by the extremities (15.7%) and the trunk (4.9%) [5]. The majority of children are bitten in only one anatomic location [6]. The most common setting for sustaining a dog bite injury was the home [5]. A parent was present at the time of injury for almost half of the cases (43.6%) [5]. The circumstances surrounding an attack, when documented, identified 39.2% of children were playing with the dog [5]. Other scenarios included no initiated interaction (18.9%), attacks related to food, especially disturbing a dog when it is eating (13.5%), territorial encounters (9.5%), intervening between fighting animals (5.4%), playing with another person (5.4%), and disturbing a dog while asleep (4.1%) [5].

2. Trauma management/advanced trauma life saving

No matter the method of injury, Emergency Medicine (EM) physicians should always adhere to the Advanced Trauma Life Support (ATLS) protocol when initially assessing a patient. Studies have shown that patient outcomes are significantly improved when trauma teams follow the ATLS guidelines [7, 8]. Beginning with the primary survey, physicians should immediately assess the most vital and basic aspects of the patient's status [7, 8].

Airway: Determine the patency of the airway. Be aware of any tongue swelling, blood, or other possible causes of occlusions. Injuries or deformities of the neck and foreign bodies embedded in the soft tissue can also cause obstruction. Placement of a hard cervical collar if deemed necessary. Consider intubation if significantly occluded and all attempts to alleviate obstruction fail (jaw thrust maneuver, manual removal of any foreign body, etc) and bag-valve-mask technique is partial or ineffective. Preparation for a surgical airway may be indicated.

Breathing: Assess for difficulties with respiration as this may indicate an injury to the chest wall or pneumothorax. Palpate and visually inspect the chest wall for tenderness, crepitus, or deformity. If stable, consider imaging of the lung fields during the secondary survey.

Cardiovascular: Check central and peripheral pulses. Inspect the skin for color, warmth, and compromised blood flow. If there is an openly bleeding wound, apply pressure and/or tourniquet. During the primary survey, consider an ultrasound per FAST exam protocol. Follow the Advanced Cardiac Life Support (ACLS) protocol if the cardiac injury is suspected.

Disability: Using the Glasgow Coma Scale (GCS), determine the neurologic status of the patient. Assess the pupillary size, pupillary response, and consider Head/Cervical Spine CT (computer tomography) if concerns are present. Consult neurosurgery if there are alterations from baseline or alarming findings (Cushing's triad, asymmetric pupils, focal neurologic deficits).

Exposure: Remove all articles of clothing to obtain full inspection of any deformities, lacerations, bruising, or excoriations. Ensure the patient's core temperature remains stable.

Once the primary survey has been completed, the secondary survey can begin. The provider can gather specific details about the event, particularly involving the history of both the dog and patient. For the patient, ask questions about the medical history, surgical history, and immunization status. In particular, when did the patient receive their last tetanus vaccine, and if they have ever been vaccinated against rabies. Determine if the patient has any comorbidities including immunodeficiency, immunocompromised status, vaccine status, surgical/dental implants, or diabetes mellitus. Lastly, inquire about drug allergies, particularly to penicillin, given antibiotics are often required. Other necessary questions include the events leading up to the attack, was it provoked or unprovoked, how many dogs were present, time of injury, how much time has elapsed since the bite, what was done before presenting to the ED to clean the wound, the last time they ate/drank, and the location of the attack (for example, was it in a home, at a park, etc). If available, determine the dog breed, rabies vaccine status, and if the dog has a previous record of biting humans.

3. Basic wound management

Determining whether a wound should have primary versus delayed closure remains controversial [3, 9]. Traditionally, it was suggested that wounds should be left open for fear of the increased risk of wound infection when sutured closed [3, 9]. Treatment initially involved daily dressings with antibacterial ointment or hydrogen peroxide, followed by secondary closure 2–7 days later [3]. However, other more recent studies have found that there was no significant difference in infection rate between primary and delayed closure of dog bite wounds [3]. These studies advocate that early washout, debridement, and primary wound closure leads to similar infection rates but improvement in cosmetic and functional results [3, 9]. Two particular scenarios universally recommend delayed closure: if the bite is a puncture wound rather than a laceration, and if more than 12 hours has elapsed before the patient is seen by a medical professional [3].

3.1 Antibiotic regimen

Antibiotic prophylaxis is recommended for high-risk bites. These include presentation 8+ hours after the bite, moderate to severe wounds, patients who are immunocompromised or diabetic, deep puncture wounds, or bites involving the hand or face [3]. No prophylaxis is necessary for scratch wounds. Some studies suggest the use of antibiotic prophylaxis for infants and patients older than 50 years, irrespective of the appearance of the wound [3]. The first-line therapy (see **Table 1**) for both prophylaxis and treatment of dog bites is oral amoxicillin-clavulanate [3, 4, 9]. If the patient has a penicillin allergy, oral extended-spectrum cephalosporins (ceftriaxone, cefotaxime) or trimethoprim-sulfamethoxazole plus clindamycin is recommended [3, 4, 9]. For more severe wounds, consider intravenous ampicillin-sulbactam or meropenem [3, 4, 9]. If the patient seems to be worsening under the coverage of ampicillin-sulbactam, consider adding MRSA coverage with either trimethoprim-sulfamethoxazole or clindamycin

Injury type	Time course	Antibiotic	PCN allergy
Prophylactic	3–5 days	PO Amoxicillin-clavulanate	PO cefpodoxime or trimethoprim-sulfamethoxazole PLUS clindamycin
Cellulitis/soft tissue infection	7–10 days	PO Amoxicillin-clavulanate or IV Ampicillin-sulbactam	PO cefpodoxime or trimethoprim-sulfamethoxazole PLUS clindamycin
Severe cellulitis/soft tissue infection	10–14 days	IV Ampicillin-sulbactam + Vancomycin	IV Ceftriaxone or trimethoprim-sulfamethoxazole PLUS clindamycin OR meropenem alone

PCN, penicillin; PO, Oral; IV, Intravenous.[1]Source: Adapted from references 3, 4, and 9.

Table 1.
Antibiotic management of dog bite injuries based on type of infection[1].

based on the hospital's local resistant patterns [4]. If the patient requires hospitalization, vancomycin would be the additional antibiotic of choice for MRSA coverage [4]. The length of time recommended for prophylactic treatment is 3- to 5-days, with close follow-up in 24–48 hours to monitor for signs of developing infection [4]. For a soft tissue infection, a 7- to 10-day course of therapy is typically sufficient [4, 9]. However, a 10- to 14-day course may be warranted for more severe infections [4, 9].

3.2 Wound care

Approximately 5–25% of all dog bite wounds in children become infected [10]. The bites most likely to become infected include deep (puncture) contaminated wounds; areas marked with tissue destruction, poor perfusion, or edema; attacks to the hands, feet, face, or genitals; and wounds with joint involvement [9–11]. Wound infections after a dog bite are usually polymicrobial and consist of both aerobic and anaerobic bacteria from the mouth flora of the biting animal [9–11]. An average of 2–5 different bacterial isolates per culture were reported in a series of infected wounds caused by dog bites [9, 11]. *Pasteurella spp*. are the most common pathogen isolated and are found to have high carriage rates in the oropharynx, making bite wounds an easily transmittable method for infection [9–11]. Other pathogens identified in dog bites include, but are not limited to, *Corynebacterium* group G, *Neisseria weaveri*, *Capnocytophaga canimorsus*, *Fusobacterium nucleatum*, *Bacteroides tectus*, *Prevotella heparinolytica*, *Propionibacterium acnes*, *Peptostreptococcus anaerobius*, *Streptococcus pyogenes*, *Staphylococcus aureus*, and *Moraxella catharralis* [9, 11]. *Pasteurella* species were found to have the shortest latency period between bite and onset of infection [11]. They are also more commonly cultured from abscesses compared to the other species listed above [11]. The second most common bacterium isolated from dog bites was a tie between *Staphylococcus* and *Streptococcus* species [11]. Both were notable for being found most frequently in nonpurulent wounds, such as cellulitis and lymphangitis [11].

Signs of infection can present within hours to days of the initial bite and may include pain, erythema, and/or swelling of the affected area [9–11]. A multicenter, prospective study of 50 dog bite wounds found that the majority of infections were purulent without abscess formation (58%), followed by nonpurulent wounds with cellulitis, lymphangitis, or both (30%), and abscess formation resulting in the smallest number of presenting infections (12%) [11].

Treatment of the wound should begin with gentle irrigation using normal saline. The amount depends on the size and nature of the wound but typically ranges from 250 to 500 mL, or 50 to 100 mL/cm of laceration [4, 10, 11]. A 20 mL or larger syringe or catheter should be used to ensure enough pressure is applied to properly clean the wound [4, 10, 11]. If the wound is large or complex, surgical evaluation may be necessary to fully examine the wound for neurovascular, muscular, and soft tissue damage. A radiograph may be necessary if there is a concern for fractures or broken teeth or deeper puncture wounds concerning the development of osteomyelitis [4, 10].

3.3 Wound closure

Based upon the nature and characteristics of the injury, there are multiple options for wound closure. As previously discussed, there is intense debate surrounding primary vs. secondary closure of dog bite injuries. Once a decision has been made if or when the closure is necessary, there are several options on the technique of closure. The gold standard for wound closure is suturing [12]. Non-absorbable sutures are more applicable for partial-thickness wounds that can be easily released after healing [12]. Absorbable sutures are used for deeper or full-thickness wounds as a double-layer of closure and to decrease the tension on the primary sutures above [12]. Once the type of suture has been determined, the technique for suturing needs to be decided. Simple interrupted sutures tend to be more cosmetically appealing and allow for a better approximation of the wound edges [12]. However, if there is a need for rapid hemorrhage control or an extensive wound, running sutures allow for quick application but have a greater risk of dehiscence [12]. Finally, mattress stitches should be applied to deeper wounds due to their ability to employ deeper penetration with greater strength of wound closure [12]. In children, the use of an adhesive such as skin glue or skin tape can be considered but remains controversial in the context of dog bite wounds [12]. These options are excellent for percutaneous wounds and allow for less painful procedures, both with placement and removal. Another option for wound closure are staples, which can be placed quickly and are most useful in settings with brisk bleeding [12]. If there are multiple non-facial lacerations, staples are an efficient, cost-effective, and simple technique but may not be ideal for cosmesis.

3.4 Scar management

There are varying opinions on the appropriate recommendations for scar prevention and management. However, the initial step is to ensure proper primary suturing technique with the absence of tension on the wound and accurate approximation of the wound edges [12–15]. The wound should be closed with as little traction as possible and force should be minimized to cause further tissue damage [13–15]. Refer to **Table 2** for recommendations on when sutures should be removed for complete healing [12–16]. Skin tape can be applied to the area to continue to reduce tension and antibiotic ointment is no longer needed [12]. The following days to weeks after the initial injury, wound hydration becomes crucial [13–15]. Daily to every other-day dressing changes and cleaning with saline or tap-water is vital [13–15]. Never use alcohol or iodide solutions because of their cytotoxic nature, which inhibits healing and increases scar formation [13–15]. Silicone gel sheeting has also been shown to be effective in the treatment and prevention of scars by increasing hydration and decreasing collagen deposition [14, 15]. If there is a concern that keloid formation will occur, referral to a dermatologist for further management is recommended. There,

Location	Removal time (days)
Face*	3–5
Chest/Abdomen	8–10
Arm/Leg**	8–12
Fingertip	10–12
Foot	12–14

**Scalp removal 6–8 days.*
***Add 2–3 days if a joint is affected.*
[1]Source: adapted from reference [17].

Table 2.
Suture removal recommendations based on location of injury[1].

they may recommend intralesional steroid injections, laser therapy, or antimitotic drugs to help prevent or treat keloid and scar formation [15].

3.5 Severe wound management

When determining which patients are most likely to require hospitalization after being bitten by a dog, there are a few potential risk factors. Male children are more likely to sustain a dog bite than their female counterparts, which also makes them more likely to sustain a bite that requires hospitalization [17]. Additionally, non-Hispanic White children were more likely than their Black, Hispanic, and Asian peers to be hospitalized after a dog bite [17]. The summer months have the highest rate of dog bite hospitalization compared to any other season [17]. Of the children that were hospitalized, approximately 1/3rd required a major surgical procedure consisting of either debridement with suturing of the wound, skin grafting, plastics' surgical intervention, or tissue reconstruction [17]. Overall, the predominant description of children requiring hospitalization after a dog bite were of Caucasian ethnicity, male, less than 10 years of age, and received deep, extended, or multiple sites of injury [17].

3.5.1 Facial

A 20-year review of dog bites to the head and neck region found that 49.33% were 18 years of age or younger [18]. The majority of the lesions were sustained in the upper lip (32%), cheek (27%), and nose (20%) [18]. Periorbital or orbital wounds were rare [18]. The majority of the wounds were closed with primary methods using either sutures or adhesive strips (63%) due to their uncomplicated nature [18]. However, determining the method of closure should be based on the depth and underlying involvement of the wound. Please see the *Lackmann classification of injury* below for further details on how to classify the extent of a facial lesion. By classifying the lesion using the Lackmann system, it can help a provider to determine prognostic status and best method(s) for management of the wound. A transposition flap or reconstructive surgery was required in a small subset (6.7%) and skin grafting in an even smaller portion (3%) with more severe injuries [18]. Secondary wound infections were reported in only 2.24%, based on the theory that blood flow is enhanced to the face and neck regions leading to decreased incidence of infection [18]. However, it should be noted that prophylactic antibiotics were prescribed in 95% of cases likely contributing to the low infection rate [18].

A second review detailing the otolaryngology perspective on head and neck injuries details that 26.8–56.5% of dog bites occur to the head or neck [19]. Infection rates are reported to be as low as 5.7% due to the vascularized nature of the tissue [19]. The current recommendation is primary closure of head and neck wounds unless the results would be cosmetically displeasing [19]. ENT/OMFS and/or Plastics specialists should be consulted to help with esthetics and determination of closure technique. Additionally, current recommendations require amoxicillin-clavulanate therapy for 3–5 days whenever dog bites involve the face [19]. If signs of infection develop, the course should be extended to 7–14 days [3–4, 9, 19].

3.5.2 Lackmann classification of facial injury

i. Superficial lesion without muscular involvement

ii. Deep lesion with muscular involvement

iii. Deep lesion with muscular involvement and tissue defect

iv. Class III + vascular damage or neural lesions

v. Class III + bony damage or organ involvement

3.5.3 Orbital

The majority of periocular or orbital involvement in dog bite wounds are eyelid lacerations (**Figure 1**) or eyelid marginal lacerations [19]. Experts recommend primary closure within 24 hours and prophylactic antibiotics with amoxicillin-clavulanate [19].

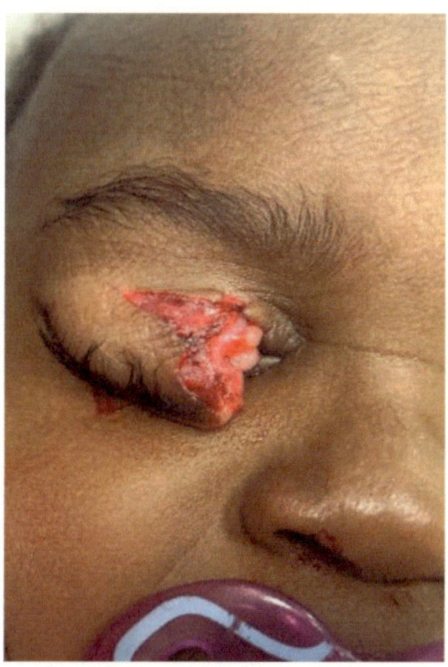

Courtesy of Jeffrey Louie, M.D.

Figure 1.
Full thickness laceration to superior eyelid. Courtesy of Jeffrey Louie, M.D.

Ensure that there is no corneal abrasion, orbital fractures, or ruptured globe associated with the injury [19, 20]. Use a woods lamp with fluorescein, unless a suspected ruptured globe is suspected, to visualize any corneal abrasions [19, 20]. If a ruptured globe is high on the differential, obtain facial CT which would show a deflated orbit if positive for globus rupture [19, 20]. Consider an additional head CT if there are further concerns for cranial injury or the patient has altered mental status [19, 20].

3.5.4 Genitalia

Copious irrigation with normal saline, debridement, and primary closure are the recommended steps in correcting dog bite lesions of the genitalia [21]. One of the biggest concerns for male genitalia wounds is the unilateral or bilateral loss of the testis. If this occurs, an ultrasound to look for torsion or hematocele formation is necessary after the attack, and an urgent urology consult is recommended [21]. Urethral injuries must also always be excluded in the cases of genitalia involvement [21]. Placement of a foley or cauterization for urine is contraindicated. Urethral endoscopy is the recommended next step after physical examination or known ureteral damage before surgical intervention [21].

3.5.5 Dental

Although not much research has been conducted on dental injuries secondary to dog attacks, it can be assumed that tooth avulsion or gingival laceration can occur [19, 22]. This is particularly relevant in cases of facial injury [19, 22]. If a patient presents with an avulsed tooth, the medium found to keep the tooth most viable is milk [23]. Current data suggest the tooth may only be viable for 30–60 minutes, thus reimplantation by the EM or dental specialist should occur as soon as possible. Gingival lacerations should always be inspected and repaired by the dental specialist.

4. Tetanus and Rabies

In addition to causing a localized infection, dog bites may also transmit pathogens that can cause a systemic illness. The most commonly considered sequelae are tetanus and rabies [4, 9, 24, 25].

4.1 Tetanus

The management of tetanus prophylaxis in dog bites is based upon the immunization status of the affected patient (see **Table 3**). If the child has received less than 3 doses of the tetanus toxoid-containing vaccine or the vaccination status is unknown, human tetanus immunoglobulin should be administered as well as a dose of tetanus toxoid-containing vaccine [24]. For those that have completed a 3-dose series, determine if/when the last dose was administered and if they have undergone any booster shots. If the last tetanus vaccine was 5 or more years ago, it is recommended that they receive a booster dose of the age-appropriate tetanus vaccine [24].

4.2 Rabies

Fortunately, rabies infections are a rare occurrence. Prevention is critical, particularly when the outcome is approximately 100% mortality when infection

Received doses of tetanus toxoid	Received doses of DTap, Tdap, or Td	Administer DTap, Tdap, or Td	Administer TIG
<3 doses or unknown		YES	YES
3 or more doses	≤ 5 years since last tetanus toxoid containing vaccine	NO	NO
	>5 years since last tetanus toxoid containing vaccine	YES	NO

[1]Source: adapted from reference 25.

Table 3.
Guideline for tetanus vaccines and immunoglobin[1].

develops [9, 25]. Post-exposure rabies prophylaxis is provided to approximately 40,000 people per year [9]. Between 1 and 3 people die per year in the United States from a rabies infection [25]. When an animal infected with rabies bites a person, the saliva containing the rabies is deposited into the tissues and incubates for 20 to 90 days [4, 25]. The virus then travels to the central nervous system where it causes the rapid development of symptoms [4, 25]. The first step in determining what type of rabies prophylaxis is needed is to evaluate the health of the dog. If the pet is healthy and able to be observed for 10 days, then prophylaxis only needs to be administered if the animal begins exhibiting signs of rabies development [9, 25]. If the dog is known or suspected to be rabid, rabies immunization and rabies immunoglobulin should be administered as soon as possible [9, 25]. The animal itself should be euthanized and tested for rabies as soon as possible [9, 25]. Immunization can be discontinued if there are negative test results [9, 25]. If the status of the animal is unknown, consult the local public health department for guidance.

Use of both active and passive prophylaxis is warranted once wound care has been completed and the patient is categorized as needing postexposure prophylaxis [9, 25]. Unvaccinated or immunocompetent children need the full 4-dose series of rabies vaccinations along with the human rabies immune globulin [9, 25]. Rabies immunoglobulin should be administered around the wound and given only on day 0 [9, 25]. The vaccinations should be scheduled on days 0, 3, 7, and 14 of wound infliction [9, 25]. Children who have previously undergone rabies vaccination should receive only a vaccine booster shot and do not require rabies immunoglobulin [9, 25]. All animal bites should be reported to the county and state health department and local animal control for record maintenance [25].

5. Further considerations

5.1 Animal control

Dog "perpetrators" are not commonly reported unless a police or animal control report is filed. A dog with multiple offenses may go undetected to law enforcement unless victims report their injuries, provide the name or address of the dog owner, and breed of dog. At our institution, all dog bites are reported to the county animal control agency. Potentially, a dog owner with a record of multiple reports could be reprimanded with fees or have their dog removed from the house.

5.2 Prevention and anticipatory guidance to dog owners

As previously discussed, the majority of dog bites are caused by household pets or animals known to the victim [2, 26]. Many of the attacks occur in or around the family home [2, 26, 27]. By nature, dogs are social animals that navigate within a pack hierarchy [26]. Communication is relayed through both vocal means and body language, which can be missed or misinterpreted by their human counterparts [26]. The posture, tail movements, facial features, and noises made by the dog can often provide information on an imminent attack [26]. Of course, this is not to say that the victim is to blame for a dog attack. Rather, dog owners should be made aware of signs of aggression and how to properly respond to them. There are plenty of resources available through the internet or local canine training programs for owners to learn techniques of de-escalating signs of aggression. Additionally, children should never be left unsupervised with a dog. Some tips to help prevent dog bites include:

- Do not disturb any dog caring for puppies, eating, or sleeping
- Never reach through or over a fence to pet a dog
- Do not run away from or chase after a dog
- Teach children to move slowly and pet gently
- Always allow the dog to sniff your hand before petting them
- Never approach an unfamiliar dog
- If an unfamiliar dog approaches, stand still with your arms at your side. Allow it to sniff you and move on. No sudden moves.

5.3 Psychological Sequelae of dog bites

Although poorly reported, the psychological impact of dog bites can range from avoidance behaviors to formally diagnosed post-traumatic stress disorder (PTSD) [27–29]. One study reports that nearly one-third of all children that suffered a dog bite injury developed a new fear or avoidance of dogs [29]. The same study found that 5% were diagnosed with PTSD at three months post-injury [29]. Symptoms of PTSD included numbness, apathy, avoidance behaviors, increased arousal, hypervigilance, and vivid recollections of the event [27–29]. These can present anywhere from immediately after the event to months later [27–29]. Additionally, an overwhelming 85% of parents whose children sustained a dog bite injury reported changes in their own emotional state [29]. Approximately two-thirds reported feelings of guilt and half reported fear and anger surrounding the event [29].

The first step toward recovery after a traumatic event is recognizing the effects it has had on the victim and those around them. Informing family members of the signs and symptoms of trauma is essential for identifying when professional help is needed [28–29]. As providers, referral to a psychiatrist or psychologist for therapeutic intervention is appropriate after any incidence of the dog attack, even if there are no apparent stress disorder symptoms [28, 29]. Particularly important for early intervention are children who sustained multiple or severe dogs bite wounds, which has been shown to increase the risk of PTSD development [29].

6. Conclusion

An estimated 4.5 million dog bites occur each year with approximately 800,000 requiring medical attention [1–3]. As the number of households with pet dogs continues to rise, the incidence of dog bite injuries will grow. Physicians must be prepared to care for children with dog bite injuries. A number of retrospective studies of dog bite injuries in children have found that the most common age to sustain a bite is 5–9 years old [4, 5]. The majority of bite wounds are inflicted by the pit bull breed and occur in the home setting [1–3]. Fortunately, mortality is rare and there were only 46 cases of death secondary to dog bite injury in the year 2020 [2]. Location of the injury has been found to correlate with age; younger children sustain bites to the head and neck while older children tend to be bitten on the hands and upper extremities [5, 6]. The most extreme injuries requiring surgical intervention tend to occur in children less than 3 years of age [5, 6].

When acutely managing a dog bite, the first step is to follow the Advanced Trauma Life Saving (ATLS) guidelines. Begin with a primary survey of the airway, breathing, and circulation [7, 8]. Additionally, determine the neurologic status of the patient and determine any required immediate interventions. After stabilization, complete a secondary survey to gather specific details of the event and the medical history of the patient. In order to address the wounds, decide whether primary vs. secondary closure is warranted. As stated previously, there continues to be controversy over primary vs. delayed closure but recent studies have found that there is no significant difference in infection rate between the two methods [3]. Cosmetic and functional results can help to drive the decision, as well as any professional input from plastic surgery, otolaryngology, or dermatology. No matter which method of closure is decided upon, begin by irrigating the wound with normal saline using 250 mL–500 mL with a 20 mL syringe to ensure adequate pressure. Debride any necrotic tissue. Contact surgery for large, complex wounds.

Antibiotic prophylaxis is warranted for any high-risk bites, such as presentation 8+ hours after the bite, moderate to severe wounds, patients who are immunocompromised or diabetic, deep puncture wounds, or bites involving the hand or face [3]. Wound infections are usually polymicrobial, with the most common bacteria being *Pasteurella* spp. [9–11]. The first-line therapy for both prophylaxis and treatment of an infected dog bite is oral amoxicillin-clavulanate or parenteral ampicillin-sulbactam, depending on the severity [3, 4, 9]. If the patient has a penicillin allergy, oral extended-spectrum cephalosporins (ceftriaxone, cefotaxime) or trimethoprim-sulfamethoxazole plus clindamycin is recommended [3, 4, 9]. The prophylactic treatment course is 3–5 days; soft tissue infections should be treated for 7–10 days [3, 4, 9]. A 10–14 day course of therapy may be necessary for more severe infections, and up to 6 weeks for osteomyelitis [3, 4, 9].

In addition to localized infection, physicians should think about other possible sequelae of dog bites: tetanus and rabies. The management of tetanus prophylaxis and the decision to provide post-exposure rabies prophylaxis can be determined using the CDC guidelines or as stated above [9, 24, 25]. If the rabies vaccination status of the dog is unknown, contact a veterinarian or department of health agency for further guidance.

In conclusion, dog bite injuries to children are a common and potentially fatal issue. Physicians must know how to stabilize and treat these injuries, as well as methods of preventing dog bites. Each family, with or without a pet dog, should have a brief discussion regarding dog bite prevention in the primary care setting. If a bite has occurred, both family members and physicians should be aware of the potential psychological sequelae of dog bites and how to treat them.

Conflict of interest

The authors declare no conflict of interest.

Author details

Katlin VanDerhoef and Jeffrey P. Louie*
Division of Emergency Medicine, Department of Pediatrics, University of Minnesota Masonic Children's Hospital, Minneapolis, Minnesota, United States of America

*Address all correspondence to: matts532@umn.edu

References

[1] U.S. Pet Ownership Statistics. 2017-2018 U.S. Pet Ownership & Demographics Sourcebook. American Veterinary Medical Association, Veterinary Economics Division Schaumburg, IL; 2017-2018. Available from: https://www.avma.org/resources-tools/reports-statistics/us-pet-ownership-statistics

[2] Dog Bite Fatality Statistics. 2020. Dogsbite.org. Available from: https://www.dogsbite.org/dog-bite-statistics-fatalities-2020.php

[3] Aziz H, Rhee P, et al. The current concepts in management of animal (dog, cat, snake, scorpion) and human bite wounds. Journal of Trauma and Acute Care Surgery. 2015;**78**(3):641-648

[4] Bula-Rudas F, Olcott J. Human and Animal Bites. Pediatrics in Review. 2018;**39**(10):490-500. DOI: 10.1542/pir.2017-0212

[5] Abraham J, Czerwinski M. Pediatric dog bite injuries in central Texas. Journal of Pediatric Surgery. 2019;**54**(7):1416-1420

[6] Golinko M, Arslanian B, Williams J. Characteristics of 1616 consecutive dog bite injuries at a single institution. Sage Journals: Clinical Pediatrics. 2017;**56**(4):316-325

[7] Carter E, Waterhouse L, et al. Adherence to ATLS primary and secondary surveys during pediatric trauma resuscitation. Resuscitation. 2013;**84**(1):66-71. DOI: 10.1016/j.resuscitation.2011.10.032

[8] James D, Pennardt A. Trauma Care Principles. Treasure Island, FL: StatPearls Publishing LLC; 2021. Available from: https://www.ncbi.nlm.nih.gov/books/NBK547757/

[9] Hurt J, Maday K. Management and treatment of animal bites. Journal of the American Academy of Physician Assistants. 2018;**31**(4):27-31. DOI: 10.1097/01.JAA.0000531049.59137.cd

[10] Rothe K, Tsokos M, et al. Animal and human bite wounds. Deutsches Arzteblatt International Journal. 2015;**112**(25):433-443. DOI: 10.3238/arztebl.2015.0433

[11] Abrahamian F, Goldstein E. Microbiology of animal bite wound infections. Clinical Microbiology Reviews. 2011;**24**(2):231-246. DOI: 10.1128/CMR.00041-10

[12] Azmat C, Council M. Wound Closure Techniques. Treasure Island, FL: StatPearls Publishing LLC; 2021 Available from: https://www-ncbi-nlm-nih-gov.ezp1.lib.umn.edu/books/NBK470598/

[13] Son D, Harijan A. Overview of surgical scar prevention and management. Journal of Korean Medical Science. 2014;**29**(6):751-757. DOI: 10.3346/jkms.2014.29.6.751

[14] Grabowski G, Pacana M, et al. Keloid and hypertrophic scar formation, prevention, and management: standard review of abnormal scarring in orthopaedic surgery. Journal of the American Academy of Orthopaedic Surgeons. 2020;**28**(10):408-414. DOI: 10.5435/JAAOS-D-19-00690

[15] Kerwin L, El Tal A, et al. Scar prevention and remodeling: A review of the medical, surgical, topical, and light treatment approaches. International Journal of Dermatology. 2014;**53**(8):922-936. DOI: 10.1111/ijd.12436

[16] Trott A. Wounds and Lacerations: Emergency Care and Closure. 4th ed. Saunders. Philadelphia, PA: Elsevier; 2012

[17] McLoughlin R, Cournoyer L, et al. Hospitalizations for Pediatric Dog Bite Injuries in the United States. Journal of Pediatric Surgery. 2020;**55**(7):1228-1233. DOI: 10.1016/j.jpedsurg.2019.06.025

[18] Piccart F, Dormaar J, et al. Dog bite injuries in the head and neck region: A 20-year review. Craniomaxillofacial Trauma Reconstruction. 2019;**12**(3):199-204. DOI: 10.1055/s-0038-1660441

[19] Mendoza J, Chi J. Reconstruction of animal bite injuries to the head and neck. Current Opinion in Otolaryngology & Head & Neck Surgery. 2019;**27**(5):407-412. DOI: 10.1097/MOO.0000000000000564

[20] Lackmann G, Draf W, et al. Surgical treatment of facial dog bite injuries in children. Journal of Craniomaxillofacial Surgery. 1992;**20**(2):81-86. DOI: 10.1016/S1010-5182(05)80472-X

[21] Bertozzi M, Appignani A. The Management of Dog Bite Injuries of Genitalia in Pediatric Age. African Journal of Pediatric Surgery. 2013;**10**(3):205-210

[22] Mannion C, Graham A, et al. Dog bites and maxillofacial surgery: What can we do? British Journal of Oral and Maxillofacial Surgery. 2015;**53**(6):522-525. DOI: 10.1016/j.bjoms.2015.02.022

[23] Adnan S, Lone M, et al. Which is the most recommended medium for the storage and transport of avulsed teeth? A systematic review. Dental Traumatology. 2018;**34**(2):59-70. DOI: 10.1111/edt.12382

[24] Tetanus: For Clinicians. Centers for Disease Control and Prevention, National Center for Immunization and Respiratory Diseases, Division of Bacterial Diseases. Atlanta, GA: US Department of Health and Human Services; 2020. Available from: https://www.cdc.gov/tetanus/clinicians.html

[25] Rabies H. Centers for Disease Control and Prevention. National Center for Emerging Zoonotic and Infectious Diseases, Division of High-Consequence Pathogens and Pathology. Atlanta, GA; 2021. Available from: https://www.cdc.gov/rabies/location/usa/surveillance/human_rabies.html

[26] Munnynck K, Van de Voorde W. Forensic approach of fatal dog attacks: A case report and literature review. International Journal of Legal Medicine. 2002;**116**:295-300. DOI: 10.1007/s00414-002-0332-9

[27] Dixon C, Mistry R. Dog bites in children surge during coronavirus disease-2019: A case for enhanced prevention. Journal of Pediatrics. 2020;**225**:231-232. DOI: 10.1016/j.jpeds.2020.06.071

[28] Jakeman M, Oxley J, et al. Pet dog bites in children: management and prevention. The BMJ: Pediatrics Open. 2020;**4**:1. DOI: 10.1136/bmjpo-2020-000726

[29] Peters V, Souttiax M, et al. Posttraumatic Stress Disorder After Dog Bites in Children. The Journal of Pediatrics. 2004;**144**(1):121-122. DOI: 10.1016/j.jpeds.2003.10.024

Chapter 6

Stevens-Johnson Syndrome and Toxic Epidermal Necrolysis

Thi Huyen Tran

Abstract

Stevens-Johnson syndrome (SJS) and toxic epidermal necrolysis (TEN) are severe cutaneous adverse drug reactions (SCARs). The most common causative drugs of SJS/TEN are allopurinol, carbamazepine, abacavir, phenytoin, and lamotrigine. SJS/TEN are categorized based on the percentage of epidermal detachment area: (i) SJS: less than 10%, (ii) TEN: greater than 30%, (iii) and overlapping SJS/TEN: 10–30%. The pathogenesis of SJS/TEN is not fully understood, but some immunological and genetic factors are believed to be involved. There is a strong association between some specific HLA haplotypes and drug-induced SJS/TEN, for example, HLA-B*15:02 and carbamazepine-, HLA-B*58:01 and allopurinol. CD8+ cytotoxic T cells and natural killer (NK) cells play an important role in the pathogenesis of SJS/TEN, and upon the activation, they produce cytokines, chemokines, and cytotoxic proteins, that cause extensive keratinocytes apoptosis. Systemic corticosteroid and cyclosporine are still used as the first line in the treatment of SJS/TEN, in combination with care support.

Keywords: Stevens-Johnson syndrome, toxic epidermal necrolysis, severe cutaneous adverse drug reactions, HLA-B*15:02, HLA-B*58:01, granulysin

1. Introduction

Stevens-Johnson syndrome (SJS) and toxic epidermal necrolysis (TEN) belong to severe cutaneous adverse drug reactions (SCARs). Although their incidence is rare, around 2–3 per million per year, their mortality rate can be up to 5–30%. These reactions are life-threatening due to internal organ failures, disseminated skin detachment, and necrolysis. The most common causative medicines inducing SJS/TEN are allopurinol, carbamazepine, sulfamethoxazole, and other antibiotics, even traditional medicine. The pathogenesis of SJS/TEN is not fully understood, but some immunological and genetic factors are believed to be involved. The treatment of SJS/TEN is still controversial in which several studies showed variable results, including systemic corticosteroid, cyclosporine, intravenous immunoglobulin (IVIG), etanercept, thalidomide, and plasmapheresis.

2. Concepts, terms, and classification

In the SCARs group, in addition to SJS/TEN, there are other forms of drug allergy such as drug reaction with eosinophilia and systemic symptoms (DRESS syndrome), acute generalized exanthematous pustulosis (AGEP), drug-induced hypersensitivity syndrome (DIHS), maculopapular exanthema (MPE).

Previously, the classification between erythema multiforme (EM), SJS, and TEN was still inconsistent due to unclear pathogenesis. There are different opinions on the differential diagnosis of severe EM from SJS/TEN. Since 1983, SJS has been considered synonymous with severe EM, both with the involvement of more than one mucosa with skin involvement [1]. In 1993–1994, Bastuji-Garin and Roujeau proposed the distinction of the two diseases based on clinical and etiological factors. In severe EM, there are mucosal lesions, bullae, skin lesions less than 10% of body surface area [2]. But unlike SJS, the skin lesions in severe EM are typical and/or atypical target lesions that are prominent compared to normal skin, distributed mainly in the extremities. Stevens-Johnson syndrome is characterized by widespread blisters due to drug reactions, which appear on the background of erythema, necrosis, and pruritus, concentrated mainly on the face and trunk. Etiologically, EM is often associated with herpes simplex virus reactivation, rarely drug-induced, SJS/TEN mainly drug-induced, rarely infection [3, 4]. There are few reports of stomatitis caused by *Mycoplasma pneumonia*, mostly in young people, characterized by primary mucosal lesions, with little or no skin lesions. This form is called *Mycoplasma pneumonia*-related mucositis [5]. Today, EM is considered as a separate disease, separate from the SJS/TEN group, with specific clinical, epidemiological, and pathophysiological features. Due to the similarity in clinical and histopathological characteristics and epidermal detachment and necrosis, SJS and TEN are classified into a spectrum of diseases, abbreviated as SJS/TEN [1, 6, 7].

Based on the area of epidermal detachment (blister, erosion), Bastuji-Garin classified the spectrum of SJS/TEN into SJS, overlapping SJS/TEN and TEN. According to this classification, there are four subgroups as follows: (1) SJS with an epidermal detachment of less than 10% of the body area, red, pruritic, atypical target macules that are flat with normal skin; (2) overlap SJS/TEN with 10–30% epidermal detachment; (3) TEN with spots (spots) when the lesions are epidermal detachment over 30% of the body area, with red, widespread pruritus, atypical target macules; (4) TEN without spot with epidermal detachment lesions of more than 30% of the body area, no individual macules, no atypical target lesions [1, 2].

3. Etiology and pathogenesis of SJS/TEN

3.1 Etiology

Several microorganisms are considered to be the cause of SJS/TEN. For example, SJS/TEN can occur after vaccination with chickenpox, measles [8], *Mycoplasma pneumonia* [9], dengue virus [10], it is also associated with cytomegalovirus reactivation [11], currently, SJS may be related with Covid 19 [12] or Covid 19 vaccination [13, 14]. Other causes include serum injection, host graft rejection [15]. Chung's study showed that a novel variant of *Coxsackievirus A6* can induce severe mucosal bullous reactions, mainly mediated by granulysin-expressing T lymphocytes and NK cells. The clinical symptoms in that group of patients resembled severe EM or SJS [16]. A classic example of the role of viruses in drug response: in DIHS, human herpesvirus 6 (HHV6) plays an important role. HHV6 reactivation in DIHS patients may increase T-cell activity after the onset of drug response, induce the synthesis of proinflammatory cytokines including TNF-α and IL-6 that are capable of regulating T cell-mediated responses [17].

The majority of cases of SJS/TEN were related to drug hypersensitivity. Some studies show that in people infected with HIV, the prevalence of the disease is about 1 in 1000, which is a thousand times higher than in the population without HIV [6]. In sub-Saharan Africa, where HIV prevalence is high, there is an association between SJS/TEN and HIV due to the use of antiretroviral and anti-tuberculosis drugs [18]. The drugs most commonly causing SJS/TEN are nevirapine, lamotrigine, carbamazepine, phenytoin, phenobarbital, cotrimoxazole, sulfonamides, sulfasalazine, allopurinol, and non-steroidal anti-inflammatory drugs (oxicam group) [6, 19]. Other less common drugs are aminopenicillin, cephalosporin, quinolone. In Asian countries, traditional medicine can also be a causative drug of SJS/TEN [20]. Currently, SJS/TEN is reported to be associated with pembrolizumab [21], and itraconazole [22]. Patch test, lymphocyte transformation test, and enzyme-linked immunospot can be used to detect culprit drugs in SJS/TEN but none of them is considered as standard [1, 23].

Sassolas et al. developed an algorithm for drug causality for epidermal necrolysis (ALDEN). This algorithm rates each drug with a score of −12 to 10 based on six criteria: (1) delay from initial drug component intake to the onset of reaction (index day); (2) drug present in the body on the index day; (3) pre-challenge/rechallenge; (4)dechallenge; (5) type of drug (notoriety); (6) other cause. Allergenic possibilities are given based on the following total score: ≥ 6: very probable; 4–5: probable; 2–3: possible; 0–1: unlikely; < 0: very unlikely [19].

Stevens-Johnson syndrome and TEN are equally common in men and women. The frequency of the disease increases with age, peaking in people over 50 years of age [24, 25]. In the population of people living with HIV/AIDS, the prevalence of SJS/TEN is higher than in the general population [6].

3.2 Pathogenesis

In SJS/TEN, keratinocytes are necrotic to varying degrees. The pathogenesis of SJS/TEN is related to the mechanism of death of keratinocytes [26–28]. These cells undergo apoptosis or necroptosis, causing the entire epidermal structure to necrosis, detachment, form blisters [26, 28].

3.2.1 Immune mechanisms in SJS/TEN

Toxic epidermal necrolysis is a T-cell-mediated disease, TCD8+ lymphocytes are found in bullous fluid [29–31], perivascular in the superficial dermis [6, 32]. TCD8+ lymphocytes together with NK cells are considered to be the main agents of apoptosis of keratinocytes [29–31]. TCD4+ lymphocytes and other immune cells such as dendritic cells and mast cells also play an important role in TEN [6]. Caproni's study of cell infiltration in the skin of TEN patients showed a high density of CD40 ligand (CD40L) staining cells in the dermis, some infiltrating the epidermis [32]. CD40L is a molecule expressed on the surface of activated CD4+ T cells, and is a co-stimulator of macrophages, dendritic cells, B lymphocytes, and endothelial cells, leading to the release of tumor necrotic factor-alpha (TNF-α), nitric oxide (NO), interleukin (IL)-8, and cell adhesion molecules. Soluble CD40L is elevated in the serum of TEN patients. The TCD4+ lineage in the epidermis and dermis of TEN patients has a balance between T helper (Th) 1 and Th2 as well as cytokine levels from these two cell types [33].

Macrophages, neutrophils, and NK cells are also involved in the pathogenesis of TEN, and studies have shown that macrophages infiltrate in predominant numbers in skin samples [32, 33]. Tohyama noted the presence of CD14+ CD16+ monocytes in the epidermis and the dermal-epidermal junction in skin lesions of SJS/TEN patients. This reinforces the proliferation and cytotoxicity of TCD8+ lymphocytes through the CD137/CD137L system. Monocytes and macrophages contribute to apoptosis through the production of TNF-α, TNF-related apoptosis ligands [34]. Neutrophils and dendritic cell factor XIIIa+ were also found in these skin samples, but their role in TEN has not been elucidated [32, 33, 35]. NK cells are present in the bullous fluid along with highly cytotoxic T cells that express the NK cell CD56 receptor. Both of these cell types are considered to be major contributors to keratinocyte apoptosis [30]. The important role of TCD8+ lymphocytes in the pathogenesis of TEN has been recently demonstrated with the murine model of TEN, which tends to resemble that of humans [36].

T cells are hyperactive due to decreased T regulatory (Treg) cell function and upregulation by monocytes. CD8+ T cells themselves are not specific for TEN; they are also present in other drug-induced reactions. Treg's function in increasing TCD8+ activity is an important factor in TEN, which causes epidermal injury. The mechanism by which Treg cells degrades function is unknown, but the loss of TCD8+ inhibition has been documented. Treg cells from the peripheral blood of TEN patients do not inhibit T cells. Treg cell counts in TEN patients do not differ from that in normal subjects, but their function is impaired during the acute phase of TEN [37].

Th17 cells, which are subtypes of TCD4+ cells, are present in SJS/TEN at a higher rate than other ordinary drug skin reactions (ODSRs), producing IL-17 and IL-22. In SJS/TEN patients, there are more IL-17-producing CD4+ T cells than in EM patients and healthy subjects. As the disease improves, the Th17 cell count decreases. They can regulate the mobilization of neutrophils and other inflammatory leukocytes, causing inflammation and skin damage. Furthermore, neutropenia, a cause of death in TEN, may be due to the action of Th17 [37].

3.2.2 Role of human leukocyte antigen (HLA) class I in SJS/TEN and SCARs

Many studies show an association between HLA class I and SCARs. In Han Chinese patients with SJS/TEN, there is a strong association between antiepileptic aromatics such as carbamazepine, phenytoin, oxcarbazepine, and lamotrigine with HLA-B*15:02 [38], and between allopurinol and HLA-B* 58:01 [39, 40]. An association between HLA-B*15:02 and carbamazepine was also seen in Thai, Vietnamese, Malaysian, and South Indian SJS/TEN patients, but not in Japanese, Korean, or European populations [41]. In patients of European descent, there was an association between HLA-B*57:01 and abacavir-induced SJS/TEN [42], and between HLA-A*31:01 and carbamazepine-induced SJS/TEN [43]. A study in Japan showed that the HLA-B*15:11 allele is a risk factor for carbamazepine-induced SJS/TEN, with an association between HLA-A*02:06 and acetaminophen-induced SJS/TEN [44]. The significant association between SJS/TEN and certain HLA haplotypes has led to speculation that these haplotypes play a role in the pathogenesis of TEN [45]. This concept was proposed when investigating the role of HLA-B*57:01 in the pathogenesis of abacavir-induced DIHS [46]. From the above studies, it is recommended to screen for some HLA alleles before prescribing some drugs that cause allergies, related to HLA. For example, HLA-B*58:01 allele carriers should not take allopurinol, and HLA-B*15:02 allele carriers should not take carbamazepine [41, 43].

3.2.3 Mechanism of death of keratinocytes in SJS/TEN

3.2.3.1 Mechanism of apoptosis of keratinocytes

In SJS/TEN, keratinocytes undergo massive, widespread necrosis. The main reason is due to the apoptosis mechanism. There are many cytotoxic proteins and molecules involved in apoptosis initiation in SJS/TEN, of which granulysin has been shown to play a major role. Other factors including FasL, TNF-α, perforin, granzyme B, and NO also play a certain role [6, 26, 47].

3.2.3.1.1 Granulysin

Granulysin is a molecule found in the granules of cytotoxic cells (along with granzyme B and perforin) such as TCD8+, NK, and natural killer T cells, that act as a tumor killer and kills bacteria. When there is an interaction between the drug and the specific HLA and T cell receptor of TCD8+, granulysin is released from the granules of TCD8+, causing apoptosis of keratinocytes. Granulysin can cut through the target cell membrane, causing ion imbalance, damage to mitochondria, releasing oxidants and caspase cascade, causing apoptosis [48].

To investigate the role of granulysin in TEN, Chung et al. compared the gene expression of bullous fluid cells. The results showed that the expression of the granulysin gene of bullous cells increased 10–20 times, granzyme B increased 8 times, perforin increased 3 times, serum FasL increased 2 times [26]. When measuring granulysin concentrations in bullous fluid following a similar pattern, granulysin levels were 2–4 times higher than perforin, granzyme B, and soluble FasL, which correlated with disease severity. On immunohistochemical staining, the skin tissues of patients with TEN were strongly stained with granulysin, while the skin tissues of patients with ODSRs were weakly stained [26]. Abe showed that serum granulysin levels were elevated in 4 out of 5 patients with SJS/TEN before epidermal detachment or mucosal lesion. Meanwhile, this concentration increased only in 1 in 24 patients with ODSRs [49].

The above studies demonstrate that granulysin is an important cause of apoptosis in TEN, it is also a marker for early diagnosis and prognosis of disease severity [24, 26].

3.2.3.1.2 Fas-FasL

Fas ligand (FasL) is a transmembrane protein of the TNF family, found on the surface of cytotoxic T cells, NK cells. When these cells are activated, FasL is expressed, binds to its receptor on the target cell, and activates the intracellular caspase, leading to uncontrolled destruction of the target cell. In addition, Fas can be separated from the cell membrane by metalloproteinase enzymes, producing soluble Fas from FasL, still maintaining the ability to bind to Fas receptors, causing apoptosis [6, 50].

The Fas receptor has a region of repeat cysteines and an intracellular region of 80 amino acids, identical to the region in TNF-R1, named the death domain. This region is required for Fas to induce apoptosis. Mutations in this region destroy apoptosis induction. The only known physical Fas ligand is FasL (CD95L), which belongs to the family of TNF-related cytokines. Like its relatives, FasL is synthesized as transmembrane and trimer-soluble forms, by the enzyme metalloprotease. Fas signaling plays a decisive role in lymphocyte homeostasis. Repeated activation of antigen receptors on T cells induces FasL expression, leading to apoptosis via Fas signaling. When this process fails, due to mutations in Fas or FasL, lymphomas and autoimmune diseases occur [51]. FasL induces apoptosis by binding to the Fas receptor, causing activation of caspases [52]. Fas is expressed mainly on activated T lymphocytes and NK cells. Viard showed that FasL is also expressed in keratinocytes in TEN lesions [27]. Serum soluble FasL levels are elevated in patients with SJS/TEN before skin detachment, mucosal lesion, or both [53].

3.2.3.1.3 Granzyme B and perforin

Granzyme B and perforin have roles in the apoptosis of keratinocytes and endothelial cells [52]. Cytotoxic T cells, once activated, secrete perforin and granzyme B, create channels on target cell membranes, and activate apoptosis-inducing caspase [6]. In TEN, monocytes from bullous fluid induce apoptosis in the presence of anti-Fas antibodies, but not apoptosis in the presence of perforin/granzyme B inhibitors, indicating perforin/granzyme B is the causative agent of apoptosis [30, 31, 50]. The concentrations of these molecules correlate with the severity of the drug reactions. Therefore, testing for perforin and granzyme B may help differentiate TEN from other drug reactions [47]. Recent studies on skin biopsies of TEN patients showed that endothelial cells were apoptosis, and immunohistochemical staining showed granzyme B and TNF-α around the dermis vessels. Although not found on biopsies, the possibility that soluble FasL is the cause of apoptosis of endothelial cells cannot be excluded. The reason is that the biopsy samples were taken 2–4 days after the onset of the disease when the soluble FasL concentration was greatly reduced [54, 55].

3.2.3.1.4 Other factors

Other molecules, cytokines such as TNF-α and NO have certain roles in apoptosis. TNF-α acts on the "death receptor" TNF-R1, causing activation of caspases, causing cell death. TNF-α is elevated in the bullous fluid, skin, and serum of patients with TEN. Its role, though, is unclear. In addition to its ability to induce apoptosis, TNF-α also has a protective role by activating the anti-apoptosis pathway with nuclear factor-kappaB (NF-κB). This may explain why the mortality of TEN is increased with treatment with anti-TNF-α (thalidomide) [56]. NO induces apoptosis through its effect on the *p53* gene. Skin samples before blistering of patients with SJS/TEN had increased NO synthase (inducible NO synthase, iNOS) enzyme. IFN-α and TNF-α secreted from activated T cells can induce iNOS expression, which downregulates NO-dependent FasL, especially apoptosis in keratinocytes. Thus, IFN-α, TNF-α, and iNOS are potential molecular bridges between the immune response to drugs and the expression of proapoptotic molecules. The combination of IFN-α, NO, and an increase in reactive oxygen species causes oxidative stress, disrupts the intracellular machinery and cell membranes, leading to apoptosis [6].

3.2.3.2 Mechanism of necroptosis of keratinocytes

Cell death resembles necrosis but is regulated by a specific intracellular program known as necroptosis [57]. Experimental studies by Saito et al. showed that apoptosis is not the only mechanism of keratinocyte death in SJS/TEN. When pan-caspase inhibitors were added to the supernatant cultures of peripheral blood monocytes (PBMCs) of patients with SJS/TEN, incubated with keratinocytes, cell death still occurs. Thus, the PBMCs cultures of patients with SJS/TEN contain a specific molecule that causes the death of keratinocytes, which is independent of the apoptosis mechanism. The authors found that the concentration of annexin A1 protein in PBMCs cultures was significantly higher in SJS/TEN patients than in ODSR patients. Anti-annexin A1 antibody inhibits the death of keratinocytes [28]. Annexin A1 is a member of the family of 13 annexin proteins, which bind to acidic phospholipids with high affinity in the presence of Ca^{2+} ions [58]. When annexin A1 binds to the formyl peptide receptor 1 (FPR1) receptor on the cells, it causes necroptosis. The level of FPR1 expression was significantly different between the SJS/TEN group and the ODSR group. Therefore, it can determine the probability of SJS/TEN or ODSRs. Although there is no gene difference in the FPR1 promoter region between SJS/TEN, ODSRs, and healthy subjects, the annexin A1-FPR1 interaction may predict the occurrence of SJS/TEN and hold promise for targeted therapy in which necrosulfonamide inhibits the necroptosis pathway related to the annexin A1-FPR1 complex [28, 52].

4. Clinical and paraclinical characteristics of SJS/TEN

4.1 Clinical characteristics

Stevens-Johnson syndrome and TEN develop acutely, with epidermal necrosis, mucositis at multiple sites, accompanied by systemic and other organ changes [1, 2]. In general, the first symptoms are fever, fatigue, discomfort in the upper respiratory tract, appearing a few days before skin and mucosal lesions [1, 6]. Often, it is difficult to diagnose ODSRs and predict the likelihood of progression to SJS/TEN at this stage. Many patients have EM-like lesions with atypical target lesions. However, according to Abe's study, serum granulysin levels were elevated during this time, based on which could predict the possibility of SJS/TEN [49], helping to treat early avoid complications, and reduce the risk of death.

The time from taking a suspected drug to the onset of symptoms varies widely, ranging from a few days to two months. Therefore, it is necessary to carefully review all drugs used by the patient within the previous two months, including over-the-counter drugs and dietary supplements [1].

Lesions of the ocular mucosa may precede skin lesions. Manifestations include eye discomfort, conjunctivitis, and scleritis. After a few days, the conjunctiva becomes ulcerated, oozing. Lesions on the ocular mucosa may occur concurrently with lesions of the oral mucosa and genital mucosa [1]. According to Revuz's research, 97% of SJS/TEN patients had mucosal lesions, of which, oral mucosal lesions were found in 93% of patients, ocular mucosa 78%, genital mucosa 63%, and other mucous membranes 66% [59].

Skin pain is an early symptom in SJS/TEN, the presence of which signals an epidermal necrolysis event [1]. There are many types of skin lesions with varying degrees of severity. The earliest lesions are atypical target lesions and/or itchy erythematous macules. The first sites where lesions appear are usually the upper half of the body, the head near the extremities, and the face. After that, the skin lesions spread to the rest of the body and distal extremities. Lesions on the palms and soles of the feet are quite prominent. In many patients, the first symptom is an intensely red, erythematous rash on the palms of the hands. In severe cases, the erythema may coalesce into large macules. The skin becomes tender, vulnerable, and mild pressure can cause epidermal detachment (positive Nikolsky test). The maximum extent of skin lesions after onset is 5–7 days. Necrotic blisters appear when the necrotic epidermal detachment separates from the underlying skin [1, 59]. Extensive necrosis epidermal detachment leaves open dermis, serous exudates, susceptible to infection and bleeding (see **Figures 1–4**) [60].

Multiple organs are affected in SJS/TEN, with necrosis and erosion occurring in the conjunctiva, trachea, bronchi, kidneys, and intestines [52]. There have been reports of acute renal failure with increased microalbuminuria, renal tubular enzymes in the urine, demonstrating glomerular and proximal tubular damage. Lung and respiratory

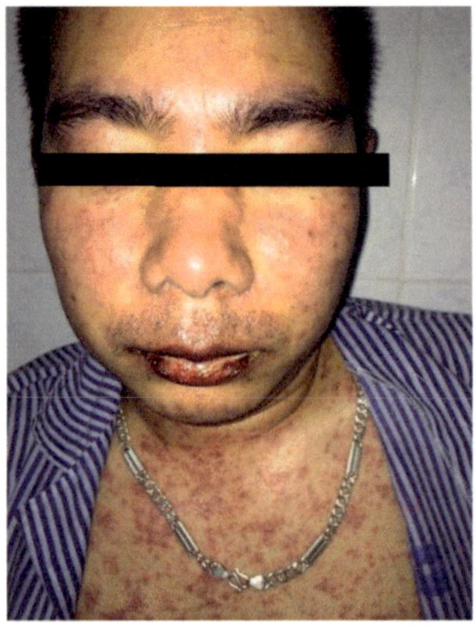

Figure 1.
A male patient with carbamazepine-induced SJS. He had erosions and dark crust on the lips, pruritic erythematous lesions on the face and the upper trunk. (photo: Tran Thi Huyen).

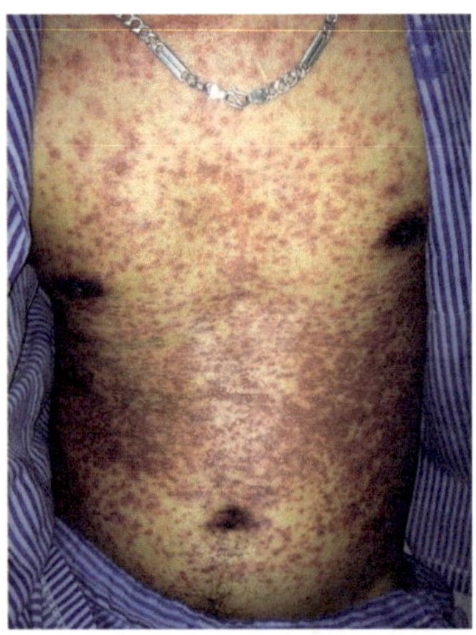

Figure 2.
A lot of blisters were formed on the dark erythematous rashes on the trunk of the patient with carbamazepine-induced SJS. (photo: Tran Thi Huyen).

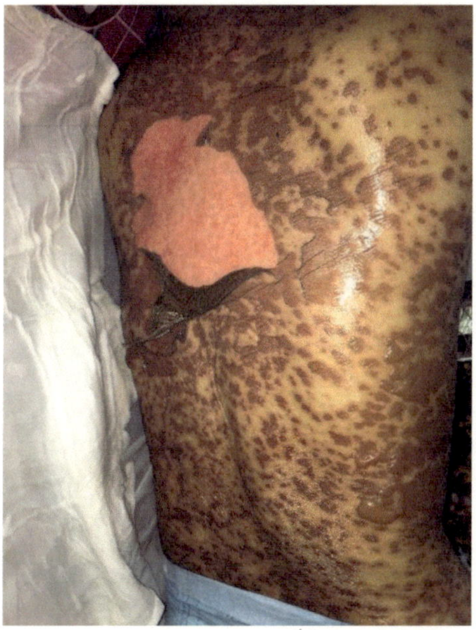

Figure 3.
Epidermal detachments, blisters, and necrotic rashes on the trunk of a patient with allopurinol-induced TEN (photo: Tran Thi Huyen).

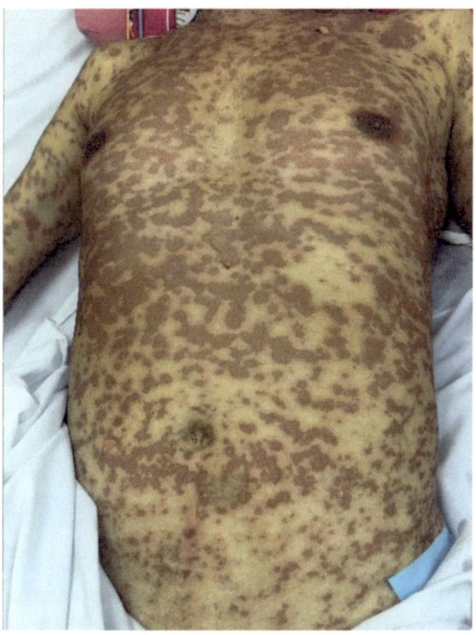

Figure 4.
The extensive epidermal necrosis in a patient with allopurinol-induced TEN (photo: Tran Thi Huyen).

lesions include tracheobronchitis, subcutaneous emphysema, dyspnea, and respiratory failure. Other systemic manifestations may include anemia, leukopenia, hepatitis, abdominal pain, diarrhea, transient elevation of liver enzymes, hypoalbuminemia, hyponatremia, and myocarditis [1].

4.2 Paraclinical characteristics

4.2.1 Histopathology

The diagnosis of SJS/TEN is mainly clinical. However, skin biopsy for histopathology is necessary to further confirm the diagnosis and rule out other bullous skin diseases [1]. On histopathology, there are different degrees of epidermal lesions, the keratinocytes are necrotic individually or in plaques, forming blisters. Appendical structures such as sweat ducts and hair follicles may be affected. The dermis has an inflammatory infiltrate (mainly perivascular) of lymphocytes, histocytes, and a few eosinophils [61]. In addition, there may be liquid degeneration of the basal layer, squamous separation, and spongiosis [62]. Depending on the stage of the disease, the histopathological picture can be different. In the early stages, a histopathological picture is a group of necrotic keratinocytes with some inflammatory cells (monocytes and neutrophils). In the late and severe stages, the keratinocytes are more necrotic, the basal epithelial cells degenerate, leading to the separation of the epidermis from the dermis, the entire layers of keratinocytes of the epidermis are necrotic, only intact horny layer. In some cases, the superficial layer of the epidermis is more necrotic than the deeper layers, forming slits between the two layers of the epidermis [29]. Monocytes and neutrophils can infiltrate areas of necrosis [29, 62].

In the early stages of SJS/TEN, necrotic keratinocytes are scattered in the lower epidermis, similar to those seen in severe EM: extensive necrotic keratinocytes with vacuoles at the dermal-epidermal junction [6, 61]. When SJS/TEN is evident, the entire epidermis is necrotic, forming subepidermal bullae. Meanwhile, in severe EM, the epidermis is less necrotic, the change occurs mainly in the basal layer. The Japanese diagnostic criteria suggested that in SJS/TEN at least 10 necrotic keratinocytes were seen at 200x magnification [63]. In the superficial dermis, perivascular inflammatory infiltration and exocytosis are usually absent. In SJS/TEN, inflammation in the dermis occurs less frequently than in severe EM [61]. The degree of inflammation correlates with the disease severity, the number of infiltrating mononuclear cells in the dermis has the same prognostic value as the SCORe for TEN (SCORTEN) index to assess the severity of TEN [35].

4.2.2 Microbiological tests

Serology for diagnosis of *Mycoplasma pneumonia* [64], herpes simplex virus, Epstein-Barr virus, cytomegalovirus, ... to rule out microbial causes of mouth ulcers and skin lesions [1, 6].

4.2.3 Biochemistry and hematology tests

In SJS/TEN, the blood count may be normal or there may be disorders such as leukocytosis, leukopenia, and anemia. Many patients have a transient elevation of liver enzymes, increased urea, creatinine, blood bicarbonate, blood glucose, C-reactive protein, procalcitonin.

4.3 Prognosis and complications

4.3.1 Prognostic factors

In severe cases of SJS/TEN, acute systemic disorders can lead to multi-organ failure and death. In 2000, Bastuji-Garin et al. published a valuable prognostic score for

Risk factors	0 point	1 point
1. Age	<40	≥ 0
2. Have a malignancy	No	Yes
3. Heart rate (beats/minute)	<120	≥120
4. Area of skin detachment	<10%	≥10%
5. Blood urea (mmol/l)	≤10	>10
6. Blood glucose (mmol/l)	≤14	>14
7. Blood bicarbonate (mmol/l)	≥20	<20

Risk of death by score: 0–1 point: 3.2%; 2 points 12.1%; 3 points 35.3%; 4 points 58.3%, 5–7 points: 90%.

Table 1.
SCORTEN score for Stevens-Johnson syndrome/toxic epidermal necrolysis and risk of in-hospital mortality based on the SCORTEN [1, 65].

SJS/TEN, called SCORTEN, which used seven clinical factors to predict in-hospital mortality. Each factor is worth one point, the higher the total score, the higher the risk of death [65]. Several studies have shown a gradual increase in SCORTEN scores during patient hospitalization, with a significant change observed on day 1 and day 4 (see **Table 1**) [66].

4.3.2 Complications

It is a disease with a high risk of death, but with time management and treatment, SJS/TEN can be cured. However, it is necessary to note visceral complications (liver, kidney) [52], eye complications, nail disorders [67], skin pigmentation changes after the disease as well as the psychological trauma of the patient. Among them, eye complications are noted the most, with different degrees [68]. Mild degree with eyelid edema, conjunctivitis; a moderate degree of membranous conjunctivitis, corneal epithelial loss, corneal ulceration, corneal infiltrates; in severe cases, there is the irreversible loss of corneal epithelium, loss of vision [1, 68, 69].

5. Differential diagnosis

Erythema multiforme.
Generalized fixed drug eruption.
Staphylococcal scalded skin syndrome.
Graft versus host disease.
Mycoplasma pneumonia-related mucositis.
Pemphigus Vulgaris.
Other bullous autoimmune diseases.

6. Treatment

6.1 General principles

Experts recommend that patients with more than 10% of their body area peeled off should be treated in an emergency care unit with doctors and nurses in a variety of specialties. Some patients are treated and cared for as burn patients. Many studies have shown that prompt admission to burn centers improves survival, while delay increases mortality [70, 71]. In the ward, room temperature should be maintained to reduce the patient's energy consumption. Energy consumption is increased to 40% of basal metabolic rate when the area of skin loss is 10%, increasing to 120% when the area of skin loss is 80% [72]. The patient's drug history should be taken, and possible tests performed to identify and discontinue the allergen. Limit the use of drugs during the treatment of SJS/TEN.

6.2 Care support

Medical staff should use protective equipment when in contact with patients to avoid oral and respiratory infections. It is important to avoid holding or pulling the patient strongly and to limit injury to the epidermis (blood pressure measuring tape, electrocardiogram) [73]. Bacteria, viruses, and Candida fungi from three skin lesions should be cultured. Herpes infection should be excluded, especially in the case of severe mucous membrane lesions. Systemic antibiotics should be used if there is evidence of infection. In patients who have diarrhea or are unable to move, avoid getting dirty stools into skin lesions. Pay attention to using pain relievers if the pain is severe [1, 74].

Skin lesions should be washed with sterile warm water or physiological saline or with an antiseptic solution such as chlorhexidine (1/5000). A moisturizer with fatty properties such as vaseline, paraffin all over the skin, including the area that is growing granules should be applied. Scaly skin could be improved with topical antimicrobial drugs. Peeled epidermal fragments should be kept as a bio-bandage. The blisters should be aspirated and drained. Areas of skin that have lost the epidermis should be covered with non-stick gauze. Necrotic and infected epidermal fragments should be removed.

Eye mucosa is often damaged in SJS/TEN, if not detected, timely treatment can leave complications such as corneal ulceration, eye corner adhesions, pterygium adhesions, blindness [68]. Patients with SJS/TEN should be examined, treated, and monitored by an ophthalmologist from the acute stage of the disease until the disease has recovered. The mucous membrane of the vulva, vagina needs to be regular check-ups and cleaning with antiseptic solutions, moist gauze. Topical corticosteroids can reduce inflammation [75]. Oral mucosa needs to be cleaned with antiseptic solutions such as chlorhexidine. Lips and mouth should be covered with moist gauze, corticosteroid solution can be applied to rinse the mouth, oral hemorrhages need to be controlled [76].

Peripheral and central lines should be placed in preserved areas. The fluid balance will be monitored by a catheter. The amount of fluid to compensate could be calculated by referring to the formula of Shiga and Cartotto [77]:2 ml kg^{-1} body weight/% of epidermal area detachment, necrotic.

If the patient can drink, oral rehydration should be maintained. Patients with SJS/TEN need more nutrition than usual. If the mouth is severely damaged, eating is difficult, a nasogastric tube should be placed or parenteral nutrition. In the acute phase, the required calorie intake is 20–25 kcal kg^{-1} per day. During the recovery phase, the calorie requirement is 25–30 kcal kg^{-1} per day [1].

Patients with SJS/TEN have pain in the skin, especially at epidermal detachment sites. There are no studies on analgesic regimens in SJS/TEN. Therefore, analgesics according to the World Health Organization tiers can be used. Paracetamol or synthetic opiate pain relievers (tramadol) should be used, but not non-steroidal anti-inflammatory analgesics because of the risk of kidney and stomach damage. Some care procedures such as bathing and changing clothes require the use of analgesics.

Other treatments including proton pump inhibitors, anticoagulants, and drugs to treat leukopenia, anemia (granulocyte colony-stimulating factor, G-CSF) should be used appropriately.

6.3 Specific medicines

6.3.1 Intravenous immunoglobulin

The basis for the use of IVIG in SJS/TEN are studies that show the role of Fas-FasL interaction in the mechanism of apoptosis of squamous cells [78]. FasL is a transmembrane protein of the TNF family that is expressed on the surface of cytotoxic T cells and natural killer cells. When cytotoxic T cells are activated, FasL is expressed, binds to its receptor on the target cell, activates the intracellular caspase, leading to uncontrolled destruction of the target cell. In addition, Fas can be separated from the cell membrane by metalloproteinase enzymes, producing soluble Fas from FasL, still maintaining the ability to bind to Fas receptors, causing apoptosis [6, 79]. High concentrations of normal immunoglobulin inhibit Fas-Fas ligand and apoptosis interactions through activation of anti-Fas antibodies.

In a systematic review and meta-analysis published by Huang in 2012 (all studies included at least 8 IVIG-treated SJS/TEN patients), cumulative estimates of risk mortality were determined, comparing IVIG and supportive care alone in patients with TEN and overlapping SJS/TEN. Statistical analysis was performed on the raw data to compare the clinical differences between high- and low-dose treatment in adult patients, and between pediatric and adult patients receiving IVIG. The mortality rate in the group of TEN and overlapping SJS/TEN patients treated with IVIG was 19.9%. Pediatric patients treated with IVIG had a lower mortality rate than adults (0% vs. 21.6%, $p = 0.01$). Adult patients treated with high dose IVIG had a lower mortality rate than those treated with low dose (18.9% vs. 50%, $p = 0.02$). However, the multivariable logistic regression model showed that IVIG dose was not correlated with mortality. But these results should be interpreted with caution due to limitations in the study design [79]. Following Huang's publication, a further study performed by Firoz et al. including 23 TEN patients treated with IVIG, demonstrated that IVIG did not improve survival compared with supportive care simply [80]. In 2013, Lee et al. published a retrospective analysis of 64 patients with overlapping SJS/TEN and TEN receiving IVIG. Based on the actual mortality compared with the SCORTEN estimated mortality, IVIG therapy showed no benefit. In addition, there was no difference between the high dose (>3 g/kg) and the low dose (<3 g/kg) [81].

6.3.2 Systemic corticosteroid therapy

Corticosteroids have been used to treat SJS/TEN for many years. Advocates emphasize the anti-inflammatory role of high doses of corticosteroids in the early stages of the disease. Opponents argue that systemic corticosteroids increase the risk of infection. Retrospective analysis of EuroSCAR data showed a lower mortality rate in the German group of patients receiving corticosteroids than in the supportive care group alone. To limit the side effects of long-term corticosteroid use, some authors use very high doses for a short time (pulse therapy) [82]. In the study by Kardaun and

Jonkman, 12 patients treated with intravenous dexamethasone 100 mg or 1.5 mg/kg for 3 days had a lower mortality rate compared with the estimated mortality according to the SCORTEN [83]. Hirahara et al. had 8 patients with SJS/TEN treated with intravenous methylprednisolone 1000 mg for three consecutive days, followed by dose reduction with oral prednisolone or 2 days of methylprednisolone at half the initial dose. No patient died although the SCORTEN estimated mortality was 1.6. Serum biomarkers IFN-γ, TNF-α, IL-6, and IL-10 were measured in 5/8 patients. On the fourth day post-treatment, the mean concentrations of these cytokines decreased compared with pre-treatment, but only significantly changed for interferon-gamma (IFN-γ) and IL-6. On day 19, there was a significant reduction in both IFN-γ, TNF-α, and IL-6, whereas IL-10 levels were higher than before treatment [84].

6.3.3 Cyclosporine

Cyclosporine is an immunosuppressive drug, indicated in many diseases such as rheumatoid arthritis, psoriasis, Crohn's disease, nephrotic syndrome, anti-rejection in organ transplantation. The mechanism of action of the drug is to reduce the function of lymphocytes by forming a complex with cyclophilin to inhibit the activation of calcium channel phosphatase, thereby reducing the production of cytokines by T lymphocytes.

Its inhibitory effect on lymphocytes defines cyclosporine as the theoretical standard drug of action in SJS/TEN [1]. A study by Valeyrie-Allanore showed that in 29 SJS/TEN patients treated with cyclosporine (1.5 mg/kg/day in 2 divided doses for the first 10 days, then reduced to 1 mg/kg/day days for the next 10 days, the last 10 days is 0.5 mg/kg/day) is effective. No patient died, although the SCORTEN estimated number of deaths was 2.75/29 [85]. Singh reported 11 patients with SJS/TEN who were treated with cyclosporine 3 mg/kg/day for 7 days, followed by dose reduction. This group was compared with 6 corticosteroid-treated SJS/TEN patients. In the cyclosporine group with a shorter hospital stay, the epithelialization rate was faster. Cyclosporine was more effective than corticosteroids when comparing SCORTEN estimated mortality. Kirchhof retrospectively studied 64 SJS/TEN patients treated with cyclosporine or IVIG (dose varied from patient to patient). Comparison of SCORTEN estimated mortality with actual mortality suggests a benefit of cyclosporine over IVIG [86]. Cyclosporine is well-tolerated, despite treatment in patients prone to hemodynamic instability and prerenal hypovolemia. It contributed to improved patient survival. Disease progression was slow and halting in the majority of patients [85, 87].

6.3.4 Other methods of treatment

Other therapies were used in SJS/TEN but in small sample sizes, no comparisons were made. Plasmapheresis is used in difficult-to-treat cases, and some reports have shown it to be effective [88, 89]. The immunoregulatory and regenerative role of G-CSF is used in the treatment of SJS/TEN (helps to stop hypersensitivity, stimulate epithelialization, control neutropenia) [90]. Biologics such as TNF-alpha antagonists have been conducted to improve the prognosis of SJS/TEN [23, 52]. Paradisi reported 10 patients with SJS/TEN treated with etanercept with a single dose of 50 mg subcutaneously. The study did not have a control group. All patients responded with a mean time of epithelialization of 8.5 days. Although the SCORTEN estimated mortality rate was 50%, no patient died [91].

6.3.5 Follow-up after patient discharge

Notes on suspected culprit drugs. Advise patients to avoid over-the-counter medications if the cause of SJS/TEN is unknown. If the patient has damage to the ocular mucosa, an ophthalmologist should be examined a few weeks after discharge from the hospital. Monitor for complications after discharge such as skin, oral, urogenital, respiratory, digestive, and psychological problems.

7. Conclusion

Stevens-Johnson syndrome and TEN have aggressive, acute, severe clinical manifestations, diagnosis is mainly based on clinical characteristics. Tests are mainly used to find probable etiology, assess severity, and differentiate from other bullous skin diseases. Treatment includes discontinuation of the suspected allergen/drug, supportive care, and/or a combination of specific drugs such as corticosteroids, cyclosporine, IVIG, and others.

Acknowledgements

We sincerely thank the medical staff and the Board of Directors of National Hospital of Dermatology and Venereology, Hanoi, Vietnam for supporting this manuscript.

Conflict of interest

The author declares no conflict of interest.

Abbreviations

ALDEN	algorithm for drug causality for epidermal necrolysis
CD	cluster of differentiation
DIHS	drug-induced hypersensitivity syndrome
EM	erythema multiforme
FasL	Fas ligand
FPR1	formyl peptide receptor 1
G-CSF	granulocyte colony-stimulating factor
HHV 6	human herpesvirus 6
HIV	human immunodeficiency virus
HLA	human leukocyte antigen
IFN-γ	interferon-gamma
IL	interleukin
iNOS	inducible nitric oxide synthase
IVIG	intravenous immunoglobulin
MPE	maculopapular exanthema
NK	natural killer
NO	nitric oxide

ODSRs	ordinary drug skin reactions
OR	odd ratio
PBMCs	peripheral blood monocytes
SCARs	severe cutaneous adverse drug reactions
SCORTEN	SCORe for TEN
SJS	Stevens-Johnson syndrome
TEN	toxic epidermal necrolysis
Th	T helper
TNF-α	tumor necrosis factor-alpha
Treg	T regulatory

Author details

Thi Huyen Tran
National Hospital of Dermatology and Venereology, Hanoi Medical University, Hanoi, Vietnam

*Address all correspondence to: drhuyentran@gmail.com

References

[1] Creamer D, Walsh SA, Dziewulski P, et al. U.K. guidelines for the management of Stevens-Johnson syndrome/toxic epidermal necrolysis in adults 2016. The British Journal of Dermatology. 2016;**174**(6):1194-1227. DOI: 10.1111/bjd.14530

[2] Bastuji-Garin S, Rzany B, Stern RS, Shear NH, Naldi L, Roujeau JC. Clinical classification of cases of toxic epidermal necrolysis, Stevens-Johnson syndrome, and erythema multiforme. Archives of Dermatology. 1993;**129**(1):92-96

[3] Auquier-Dunant A, Mockenhaupt M, Naldi L. Correlations between clinical patterns and causes of erythema multiforme major, Stevens-Johnson syndrome, and toxic epidermal necrolysis: The result of an international prospective study. Archives of Dermatology. 2002;**138**:1019-1024

[4] Assier H, Bastuji-Garin S, Revuz J, Roujeau JC. Erythema multiforme with mucous membrane involvement and Stevens-Johnson syndrome are clinically different disorders with distinct causes. Archives of Dermatology. 1995;**131**(5):539-543

[5] Vujic I, Shroff A, Grzelka M, et al. *Mycoplasma pneumoniae*-associated mucositis—Case report and systematic review of the literature. Journal of the European Academy of Dermatology and Venereology JEADV. 2015;**29**(3):595-598. DOI: 10.1111/jdv.12392

[6] Schwartz RA, McDonough PH, Lee BW. Toxic epidermal necrolysis: Part I. Introduction, history, classification, clinical features, systemic manifestations, etiology, and immunopathogenesis. Journal of the American Academy of Dermatology. 2013;**69**(2):173.e1-173.13; quiz 185-186. DOI: 10.1016/j.jaad.2013.05.003

[7] Grünwald P, Mockenhaupt M, Panzer R, Emmert S. Erythema multiforme, Stevens-Johnson syndrome/toxic epidermal necrolysis—Diagnosis and treatment. Journal der Deutschen Dermatologischen Gesellschaft JDDG. 2020;**18**(6):547-553. DOI: 10.1111/ddg.14118

[8] Su JR, Haber P, Ng CS, et al. Erythema multiforme, Stevens-Johnson syndrome, and toxic epidermal necrolysis reported after vaccination, 1999-2017. Vaccine. 2020;**38**(7):1746-1752. DOI: 10.1016/j.vaccine.2019.12.028

[9] Sah R, Neupane S, Khadka S, et al. A case study of Stevens-Johnson syndrome-toxic epidermal necrolysis (SJS-TEN) overlap in mycoplasma pneumoniae-associated tracheobronchitis. Case Reports in Infectious Diseases. 2019;**2019**:5471765. DOI: 10.1155/2019/5471765

[10] Grieb G, Alazemi M, Das R, Dunda SE, Fuchs PC, Pallua N. A rare case of toxic epidermal necrolysis with unexpected fever resulting from dengue virus. Case Reports in Dermatology. 2010;**2**(3):189-194. DOI: 10.1159/000322963

[11] Tagajdid MR, Doblali T, Elannaz H, Hammi S, Belfequih B, Mrani S. Reactivation of cytomegalovirus in a patient with Stevens-Johnson syndrome-toxic epidermal necrolysis. Iran Journal of Medical Sciences. 2013;**38**(Suppl. 2):195-197

[12] Muhd Besari A, Lim JA, Vellaichamy PT, Hussain FA, Kamaludin Z, Nor M. Stevens-Johnson

syndrome as a primary skin manifestation of COVID-19. Postgraduate Medical Journal. 2021. DOI: 10.1136/postgradmed-2021-140778. Available from: https://pubmed.ncbi.nlm.nih.gov/34670852/

[13] Dash S, Sirka CS, Mishra S, Viswan P. COVID-19 vaccine-induced Stevens-Johnson syndrome. Clinical and Experimental Dermatology. 2021;**46**(8):1615-1617. DOI: 10.1111/ced.14784

[14] Mansouri P, Chalangari R, Martits-Chalangari K, Mozafari N. Stevens-Johnson syndrome due to COVID-19 vaccination. Clinical Case Reports. 2021;**9**(11) e05099. DOI: 10.1002/ccr3.5099

[15] Chung WH, Wang CW, Dao RL. Severe cutaneous adverse drug reactions. The Journal of Dermatology. 2016;**43**(7):758-766. DOI: 10.1111/1346-8138.13430

[16] Chung WH, Shih SR, Chang CF, et al. Clinicopathologic analysis of coxsackievirus a6 new variant induced widespread mucocutaneous bullous reactions mimicking severe cutaneous adverse reactions. The Journal of Infectious Diseases. 2013;**208**(12):1968-1978. DOI: 10.1093/infdis/jit383

[17] Yoshikawa T, Fujita A, Yagami A, et al. Human herpesvirus 6 reactivation and inflammatory cytokine production in patients with drug-induced hypersensitivity syndrome. Journal of Clinical Virology Offical Publications Pan American Society Clinical Virology. 2006;**37**(Suppl. 1):S92-S96. DOI: 10.1016/S1386-6532(06)70019-1

[18] Saka B, Barro-Traoré F, Atadokpédé FA, et al. Stevens-Johnson syndrome and toxic epidermal necrolysis in sub-Saharan Africa: A multicentric study in four countries. International Journal of Dermatology. 2013;**52**(5):575-579. DOI: 10.1111/j.1365-4632.2012.05743.x

[19] Sassolas B, Haddad C, Mockenhaupt M, et al. ALDEN, an algorithm for assessment of drug causality in Stevens-Johnson syndrome and toxic epidermal necrolysis: Comparison with case-control analysis. Clinical Pharmacology and Therapeutics. 2010;**88**(1):60-68. DOI: 10.1038/clpt.2009.252

[20] Yang L, Shou YH, Li F, Zhu XH, Yang YS, Xu JH. Retrospective study of 213 cases of Stevens-Johnson syndrome and toxic epidermal necrolysis from China. Burns Journal of International Society Burn Injections. 2019;**46**(4):959-969. DOI: 10.1016/j.burns.2019.10.008

[21] Cai ZR, Lecours J, Adam JP, et al. Toxic epidermal necrolysis associated with pembrolizumab. Journal of Oncology Pharmacy Practice Offical Publications International Society Oncology Pharmacy Practices. 2020;**26**(5):1259-1265. DOI: 10.1177/1078155219890659

[22] Das A, Sil A, Mohanty S. Itraconazole-induced Stevens-Johnson syndrome and toxic epidermal necrolysis overlap: Report of a rare incident. Dermatologic Therapy. 2020;**33**(6):e14311. DOI: 10.1111/dth.14311

[23] Lin CC, Chen CB, Wang CW, Hung SI, Chung WH. Stevens-Johnson syndrome and toxic epidermal necrolysis: Risk factors, causality assessment, and potential prevention strategies. Expert Review of Clinical Immunology. 2020;**16**(4):373-387. DOI: 10.1080/1744666X.2020.1740591

[24] Su SC, Mockenhaupt M, Wolkenstein P, et al. Interleukin-15 is associated with severity and mortality

in Stevens-Johnson syndrome/toxic epidermal necrolysis. The Journal of Investigative Dermatology. 2017;**137**(5):1065-1073. DOI: 10.1016/j.jid.2016.11.034

[25] Nguyen DV, Chu HC, Nguyen DV, et al. HLA-B*1502 and carbamazepine-induced severe cutaneous adverse drug reactions in Vietnamese. Asia Pacific Allergy. 2015;**5**(2):68-77. DOI: 10.5415/apallergy.2015.5.2.68

[26] Chung WH, Hung SI, Yang JY, et al. Granulysin is a key mediator for disseminated keratinocyte death in Stevens-Johnson syndrome and toxic epidermal necrolysis. Nature Medicine. 2008;**14**(12):1343-1350. DOI: 10.1038/nm.1884

[27] Viard-Leveugle I, Gaide O, Jankovic D, et al. TNF-α and IFN-γ are potential inducers of Fas-mediated keratinocyte apoptosis through activation of inducible nitric oxide synthase in toxic epidermal necrolysis. The Journal of Investigative Dermatology. 2013;**133**(2):489-498. DOI: 10.1038/jid.2012.330

[28] Saito N, Qiao H, Yanagi T, et al. An annexin A1-FPR1 interaction contributes to necroptosis of keratinocytes in severe cutaneous adverse drug reactions. Science Translational Medicine. 2014;**6**(245):245ra95. DOI: 10.1126/scitranslmed.3008227

[29] Paquet P, Piérard GE, Quatresooz P. Novel treatments for drug-induced toxic epidermal necrolysis (Lyell's syndrome). International Archives of Allergy and Immunology. 2005;**136**(3):205-216. DOI: 10.1159/000083947

[30] Nassif A, Bensussan A, Dorothée G, et al. Drug specific cytotoxic T-cells in the skin lesions of a patient with toxic epidermal necrolysis. The Journal of Investigative Dermatology. 2002;**118**(4):728-733. DOI: 10.1046/j.1523-1747.2002.01622.x

[31] Nassif A, Bensussan A, Boumsell L, et al. Toxic epidermal necrolysis: Effector cells are drug-specific cytotoxic T cells. The Journal of Allergy and Clinical Immunology. 2004;**114**(5):1209-1215. DOI: 10.1016/j.jaci.2004.07.047

[32] Caproni M, Torchia D, Schincaglia E, et al. The CD40/CD40 ligand system is expressed in the cutaneous lesions of erythema multiforme and Stevens-Johnson syndrome/toxic epidermal necrolysis spectrum. The British Journal of Dermatology. 2006;**154**(2):319-324. DOI: 10.1111/j.1365-2133.2005.07023.x

[33] Paquet P, Paquet F, Al Saleh W, Reper P, Vanderkelen A, Piérard GE. Immunoregulatory effector cells in drug-induced toxic epidermal necrolysis. The American Journal of Dermatopathology. 2000;**22**(5):413-417. DOI: 10.1097/00000372-200010000-00005

[34] Tohyama M, Hashimoto K. Immunological mechanisms of epidermal damage in toxic epidermal necrolysis. Current Opinion in Allergy and Clinical Immunology. 2012;**12**(4):376-382. DOI: 10.1097/ACI.0b013e328355b865

[35] Quinn AM, Brown K, Bonish BK, et al. Uncovering histologic criteria with prognostic significance in toxic epidermal necrolysis. Archives of Dermatology. 2005;**141**(6):683-687. DOI: 10.1001/archderm.141.6.683

[36] Saito N, Yoshioka N, Abe R, et al. Stevens-Johnson syndrome/toxic epidermal necrolysis mouse model generated by using PBMCs and the skin of patients. The Journal of Allergy and Clinical Immunology. 2013;**131**(2):434-441.e1-9. DOI: 10.1016/j.jaci.2012.09.014

[37] Kinoshita Y, Saeki H. A review of the pathogenesis of toxic epidermal necrolysis. Journal of Nippon Medicine School Nippon Ika Daigaku Zasshi. 2016;**83**(6):216-222. DOI: 10.1272/jnms.83.216

[38] Man CBL, Kwan P, Baum L, et al. Association between HLA-B*1502 allele and antiepileptic drug-induced cutaneous reactions in Han Chinese. Epilepsia. 2007;**48**(5):1015-1018. DOI: 10.1111/j.1528-1167.2007.01022.x

[39] Hung SI, Chung WH, Liou LB, et al. HLA-B*5801 allele as a genetic marker for severe cutaneous adverse reactions caused by allopurinol. Proceedings of the National Academy of Sciences of the United States of America. 2005;**102**(11):4134-4139. DOI: 10.1073/pnas.0409500102

[40] Chung WH, Hung SI, Hong HS, et al. Medical genetics: A marker for Stevens-Johnson syndrome. Nature. 2004;**428**(6982):486. DOI: 10.1038/428486a

[41] Fricke-Galindo I, Lerena A, López-López M. An update on HLA alleles associated with adverse drug reactions. Drug Metabolism and Personalized Therapy. 2017;**32**(2):73-87. DOI: 10.1515/dmpt-2016-0025

[42] Mounzer K, Hsu R, Fusco JS, et al. HLA-B*57:01 screening and hypersensitivity reaction to abacavir between 1999 and 2016 in the OPERA® observational database: A cohort study. AIDS Research and Therapy. 2019;**16**(1):1. DOI: 10.1186/s12981-019-0217-3

[43] Phillips EJ, Sukasem C, Whirl-Carrillo M, et al. Clinical pharmacogenetics implementation consortium guideline for HLA genotype and use of carbamazepine and oxcarbazepine: 2017 update. Clinical Pharmacology and Therapeutics. 2018;**103**(4):574-581. DOI: 10.1002/cpt.1004

[44] Kaniwa N, Saito Y, Aihara M, et al. HLA-B*1511 is a risk factor for carbamazepine-induced Stevens-Johnson syndrome and toxic epidermal necrolysis in Japanese patients. Epilepsia. 2010;**51**(12):2461-2465. DOI: 10.1111/j.1528-1167.2010.02766.x

[45] Yang CWO, Hung SI, Juo CG, et al. HLA-B*1502-bound peptides: Implications for the pathogenesis of carbamazepine-induced Stevens-Johnson syndrome. The Journal of Allergy and Clinical Immunology. 2007;**120**(4):870-877. DOI: 10.1016/j.jaci.2007.06.017

[46] Chessman D, Kostenko L, Lethborg T, et al. Human leukocyte antigen class I-restricted activation of CD8+ T cells provides the immunogenetic basis of systemic drug hypersensitivity. Immunity. 2008;**28**(6):822-832. DOI: 10.1016/j.immuni.2008.04.020

[47] Posadas SJ, Padial A, Torres MJ, et al. Delayed reactions to drugs show levels of perforin, granzyme B, and Fas-L to be related to disease severity. The Journal of Allergy and Clinical Immunology. 2002;**109**(1):155-161. DOI: 10.1067/mai.2002.120563

[48] Krensky AM, Clayberger C. Biology and clinical relevance of granulysin. Tissue Antigens. 2009;**73**(3):193-198. DOI: 10.1111/j.1399-0039.2008.01218.x

[49] Abe R, Yoshioka N, Murata J, Fujita Y, Shimizu H. Granulysin as a marker for early diagnosis of the Stevens-Johnson syndrome. Annals of Internal Medicine. 2009;**151**(7):514-515. DOI: 10.7326/0003-4819-151-7-200910060-00016

[50] Abe R, Shimizu T, Shibaki A, Nakamura H, Watanabe H, Shimizu H.

Toxic epidermal necrolysis and Stevens-Johnson syndrome are induced by soluble Fas ligand. The American Journal of Pathology. 2003;**162**(5):1515-1520. DOI: 10.1016/S0002-9440(10)64284-8

[51] Siegel RM, Fleisher TA. The role of Fas and related death receptors in autoimmune and other disease states. The Journal of Allergy and Clinical Immunology. 1999;**103**(5 Pt 1):729-738. DOI: 10.1016/s0091-6749(99)70412-4

[52] Hasegawa A, Abe R. Recent advances in managing and understanding Stevens-Johnson syndrome and toxic epidermal necrolysis. F1000 Research. 2020;**9**:F1000. Faculty Rev-612. DOI: 10.12688/f1000research.24748.1

[53] Murata J, Abe R, Shimizu H. Increased soluble Fas ligand levels in patients with Stevens-Johnson syndrome and toxic epidermal necrolysis preceding skin detachment. The Journal of Allergy and Clinical Immunology. 2008;**122**(5):992-1000. DOI: 10.1016/j.jaci.2008.06.013

[54] Verneuil L, Ratajczak P, Allabert C, et al. Endothelial cell apoptosis in severe drug-induced bullous eruptions. The British Journal of Dermatology. 2009;**161**(6):1371-1375. DOI: 10.1111/j.1365-2133.2009.09357.x

[55] Verneuil L, Leboeuf C, Vidal JS, et al. Endothelial damage in all types of T-lymphocyte-mediated drug-induced eruptions. Archives of Dermatology. 2011;**147**(5):579-584. DOI: 10.1001/archdermatol.2011.104

[56] Wolkenstein P, Latarjet J, Roujeau JC, et al. Randomised comparison of thalidomide versus placebo in toxic epidermal necrolysis. Lancet London England. 1998;**352**(9140):1586-1589. DOI: 10.1016/S0140-6736(98)02197-7

[57] Weinlich R, Oberst A, Beere HM, Green DR. Necroptosis in development, inflammation, and disease. Nature Reviews. Molecular Cell Biology. 2017;**18**(2):127-136. DOI: 10.1038/nrm.2016.149

[58] Perretti M, D'Acquisto F. Annexin A1 and glucocorticoids as effectors of the resolution of inflammation. Nature Reviews. Immunology. 2009;**9**(1):62-70. DOI: 10.1038/nri2470

[59] Revuz J, Penso D, Roujeau JC, et al. Toxic epidermal necrolysis. Clinical findings and prognosis factors in 87 patients. Archives of Dermatology. 1987;**123**(9):1160-1165. DOI: 10.1001/archderm.123.9.1160

[60] Mahajan R, Kanwar AJ. Use of granulocyte colony-stimulating factor in the treatment of toxic epidermal necrolysis—Experience with 3 patients. Skinmed. 2013;**11**(5):269-271

[61] Rzany B, Hering O, Mockenhaupt M, et al. Histopathological and epidemiological characteristics of patients with erythema exudativum multiforme major, Stevens-Johnson syndrome and toxic epidermal necrolysis. The British Journal of Dermatology. 1996;**135**(1):6-11

[62] Breathnach SM. Erythema Multiforme, Stevens-Johnson Syndrome and Toxic Epidermal Necrolysis. 8th ed. Vol. 1. Rook's Textbook of Dermatology. Wiley-Blackwell; 2010

[63] Orime M. Immunohistopathological findings of severe cutaneous adverse drug reactions. Journal of Immunology Research. 2017;**2017**:6928363. DOI: 10.1155/2017/6928363

[64] Russell E, Walker S, McPherson T. Diagnosis of mycoplasma etiology in Stevens-Johnson syndrome/toxic

epidermal necrolysis. The British Journal of Dermatology. 2021;**184**(1):176-178. DOI: 10.1111/bjd.19458

[65] Bastuji-Garin S, Fouchard N, Bertocchi M, Roujeau JC, Revuz J, Wolkenstein P. SCORTEN: A severity-of-illness score for toxic epidermal necrolysis. The Journal of Investigative Dermatology. 2000;**115**(2):149-153. DOI: 10.1046/j.1523-1747.2000.00061.x

[66] Guégan S, Bastuji-Garin S, Poszepczynska-Guigné E, Roujeau JC, Revuz J. Performance of the SCORTEN during the first five days of hospitalization to predict the prognosis of epidermal necrolysis. The Journal of Investigative Dermatology. 2006;**126**(2):272-276. DOI: 10.1038/sj.jid.5700068

[67] Lian SB, Oh CC, Yeo YW, Lee HY. The spectrum of nail sequelae in Stevens-Johnson syndrome and toxic epidermal necrolysis. JAMA Dermatology. 2021;**157**(1):117-119. DOI: 10.1001/jamadermatol.2020.4664

[68] Ueta M. Stevens-Johnson syndrome/toxic epidermal necrolysis with severe ocular complications. Expert Review of Clinical Immunology. 2020;**16**(3):285-291. DOI: 10.1080/1744666X.2020.1729128

[69] Chronopoulos A, Mockenhaupt M, Pleyer U. Ocular involvement in Stevens-Johnson syndrome and toxic epidermal necrolysis. Ophthalmol Z Dtsch Ophthalmol Gestrology. 2021;**118**(5):519-532. DOI: 10.1007/s00347-021-01351-2

[70] Schulz JT, Sheridan RL, Ryan CM, MacKool B, Tompkins RG. A 10-year experience with toxic epidermal necrolysis. The Journal of Burn Care & Rehabilitation. 2000;**21**(3):199-204. DOI: 10.1097/00004630-200021030-00004

[71] McGee T, Munster A. Toxic epidermal necrolysis syndrome: Mortality rate reduced with early referral to a regional burn center. Plastic and Reconstructive Surgery. 1998;**102**(4):1018-1022. DOI: 10.1097/00006534-199809040-00014

[72] Herndon DN, Tompkins RG. Support of the metabolic response to burn injury. Lancet London England. 2004;**363**(9424):1895-1902. DOI: 10.1016/S0140-6736(04)16360-5

[73] Hanson LM, Bettencourt AP. Stevens-Johnson syndrome and toxic epidermal necrolysis: A guide for nurses. AACN Advanced Critical Care. 2020;**31**(3):281-295. DOI: 10.4037/aacnacc2020634

[74] Woolum JA, Bailey AM, Baum RA, Metts EL. A review of the management of Stevens-Johnson syndrome and toxic epidermal necrolysis. Advanced Emergency Nursing Journal. 2019;**41**(1):56-64. DOI: 10.1097/TME.0000000000000225

[75] O'Brien KF, Bradley SE, Mitchell CM, Cardis MA, Mauskar MM, Pasieka HB. Vulvovaginal manifestations in Stevens-Johnson syndrome and toxic epidermal necrolysis: Prevention and treatment. Journal of the American Academy of Dermatology. 2021;**85**(2):523-528. DOI: 10.1016/j.jaad.2019.08.031

[76] Adams L, Creamer D. Controlling oral hemorrhages in Steven-Johnson syndrome/toxic epidermal necrolysis. Journal of the American Academy of Dermatology. 2020;**82**(1):e3-e4. DOI: 10.1016/j.jaad.2019.06.1299

[77] Shiga S, Cartotto R. What are the fluid requirements in toxic epidermal necrolysis? Journal of Burn Care Research Official Publications American Burn Association. 2010;**31**(1):100-104. DOI: 10.1097/BCR.0b013e3181cb8cb8

[78] Viard I, Wehrli P, Bullani R, et al. Inhibition of toxic epidermal necrolysis by blockade of CD95 with human intravenous immunoglobulin. Science. 1998;**282**(5388):490-493. DOI: 10.1126/science.282.5388.490

[79] Huang YC, Li YC, Chen TJ. The efficacy of intravenous immunoglobulin for the treatment of toxic epidermal necrolysis: A systematic review and meta-analysis. The British Journal of Dermatology. 2012;**167**(2):424-432. DOI: 10.1111/j.1365-2133.2012.10965.x

[80] Firoz BF, Henning JS, Zarzabal LA, Pollock BH. Toxic epidermal necrolysis: Five years of treatment experience from a burn unit. Journal of the American Academy of Dermatology. 2012;**67**(4):630-635. DOI: 10.1016/j.jaad.2011.12.014

[81] Lee HY, Lim YL, Thirumoorthy T, Pang SM. The role of intravenous immunoglobulin in toxic epidermal necrolysis: A retrospective analysis of 64 patients managed in a specialized center. The British Journal of Dermatology. 2013;**169**(6):1304-1309. DOI: 10.1111/bjd.12607

[82] Schneck J, Fagot JP, Sekula P, Sassolas B, Roujeau JC, Mockenhaupt M. Effects of treatments on the mortality of Stevens-Johnson syndrome and toxic epidermal necrolysis: A retrospective study on patients included in the prospective EuroSCAR study. Journal of the American Academy of Dermatology. 2008;**58**(1):33-40. DOI: 10.1016/j.jaad.2007.08.039

[83] Kardaun SH, Jonkman MF. Dexamethasone pulse therapy for Stevens-Johnson syndrome/toxic epidermal necrolysis. Acta Dermato-Venereologica. 2007;**87**(2):144-148. DOI: 10.2340/00015555-0214

[84] Hirahara K, Kano Y, Sato Y, et al. Methylprednisolone pulse therapy for Stevens-Johnson syndrome/toxic epidermal necrolysis: Clinical evaluation and analysis of biomarkers. Journal of the American Academy of Dermatology. 2013;**69**(3):496-498. DOI: 10.1016/j.jaad.2013.04.007

[85] Valeyrie-Allanore L, Wolkenstein P, Brochard L, et al. Open trial of ciclosporin treatment for Stevens-Johnson syndrome and toxic epidermal necrolysis. The British Journal of Dermatology. 2010;**163**(4):847-853. DOI: 10.1111/j.1365-2133.2010.09863.x

[86] Kirchhof MG, Miliszewski MA, Sikora S, Papp A, Dutz JP. Retrospective review of Stevens-Johnson syndrome/toxic epidermal necrolysis treatment comparing intravenous immunoglobulin with cyclosporine. Journal of the American Academy of Dermatology. 2014;**71**(5):941-947. DOI: 10.1016/j.jaad.2014.07.016

[87] Gilbert M, Scherrer LA. Efficacy and safety of cyclosporine in Stevens-Johnson syndrome and toxic epidermal necrolysis. Dermatologic Therapy. 2019;**32**(1):e12758. DOI: 10.1111/dth.12758

[88] Narita YM, Hirahara K, Mizukawa Y, Kano Y, Shiohara T. Efficacy of plasmapheresis for the treatment of severe toxic epidermal necrolysis: Is cytokine expression analysis useful in predicting its therapeutic efficacy? The Journal of Dermatology. 2011;**38**(3):236-245. DOI: 10.1111/j.1346-8138.2010.01154.x

[89] Koštál M, Bláha M, Lánská M, et al. Beneficial effect of plasma exchange in the treatment of toxic epidermal necrolysis: A series of four cases. Journal of Clinical Apheresis. 2012;**27**(4):215-220. DOI: 10.1002/jca.21213

[90] de Sica-Chapman A, Williams G, Soni N, Bunker CB. Granulocyte colony-stimulating factor in toxic epidermal necrolysis (TEN) and Chelsea & Westminster TEN management protocol [corrected]. The British Journal of Dermatology. 2010;**162**(4):860-865. DOI: 10.1111/j.1365-2133.2009.09585.x

[91] Paradisi A, Abeni D, Bergamo F, Ricci F, Didona D, Didona B. Etanercept therapy for toxic epidermal necrolysis. Journal of the American Academy of Dermatology. 2014;**71**(2):278-283. DOI: 10.1016/j.jaad.2014.04.044

Chapter 7

Pemphigus Vulgaris

Ozlem Su Kucuk and Nazan Taşlidere

Abstract

Pemphigus vulgaris is a life-threatening bullous disease characterized by acantholysis resulting in the formation of intraepithelial blebs in the mucous membranes and skin. It is a chronic autoimmune bullous dermatosis caused by the production of autoantibodies against desmoglein 1 and 3. It often begins with blisters and erosions on the oral mucosa, followed by lesions on other mucous membranes and drooping blisters that may spread to the skin. If there is clinical suspicion, the diagnosis can be confirmed by cytological examination, histopathological examination, direct and indirect immunofluorescence tests. Before the introduction of corticosteroids, PV was fatal due to dehydration or secondary systemic infections. The mainstay of treatment is still systemic steroids. Immunosuppressants such as azathioprine, mycophenolate mofetil and methotrexate, high-dose intravenous immunoglobulins, CD20 monoclonal antibody Rituximab treatments are used as an adjuvant with steroids in suitable patients and successful results are obtained.

Keywords: Vesiculobullous skin diseases, pemphigus, pemphigus vulgaris, desmogleins, autoimmune diseases

1. Introduction

Pemphigus vulgaris (PV) is a rare disease that causes blisters. It is the most common type of pemphigus group disease. The name of pemphigus derives from the Greek word 'pemphix'. It is a disease characterized by intraepidermal bullae of skin and mucosa that can be life-threatening.

2. Epidemiology

The incidence of pemphigus group disease is about 1 in 100,000, while PV occurs at a rate of 0.1 to 0.5 per 100,000, with a higher rate in Ashkenazi Jews and people of Mediterranean descent. In India, Malaysia, China and the Middle East, PV accounts for 70% of all pemphigus cases and is the most common autoimmune bullous disease [1].

The average age of onset is between 45- and 65 years. Pemphigus is rare under 18 years of age, except in endemic areas where 30% of patients are reported to be younger than 20 years of age [2]. All over the world, men and women are equally affected. However, adolescent girls are more affected than boys of the same age [3].

3. Predisposing factors

PV is a polygenic disease and low titers of disease-associated autoantibodies have been demonstrated in first-degree healthy relatives of patients with pemphigus [4, 5]. For many years, a strong association between Class II Human leukocyte antigen (HLA) polymorphism and pemphigus vulgaris has been known, with the highest incidence seen among Ashkenazi Jews. The interethnic variability in the occurrence of pemphigus vulgaris has been associated with genetic susceptibility. Associated HLA polymorphisms are HLA-DRB1∗ 0402, HLA-DRB1∗14, HLA-DQB1∗ 0503, HLA-DRB1∗ 0302 and HLA-DRB1∗ 08. Of these, HLA-DRB1∗ 0402, HLA-DRB1∗ 14 and HLA-DRB1∗ 08 have a statistically significant relationship with the incidence of pemphigus vulgaris [6].

Pemphigus vulgaris is associated with a variety of diseases, including other autoimmune disorders, psoriasis, neurological and psychiatric disorders, and some malignancies [7]. In addition, environmental factors may also be effective in initiating and maintaining the disease process. These causes include medications, viral infections, physical agents, contact allergens, vaccines, diet and psychological factors (**Table 1**) [8–11].

Drugs	Containing a Thiol Group	Penicillamine, Captopril, and Cephalosporin
	Containing a Phenol Group	Cephalosporin, Rifampin, and Levodopa
	Other	ACE inhibitors other than captopril, most NSAIDs, biological modifiers of the immune response (vaccine, interferons, imiquimod and other cytokines), chloroquine/hydroxychloroquine, cocaine
Viral İnfections	HSV, HHV8, and EBV	
Physical Agents	Sunburns, ionizing radiation, thermal or electrical burns, and surgical and cosmetic procedures	
Contact Allergens	Chemical exposure in those involved in photography, dry cleaning, industrial solvent work, horticulture, pesticides and intensive agriculture	
Dietary Factors	Although not proven, thiol allyl compounds in garlic, leeks and onions, as well as tannins in black pepper, red pepper, cherry, cranberry, blackberry, red wine and tea are known to cause acantholysis	

Table 1.
Trigger factors for pemphigus vulgaris.

4. Pathogenesis

Pemphigus vulgaris is an autoimmune condition that is more likely to develop in patients with certain HLA types after triggers. Central to the pathogenesis of pemphigus is the presence of immunoglobulin (Ig) antibodies against proteins on the cell surface of keratinocytes. Immunochemical and molecular cloning studies have shown that antigenic targets in PV are desmogleins. Desmogleins (Dsg) are desmosome-associated transmembrane glycoproteins that provide cell-cell adhesion in the epidermis [3]. The main antigen in PV is Dsg3 (130 kDa), but 50% of patients also have autoantibodies against Dsg1 (160 kDa). The ratio of Dsg1 and Dsg3 antibodies appear to correlate with the clinical severity of PV; those with only Dsg3 antibodies have predominantly oral lesions. IgG antibodies against Dsgs impair the adhesive function of desmosomes and inhibit cell-cell adhesion. This results in epidermal acantholysis and drooping blister formation, which is the characteristic clinical feature of pemphigus diseases [3].

The localization of blister formation and involvement of mucosal surfaces varies with the pemphigus disease subtype and can be explained by the Dsg compensation theory. This theory states that on cutaneous surfaces, Dsg 1 is expressed in all layers of the epidermis, while Dsg 3 is expressed in deeper layers. Dsg 1 expression in the mucosa is minimal, while Dsg 3 is dominant. The interpretation of the Dsg compensation theory, as it relates to the clinical manifestations in pemphigus, can be summarized as follows: Only patients with antibodies to Dsg 3 should have mucosal dominant PV because Dsg 1 compensates for the loss of Dsg 3 in the skin. Mucous membranes predominantly contain Dsg 3; low levels of Dsg 1 in the mucosa cannot replace the lost Dsg 3 and lead to epithelial acantholysis and mucosal erosions. When antibodies against both Dsg 1 and 3 develop, epidermal acantholysis occurs in both the skin and mucous membranes. It is still a matter of debate whether the Dsg compensation theory can adequately explain the complex pathogenic mechanism of pemphigus [3, 12].

Although Dsgs are the main autoantigens targeted by autoantibodies in the vast majority of pemphigus patients, antibodies against other desmosomal cadherins (e.g., desmocollins), desmoplakin and acetylcholine receptors on keratinocytes have also been detected in patients with pemphigus vulgaris [13, 14]. In recent years, the blood of some PV patients has been found to show reactivity with Dsg4, which has similar properties to Dsg1 and Dsg3, but the pathogenic nature of anti-Dsg4 is unclear [14]. In the presence of both anti-Dsg 1 and anti-Dsg 3 antibodies in PV, the entire skin should have been completely lysed. However, such a clinic is not seen in any patient. Therefore, the separation of keratinocytes may also be due to a different subset of non-Dsg pemphigus antibodies that recognize and block keratinocyte acetylcholine receptors. In this light, the earliest sign of keratinocyte separation is maintained by autoantibodies to these acetylcholine receptors located on the keratinocyte membrane, while antiDsg antibodies will only then be activated, triggering cell-cell separation [8]. Pharmacological blockade of acetylcholine receptors with muscarinic or nicotinic antagonists, atropine and mecamylamine, respectively, resulted in pemphigus-like acantholysis in monolayers of human oral and epidermal keratinocytes in both conditions. These observations suggest that PV IgGs act antagonistically to acetylcholine receptors of keratinocytes, interrupting the stimulation of these receptors by acetylcholine, thereby, altering the normal pattern of keratinocyte adhesion via cholinergic signaling that can lead to acantholysis [15].

Caspases are involved in the pathogenesis of PV through apoptosis and acantholysis. Caspases are activated through various cellular pathways to affect programmed cell death. While apoptosis via caspases is a normal process in the body, the presence of PV-IgG causes pathological activation of caspases in keratinocytes. In all studies, inhibition of caspases has been shown to reduce apoptosis and acantholysis and thus have a positive effect on cell-cell adhesion [16].

The pathogenesis of pemphigus involves the production of activated B-cells and IgG with stimulation by IL-4 by T-helper 2 (Th2) cells. Excessive activation of Th2 cells causes the production of autoantibodies required for PV. Th2 cells secrete IL-4 and multiple interleukins (IL), which are known to play an important role in pemphigus. IL-4 promotes antibody production by primed B cells and an isotype switching from IgG1 to IgG4 antibodies which are important in the active form of PV. IL-4 also causes naive CD4+ T cells to differentiate into Th2 cells, thus maintaining the disease. Production of autoantibodies and epitope binding are sufficient for the loss of adhesions directly between desmosomes [17].

Intracellular kinase signaling has been identified in the pathogenic process of PV. Intracellular kinase signaling has been identified in the pathogenic process of PV. The binding of autoantibodies in PV promotes phosphorylation of kinases. In the study in which patients with a diagnosis of PV were examined, kinases (e.g., phosphokinase C (PKC), p38 mitogen-activated protein kinase (p38MAPK), cyclin-dependent kinase (Cdk2), sarcoma-associated kinase (Src), extracellular signal-regulated kinase (ERK), Bruton tyrosine kinase (BTK), apoptosis signal regulatory kinase (ASK1), epidermal growth factor receptor kinase (EFGRK)), tyrosine kinase (TK)) were found to be phosphorylated in PV-induced models [16]. Inhibition of these pathways reduces acantholysis in vitro and in vivo. The role of p38MAPK has been highlighted in multiple studies. p38MAPK is activated after PVIgG-binding upstream of Rho kinase. In particular, p38MAPK inhibition prevents PV-IgG–induced redistribution of Dsg3 and results in PV-IgG and Dsg3 co-localizing at the cell membrane. As a result, p38MAPK inhibition has been shown to prevent both histologic and clinical blister formation in both in vivo and in vitro models. Therefore, p38MAPK plays an essential role in regulating Dsg3 internalization and must be considered as a key component in PV pathogenicity [16].

Proteases are enzymes that hydrolyze peptide bonds within proteins. Proteases have been blamed because the use of various protease inhibitors was found to be effective in inhibiting PV-associated acantholysis in studies [16]. Pemphigus antibodies (described as IgGp) may mediate acantholysis by the activation and release of non-lysosomal proteolytic enzymes from epidermal cells. Recent data indicate that the proteolytic enzyme is an activator of plasminogen. This has been demonstrated by the addition of a plasmin inhibitor such as aprotinin, which can inhibit the development of acantholysis when PV or PF IgG is added to the skin in organ cultures. Both plasminogen and IgG are required to cause acantholysis [15].

There are many mechanisms in the pathogenesis of PV that are still not understood and more studies are needed.

5. Comorbidities

In cross-sectional studies, pemphigus is associated with some diseases including psoriasis, hematological and solid organ malignancies (esophageal and laryngeal cancer), other autoimmune diseases (Sjögren's syndrome, systemic lupus erythematosus and alopecia areata), and neurological diseases (dementia, Parkinson's disease and epilepsy), Crohn disease and ulcerative colitis. Studies on the comorbidities of PV are needed.

6. Clinical features

All patients with PV develop painful erosions of the mucosal areas, especially oral mucosa. Oral lesions are the first finding in 50–70% of cases and occur during the course of the disease in 90% of patients [18]. More than half of patients also develop flaccid blisters and extensive cutaneous erosions. PV is divided into two subgroups according to the area of involvement: (1) mucosal dominant type, in which mucosal erosions are prominent and skin involvement is minimal; and (2) mucocutaneous type with extensive cutaneous bullae and erosions in addition to mucosal involvement [19].

Mucosal erosions usually precede the cutaneous manifestations of the disease. In some cases, oral ulcers may be the only manifestation of the disease. Intact bullae are rare because they are fragile and break easily. Although diffuse or widespread erosions can occur anywhere in the oral cavity, the most common sites are the buccal and palatine mucosa, lips and gingiva. Erosions are numerous and found in varying sizes and irregular shapes; they extend peripherally and there is usually a delay in re-epithelialization. Gingival involvement is seen as desquamative gingivitis. There are fissured hemorrhagic crusts that can extend up to the vermilion border in lip involvement. Involvement of the oral mucosa may impair nutrition and therefore the general condition of the patient [20]. Lesions of the nasal mucosa lead to hemorrhagic crusts. Apart from the oral and nasal mucosa, the oropharynx, esophagus, conjunctiva, larynx, urethra, vulva, vagina, penis and anus are other mucosal involvement areas.

Skin involvement may be localized or generalized. Often there are clear flaccid blisters on normal or erythematous skin. The contents of the bullae are clear at first, but over time they may become turbid, seropurulent and hemorrhagic. The bullae may coalesce and rupture quickly to form painful erosions that bleed easily. Erosions are covered with crusts that heal slowly in a short time. PV skin lesions can be seen anywhere on the body, but the involvement of the trunk, groin, axilla, scalp and face is common, while the palms and soles of the feet are usually protected.

Due to the abundance of Dsgs in the hair follicles, the scalp is a unique place for pemphigus. In the course of pemphigus, scalp involvement is observed in up to 60% of patients. Erosions, crusts and scaly plaques can sometimes lead to alopecia. Effortless removal of anagen hairs in a pull test is a sign of high disease activity [21].

The flaccid nature of the blisters seen in PV are due to intraepidermal acantholysis caused by anti-Dsg antibodies. Due to the loss of cohesion in the epidermis, it moves easily laterally in patients with active disease (Nikolsky sign) by applying light pressure or friction to the upper layers of the skin [19]. Direct Nikolsky (Asboe–Hansen sign) is the spreading of the blister to adjacent skin by applying light pressure on a blister, indirect Nikolsky is the application of rubbing to clinically normal-appearing skin to cause separation as a result of rubbing. These findings are not 100% specific for the diagnosis, but their presence suggests PV. These signs clinically represent acantholysis or loss of cell adhesion. It can also be found in other forms of pemphigus, as well as in toxic epidermal necrolysis [19, 20].

Pruritus is rare. Both mucosal and skin lesions heal without scarring, but hyperpigmentation in the affected areas may persist for months, especially in dark-skinned patients. PV is a chronic disease with periods of remission and exacerbation. Without appropriate treatment, PV can be fatal because extensive skin involvement may result in loss of epidermal barrier function and lead to loss of body fluids, malnutrition, and secondary infections. Secondary bacterial infection is one of the most common complications and can progress to septic shock [19, 20].

Among the rare clinical findings of PV; isolated crusty plaques on the face and scalp, foot ulcers, dyshidrotic eczema, macroglossia, nail dystrophy, paronychia and subungual hematomas can be counted. Nail involvement usually occurs when the disease is severe and in most cases responds partially or completely to systemic therapy [1, 19]. In the literature, two patients with cervical pemphigus vulgaris with symptoms as postmenopausal bleeding have been reported [22].

7. Disease activity assessment

Various scoring systems have been developed and validated for assessing pemphigus disease severity. The most widely used disease activity scoring system is the Pemphigus Disease Activity Index (PDAI). PDAI is based on the number of lesions found in the skin, scalp, and mucosa and the area of skin lesion. PDAI is an objective scoring method as it gives equal weight to the involvement of the skin and different mucosal areas and provides extra evaluation within the scalp. In addition, the fact that it consists of a single-page form provides ease of use. This score ranges from 0 to 263, moderate disease is defined by a PDAI score of 14 or less, major disease is defined by a PDAI score of 15 to 44, and extensive disease is defined by a PDAI score of 45 or higher [7, 23]. Another frequently used scoring method is ABSIS (Autoimmune Bullous Skin Disorder Intensity Score). It is evaluated between 0 and 206 according to the clinical severity of skin lesions, the number of areas involved in the oral mucosa, and the discomfort during feeding. When evaluating this score, ABSIS <17 is considered a mild disease, ABSIS 17–53 is considered a moderate disease, and ABSIS >53 is considered a severe disease. The advantages of this method are that it allows both objective and subjective evaluation and can be used in all bullous diseases [7, 23]. A third system, called the Pemphigus Vulgaris Activity Score (PVAS), takes into account the localization, morphology and severity of mucocutaneous lesions, as well as the presence of Nikolsky's sign [24].

8. Diagnosis

Early and accurate diagnosis is important. This is dependent on the co-detection of clinical presentation and tissue-bound and/or circulating autoantibodies.

The diagnosis of pemphigus vulgaris begins with a thorough history and physical examination. Since the presence of mucosal lesions is more common in PV than in other pemphigus, it should detect the presence of mucosal involvement. Mucosal involvement may not always be in the areas to be seen during the examination. Therefore, clinicians should question the presence of ocular symptoms, hoarseness, dysphagia and dyspareunia to assess the involvement of all mucosal surfaces [3]. Drug use should be questioned.

After a thorough history and physical examination, two separate biopsies should be obtained from the patient for both histopathological examination and DIF.

A 4 mm punch biopsy should be taken from the edge of the early lesion or erosion for hematoxylin and eosin (H&E) staining and routine histopathological examination. For direct immunofluorescence (DIF), an additional perilesional skin biopsy should be taken from normal-appearing skin 4 mm from a vesicle or erosion. Lesions of skin biopsies for DIF are more likely to be associated with false-negative results as a result of the elimination of immunoreactions involved in the inflammatory process of the underlying pemphigus disease. DIF biopsies should not be placed in formalin. Michel medium or Zeus medium should be used. Fresh specimens also may be sent to the laboratory, provided they are kept moist with saline and processing within 24 hours.

The characteristic histopathological finding in PV is acantholysis due to loss of intercellular adhesion without necrosis in keratinocytes and thus the formation of intraepidermal bullae. Although acantholysis is often located just above the basal layer (suprabasal), intraepidermal localization at the level of the stratum spinosum has also been reported to a lesser extent. There are epidermal cell clumps and acantholytic cells in the bulla cavity. Although basal keratinocytes lose their connection with the adjacent cell, they do not lose their bond with the basal membrane through hemidesmosomes, leading to the appearance of a 'tombstone pattern' [19]. Sparse inflammatory infiltrates in the dermis with eosinophils.

The gold standard in the diagnosis of PV is direct immunofluorescence (DIF) microscopy, which can detect tissue-bound autoantibodies [4]. In DIF, there is the accumulation of IgG and C3 in the intercellular space throughout the mid-lower or entire epidermis.

IIF and ELISA are serological tests that detect circulating autoantibodies that bind epithelial cell surface antigens. These tests are used to further support the diagnosis of pemphigus in patients with a positive DIF result. More than 80% of pemphigus vulgaris patients have circulating antibodies detectable by IIF. The substrate used affects the test sensitivity [25]. The monkey esophagus is the preferred substrate for the diagnosis of pemphigus vulgaris. Intercellular 'honeycomb' or 'coil wire' IgG accumulation is observed in PV [26]. The enzyme-linked immunosorbent assay (ELISA) test can be used for IgG antibodies to Dsg 1 and Dsg 3. ELISA is more sensitive and specific than IIF in the diagnosis of pemphigus vulgaris [25]. The ELISA test can also be used to monitor disease course and response to therapy in PV. In a study in which Dsg 1 and Dsg 3 autoantibody levels were followed in patients under treatment, it was found that Dsg 1 level more clearly showed the course of the disease. Dsg 3 antibody levels remained elevated during remission in some patients with mucosal pemphigus vulgaris [27]. Antibodies can be detected in patients who do not yet have clinical signs of pemphigus and can be found in patients with staphylococcal scalded skin, penicillin adverse drug reactions, toxic epidermolysis necrosis and burns [1].

Additional serological tests that may be used to diagnose pemphigus vulgaris include immunoblotting and immunoprecipitation. However, these tests are more difficult to perform than IIF and ELISA. Therefore, they are rarely used in the clinical setting.

In addition, cytological examination (Tzanck smear) stained with hematoxylin and eosin is useful for rapid demonstration of acantholytic keratinocytes of the spinous layer (abundant eosinophilic cytoplasm and rounded central nucleus) [20].

9. Differential diagnosis

Diagnosis is more difficult in patients with only oral lesions. Differential diagnoses for mucosal lesions include stomatitis secondary to herpes simplex virüs, aphthous ulcers, lichen planus, erythema multiforme, Stevens-Johnson syndrome, paraneoplastic pemphigus cicatricial pemphigoid, autoimmune diseases such as systemic lupus erythematosus or dermatitis herpetiformis [1, 19]. The differential diagnosis of cutaneous lesions includes other forms of pemphigus, bullous pemphigoid, linear Ig A bullous dermatosis, erythema multiforme, Hailey-Hailey disease and Grover's disease, epidermolysis bullosa acquisita [1, 19]. Demonstration of IgG autoantibodies against keratinocyte cell surfaces and anti-Dsg3 IgG will exclude these diseases (except drug-induced pemphigus vulgaris and paraneoplastic pemphigus). Fresh bullous pemphigoid blisters are tense due to a subepidermal division. The Hailey-Hailey disease has full-thickness acantholysis 'dilapidated brick wall' with epidermal hyperplasia and impetiginized scales, and acantholysis does not extend follicles down as in pemphigus. Transient acantholytic dermatosis exhibits only small intraepidermal foci of acantholysis [1].

10. Treatment

Prior to the use of systemic corticosteroids, pemphigus vulgaris was an often fatal disease. Most patients would die within 2–5 years from the onset of the disease. Extensive involvement of the body surface led to the loss of epidermal barrier function and increased fluid loss or secondary bacterial infections. The anti-inflammatory effects of corticosteroids have made them one of the most important drugs in the treatment of autoimmune bullae diseases, and their use has reduced the mortality rate by 60%. Without treatment, PV has a mortality rate ranging from 60 to 90% [28]. However, these agents are not without their side effects, and the mortality of PV remains significant (5–20%), largely due to complications of long-term immunosuppression. However, immunosuppressive agents remain important in the treatment of PV [29].

The first line of treatment is corticosteroids. Recommends starting prednisone treatment at doses of 0.5–1.5 mg/kg/day (mean 1 mg/kg/day, 60 mg/day) for approximately 2 weeks or more. If disease control is not achieved thereafter, the dose is increased to 2 mg/kg/day or reduced to 25% per week unless relapsed [29]. Pulse therapy in the form of 1 gr/day can also be used (with close cardiological monitoring), but it is not recommended due to the high risk of side effects.

The following should be considered when deciding which immunosuppressive drug to use in the patient. First, the patient's medical condition, general health, comorbidities, and the response of PV to corticosteroid therapy. Second, the level of steroid-sparing effect required to maintain clinical remission if the disease is under control. Third, data on remission times, the incidence of relapse, and time to relapse [29].

Adjuvant Therapies; azathioprine (AZA) is a cytotoxic drug used in many autoimmune diseases. It is the oldest and most prescribed immunosuppressive drug used for PV, and contributes to treatment by suppressing lymphocyte proliferation and antibody synthesis. AZA is an effective adjunctive immunosuppressive agent for pemphigus, with clinical remission rates of approximately 50% in retrospective studies [25]. The recommended dose of AZA in PV is 1 to 3 mg/kg/day orally in two divided doses. It should be used for four to six weeks to achieve a full therapeutic effect, which limits its use as monotherapy. In case of unsatisfactory clinical response, it is recommended to continue use for 3 months before replacing with another adjuvant [20]. Due to genetic polymorphisms that affect AZA clearance and activation, testing for thiopurine methyltransferase (TPMT) levels is strongly recommended prior to initiating therapy. In general, adults with pemphigus with high TPMT activity should be treated with a normal dose of AZA (up to 2.5 mg/kg/day), and those with moderate or low TPMT activity at a low maintenance dose (up to 0.5–1.5 mg/kg/day) should be treated with AZA therapy, should not be given to patients without TPMT activity [26]. Blood and liver enzymes should be monitored weekly for the first month of treatment and biweekly after the second month. Intervals can be increased later. Serious side effects include reversible lymphopenia, neutropenia and early pancreatitis. More commonly, gastrointestinal upset and hepatotoxicity, which can be reduced by dose adjustment, have been reported [29].

Mycophenolate mofetil (MMF) has been used as an adjuvant to corticosteroids in patients who do not respond to AZA. Several groups prefer MMF to AZA as first-line adjuvant therapy in PV because of its low hepatotoxicity and comparable efficacy. It is started at a dose of 2–3 g/day divided into two doses in combination with MMF systemic steroid. This combination therapy has been shown to provide clinical remission in an average of 9 months. Therapeutic failure should only be considered after 3 months of use at a dose of 3 g/day. Its main side effects are altered bowel habits, neutropenia, lymphopenia and myalgia. Its use is contraindicated in case of hematological dysfunction, acute and chronic infections, pregnancy and malignancy. Because it is teratogenic, contraception should be initiated in women of childbearing age before starting MMF therapy. Complete blood count and liver-kidney function tests should be performed at the start of treatment, every other week for the first 3 months, and monthly after 3 months of treatment. In addition, patients should be followed up for the development of cutaneous neoplasms and lymphoma.

Although not as frequently used as AZA or MMF, it is an alternative to methotrexate (MTX) for immunosuppressive therapy in pemphigus vulgaris. In a retrospective study of 30 PV patients treated with adjuvant methotrexate at a dose of 15 mg per week, it was shown that 84% of patients showed clinical improvement within 6 months and the steroid dose could be reduced in 21 (76.6%) and MTX was effective and safe in the treatment of PV has been reported [30]. Before starting treatment, complete blood count, liver and kidney function tests and urinalysis should be performed. It is then recommended to monitor the blood count and liver function tests once a week for the first month, monthly for the next 2 months, and then every 2–3 months. Major side effects are susceptibility to infections and liver dysfunction. Hepatotoxicity is important during drug use. In some studies, it has been stated that if the patient is not in the risk group for liver disease, liver biopsy may not be performed by monitoring the procollagen III level [29]. Side effects can be alleviated with the administration of 5–10 mg of folic acid after methotrexate treatment.

Cyclosporine is a selective inhibitor of calcineurin and acts by reducing the transcription of cytokines required for T-lymphocyte proliferation. This may suppress the autoimmune response in the pathogenesis of PV [29]. Some authors report that the efficacy of cyclosporine in the treatment of pemphigus is limited compared to AZA or MMF [31]. The standard dose is 2.5–3 mg/kg/day. Cyclosporine requires close monitoring for hypertension and renal toxicity.

Cyclophosphamide, as an alkylating agent, cross-links DNA and suppresses B and T lymphocyte responses, thereby helping PV treatment by reducing antibody production [29]. Cyclophosphamide is administered at a dose of 1–3 mg/kg/day (usually 50–200 mg/day). The most important side effects are hemorrhagic cystitis, infertility and leukopenia. Complete remission was achieved in 17 of 20 patients with PV, and treatment failed in three patients. The treatment was applied for an average of 17 months and the patients were followed for 27 months. The median time to complete remission was reported as 8.5 months. Hematuria was observed in five patients, mild infection in six patients, and transitional cell carcinoma of the bladder 15 years later in one patient. There were no deaths due to cyclophosphamide treatment [32]. In another study, weekly intravenous cyclophosphamide infusion with high-dose corticosteroids safely, effectively and quickly controlled the condition of corticosteroid-insensitive patients with resistant PV, shortened hospital stay and prevented the risk of further complications [33]. Several small case series have evaluated regimens of immunoablative intravenous cyclophosphamide with daily oral therapy (1.1–2.5 mg/kg/day), intermittent high-dose intravenous dexamethasone and cyclophosphamide with 50 mg/day oral cyclophosphamide daily. Although none of them are curative, all methods have been found to be effective in the short term. Significant adverse events, including hematuria, infection and transitional cell carcinoma of the bladder, have been observed with high-dose treatment regimens. In a study using low-dose cyclophosphamide (1.0–1.5 mg/kg/day), no significant difference in the safety profile was observed when compared with other immunosuppressive agents. With the risk of infertility, cyclophosphamide is not considered a first-line steroid-sparing agent in the treatment of PV [25].

Dapsone inhibits various inflammatory mediators, but its exact mechanism of action in PV is unknown [34]. Steroid-reducing effects have been demonstrated at doses up to 100 mg/day or ≤ 1.5 mg/kg/day [35]. In different studies, Dapsone showed a trend toward efficacy as a steroid-sparing drug in PV, but the results were not statistically significant. It can be used with other immunosuppressants, especially Rituximab. It helps in the prophylaxis of Pneumocystis pneumonia [25]. Serum glucose-6-phosphate-dehydrogenase (G6PDH) activity should be checked before starting treatment.

Plasmapheresis, the process typically involves plasma exchange to remove IgG antibodies from the serum and replace them with albumin, fresh frozen plasma, or donor plasma. Plasmapheresis is sometimes used to treat severe pemphigus or PV unresponsive to a combination of corticosteroids and immunosuppressive agents. Although one controlled study reported ineffectiveness, other studies have shown that both reduces serum autoantibody levels and controls disease activity [25]. For maximum efficacy, patients should receive immunosuppressive agents to avoid the antibody rebound phenomenon that may follow IgG removal, the most commonly used agent for this purpose is Cyclophosphamide [25, 29]. Side effects of plasmapheresis include sepsis, hypotension and depletion of clotting factors.

Immunoadsorption (IA) is an advanced technique used to remove circulating antibodies in patients with severe disease and high IgG titers. Removal of pathogenic antibodies from the circulation has been theorized to promote the migration of anti-Dsg3 antibodies from the skin to the systemic circulation, thereby minimizing autoantibody binding to antigens in the epidermis, thereby preventing the underlying pathogenesis of pemphigus. Cost and availability are major limiting factors for the use of IA [29]. The basic principles of IA are actually similar to plasmapheresis, but when the two are compared, IA does not remove plasma proteins such as albumin and clotting factors. The use of plasmapheresis in pemphigus has been largely abandoned due to the significant incidence of serious adverse events such as sepsis [36].

Pulse Corticosteroid, intravenous, pulsed administration of 250 to 1000 mg of methylprednisolone administered over approximately 3 hours per day for 4 to 5 consecutive days can achieve prolonged remission and reduce the total dose of glucocorticoids needed to control the disease. Although the goal of this therapy is to reduce the incidence of complications from long-term steroid use, it can cause cardiac arrhythmias resulting in sudden death, in addition to all the usual glucocorticoid complications, and its use remains controversial. In addition, a controlled trial showed that adjuvant oral dexamethasone pulse was not superior to standard treatment with prednisolone and AZA for PV. Simply giving lower doses of prednisone in divided doses may produce the same result with fewer side effects [25].

Rituximab; chimeric monoclonal anti-CD 20 antibodies. Rituximab binding to CD20 induces B-cell depletion by, at least, four different mechanisms:

1. Direct induction of programmed cell death, which is dependent on activation of caspases and involves intracellular molecules, including Src kinases, p38 MAPK and NFkB.

2. Complement-dependent cytotoxicity, which happens when C1s binds to Rituximab opsonized cells and trigger complement activation and formation of the membrane attack complex (MAC), which eventually induces cell lysis.

3. Antibody-dependent cytotoxicity, which consists of activation of NK cells through binding the human Fc portion of Rituximab to the FcRIII receptor: this activates NK cells to release cytotoxic mediators, including perforins and granzyme B, which induces caspases-dependent cell death in the target lymphocyte.

4. Antibody-dependent phagocytosis, in which neutrophils, monocytes and macrophages bind Rituximab opsonized B-cells through the Fcγ Receptor. Recently, a new mechanism referred to as trogocytosis, or shaving has been characterized. In trogocytosis, macrophages remove Rituximab-CD20 complexes by transferring plasma membrane; this triggers cell death through a yet-to-be identified mechanism [36].

Despite being used in the treatment of pemphigus since the early 2000s, anti-CD20 monoclonal antibodies such as rituximab are still considered third-line agents in the European Academy of Dermatology and Venereal Diseases guidelines published in 2015 [26]. Recently, anti-CD20 antibodies have been recommended as the first choice only for moderate to severe and/or resistant pemphigus. Following administration of rituximab, a rapid and sustained decrease in circulating and tissue B lymphocytes is observed, lasting at least 6 to 12 months. Recent evidence suggests that it also affects T lymphocytes [20]. Rituximab treatment reduced the total corticosteroid dose required for clinical remission, thus reducing side effects secondary to long-term high-dose corticosteroids. A recent retrospective case-control study involving 40 patients showed that patients previously treated with rituximab treated with conventional therapy were able to reduce their monthly prednisone dose by 73% from a median of 658.6 mg/month to 177.2 mg/month [12].

It should be administered IV as a slow infusion (four to 6 hours). There are no standardized protocols for the use of rituximab in autoimmune bullous diseases. There is much debate about the optimal dose of Rituximab in pemphigus. Two main protocols are used: the rheumatoid arthritis protocol, which consists of two 1,000 mg infusions two weeks apart, and the lymphoma protocol, which consists of four 500 mg once-weekly infusions [36]. No differences in percent remission and disease-free time were observed in either protocol. They can be used alone or in combination with intravenous immunoglobulin, plasmapheresis and immunoadsorption. It can also be applied to patients already taking prednisone and immunosuppressive drugs; dose reduction and suspension of the latter should be accelerated, due to the increased risk of infection [20].

Intravenous Immunoglobulin (IVIg); derived from a pool of donors, IVIg consists of human plasma-derived IgG, sugars, salts and solvents [36]. It is thought that IVIg functions by saturating the neonatal Fc receptor, thereby increasing the catabolism of the patient's serum antibodies containing pathogenic autoantibodies [25]. IVIg is mostly used in patients resistant to corticosteroid and immunosuppressive treatments. 2 gr/kg is applied in each session. In studies, it has been shown that the application of 0.4 g/kg/day for 5 consecutive days is effective in the treatment [20, 36]. It can also be combined with rituximab. Slow 5–5.5 hour infusions can minimize infusion reactions [13]. A major benefit of IVIg is its few side effects. The most common side effects are headache, dyspnea, tachycardia, and abdominal discomfort. The most serious adverse events are aseptic meningitis and cerebrovascular accidents, occurring in <1% of PV patients treated with IVIg [13]. It can be used on pregnant women.

TNF-α inhibitors; TNF-α is one of the cytokines involved in acantholysis. Although the use of Infliximab and Etanercept as a case report appears to be effective in the treatment of PV, there are conflicting results [20].

Topical treatment; PV is largely managed with systemic therapy, but skin and mucosal care are extremely important. For this purpose, topical corticosteroids and, if there is a risk of infection, antibiotic creams are often added to the treatment. It has also been reported that tacrolimus and pimecrolimus, pilocarpine gel 4%, nicotinamide gel 4%, 0.1% sulfadiazine creams are also beneficial [37].

During the treatment period, patients should be followed closely for diabetes, hypertension, heart failure, myopathy, osteoporosis, avascular bone necrosis, glaucoma, cataract due to corticosteroids, infections, especially respiratory tract infections, hepatitis, CMV reactivation or hematological abnormalities (anemia, leukopenia) as a result of immunosuppression.

Future Therapies; CAAR-T Therapy, BTK inhibitor and p38MAPK inhibitor are included.

CAAR-T Therapy; T cells expressing chimeric autoantibody receptors (CAAR-T cells) that target antibody-producing B cells are one of the latest proposed avenues for treating for autoimmune conditions.

Bruton tyrosine kinase (BTK) Inhibitor; Bruton tyrosine kinase (BTK) is expressed in B cells and innate immune cells, acting as an essential signaling element in multiple immune cell pathways. Selective BTK inhibition has the potential to target multiple immune-mediated disease pathways. Rilzabrutinib is an oral, reversible, covalent BTK inhibitor designed for immune-mediated diseases [38]. One of the new potential treatments for pemphigus, the BTK inhibitor rilzabrutinib (PRN1088) was recently tested in patients with PV in a phase II trial and controlled 50–56% of lesion activity in patients in a mean of 4 weeks [39]. Thus, inhibition of kinases such as BTK shows promising potential for future treatment of PV.

p38MAPK inhibitor (SB202190); In a murine model of pemphigus, p38MAPK inhibition prevented blister formation. On the other hand, in a study, the formation of blisters in the mucosa could not be prevented by a p38MAPK inhibitor, and they claimed that, unlike the epidermis, the ultrastructural changes of blister formation and desmosomes were independent of p38MAPK in the oral mucosa [40].

11. Prophylaxis against side effects in prolonged corticosteroid

Basic screening and prophylaxis of osteoporosis, ophthalmological evaluation, vitamin D and calcium supplementation during corticosteroid therapy, treatment with bisphosphonates (ie alendronate, risedronate) in patients at risk of developing osteoporosis (postmenopausal women and > 50 years and > 3 months on corticosteroid treatment), clinical systemic antifungals, antiviral and antibiotic therapy if needed, use of H2-blockers or proton pump inhibitors, antithrombotic prophylaxis in case of high thrombosis risk, psychological support if necessary, physiotherapy if long-term corticosteroid therapy is required [41].

12. Prognosis

The mortality rate of PV is estimated about 5–10%. Death is mainly a result of corticosteroid and immunosuppressant side effects. In particular, patients with persistent PV may develop serious infections secondary to high-dose corticosteroid use. Most patients with relapsing forms of the disease require a long course of treatment of 10 years or more [42].

13. Pemfigus vulgaris in children

PV is the most common type in the pediatric group among all pemphigus types, excluding endemic pemphigus foliaceus [43]. The pediatric variant is divided into two, childhood PV (0–12 years) and adolescent (juvenile) PV (13–18 years) [44]. Most patients have mucocutaneous involvement, both in childhood and in the juvenile form. Oral, nasal, ocular and anal mucous membranes are involved. The frequency of genital involvement is high in both groups [45]. The clinical picture is similar to that in adults. Loose bullae on intact or erythematous skin open easily and become eroded and crusted lesions. Antibody titrations can be detected in the serum in most of patients [43]. Nikolsky's sign is positive.

Systemic steroid as in adults, is the cornerstone of treatment [45]. Systemic side effects develop in two-thirds of patients treated with systemic steroids. The most common side effects are; Cushing's syndrome (65%), growth retardation (50%) and infection (50%). Prednisone dose is started at 40–60 mg/day, when new lesion growth stops, it is gradually reduced and adjuvant therapy is added. Many adjuvant agents such as AZA, dapsone, mycophenolate mofetil, cyclophosphamide, methotrexate, cyclosporine, plasmapheresis, IVIg and rituximab have been used in the treatment of children as in adults. Data on the use of rituximab therapy in pediatric patients are limited. The youngest case treated with rituximab was a 4-year-old girl [44]. There are partial and complete remission reports in the literature. There is no standard dosing regimen in children. The lymphoma protocol was used in most of the published cases. Treatments usually last 2–3 years and the prognosis is better than in adult patients [46].

14. Pemfigus vulgaris during pregnancy

PV is extremely rare in pregnancy. On the other hand, pregnancy may accelerate or increase PV, as reported in well-known autoimmune diseases such as systemic lupus erythematosus [47]. Babies of mothers with pemphigus may be affected by the disease in many different ways, from stillbirth to transient PV lesions in newborns, due to transplacental transmission of pathogenic anti-Dsg antibodies [48]. The more uncontrolled the disease in the mother and the higher the titers of Dsg antibodies in the mother's serum or umbilical cord blood, the worse the possible outcomes [48]. PV seen during pregnancy can affect the mother, delivery and fetus. While the disease exacerbates mostly in the first, second trimester and postpartum periods, it calms down in the third trimester [49]. The reason for this is probably the increase in the endogenous chorionic corticosteroid hormone and the resulting immunosuppression [50, 51]. However, no change is observed in some patients during pregnancy, and these patients may remain in remission [49]. The postpartum disease worsens in all pemphigus patients who are not treated during pregnancy [52]. If the disease worsens in the first trimester, medical termination of pregnancy may be considered. If the worsening of the disease occurs in the second or third trimester, steroids are a safe treatment option [53].

In the publications on the treatment of autoimmune bullous diseases in pregnancy, it is stated that topical/systemic steroids and AZA can be used safely. In a small number of case reports, it has been reported that rituximab, IVIg, and dapsone may also be safe [54]. AZA is the most commonly used non-steroidal immunosuppressant in pemphigus. If it is necessary to give, the lowest dose should be preferred to prevent fetal damage [55]. The pregnancy category is D. Cyclosporine is believed to be less effective in the treatment of pemphigus but is the most reliable agent in pregnancy [56]. MMF, cyclophosphamide, and methotrexate are drugs that are not preferred or even contraindicated during pregnancy [57].

15. Vaccination in pemphigus patients

Administration of live vaccines is contraindicated when using adjuvant immunosuppressants and rituximab. Vaccination against seasonal influenza, H1N1, tetanus and pneumococci are recommended in patients receiving oral corticosteroids or immunosuppressives. During systemic immunosuppression, the level of protection after vaccination raises question marks [26]. On the other hand, it has been reported in the literature that pemphigus vulgaris is seen after tetanus diphtheria, hepatitis B and influenza vaccine applications, and that the disease exacerbates after influenza vaccine use [58]. We do not have any data on which patients vaccination will cause disease reactivation [59].

Although COVID mRNA vaccines may cause autoimmune bullous disease activation, it is recommended not to abandon the vaccination and to treat the existing picture in case of disease activation [60].

Based on vaccination experience, when vaccines for COVID-19 are available, dermatologists may advise vaccination 12–20 weeks after completion of a treatment cycle with rituximab or extend dosing intervals so that a minimum time of 4 weeks precedes the next drug infusion [61].

Limited data suggest that patients with autoimmune bullous disease receiving immunomodulatory therapies are not primarily at risk for serious or fatal COVID-19 [60].

Author details

Ozlem Su Kucuk* and Nazan Taşlidere
Department of Dermatovenereology, Bezmialem Vakif University School of Medicine, Istanbul, Turkey

*Address all correspondence to: ozlemsukucuk2@yahoo.com.tr

References

[1] Venugopal SS, Murrell FD. Diagnosis and clinical features of pemphigus vulgaris. Dermatologic Clinics. 2011;**29**(3):373-380

[2] Kridin K, Schmidt E. Epidemiology of Pemphigus. JID Innovation. 2021;**1**(1):100004

[3] Malik AM, Tupchong S, Huang S, Are A, Hsu S, Motaparthi K. An updated review of pemphigus diseases. Medicina (Kaunas, Lithuania). 2021;**57**(10):1080

[4] Popescu IA, Statescu L, Vata D, Porumb-Andrese E, Patrascu AI, Grajdeanu IA, et al. Pemphigus vulgaris—Approach and management. Experimental and Therapeutic Medicine. 2019;**18**:5056-5060

[5] Torzecka JD, Woźniak K, Kowalewski C, Waszczykowska E, Sysa-Jedrzejowska A, Pas HH, et al. Circulating pemphigus autoantibodies in healthy relatives of pemphigus patients: Coincidental phenomenon with a risk of disease development? Archives of Dermatological Research. 2007;**299**:239-243

[6] Yan L, Wang JM, Zeng K. Association between HLA-DRB1 polymorphisms and pemphigus vulgaris: A meta-analysis. The British Journal of Dermatology. 2012;**167**:768-777

[7] Schmidt E, Kasperkiewicz M, Joly P. Pemphigus. Lancet. 2019; **394**(10201):882-894

[8] Ruocco V, Ruocco E, Lo Schiavo A, Brunetti G, Guerrera LP, Wolf R. Pemphigus: Etiology, pathogenesis, and inducing or triggering factors: Facts and controversies. Clinics in Dermatology. 2013;**31**(4):374-381

[9] Hannah R, Ramani P, Tilakaratne WM, Sukumaran G, Ramasubramanian A, Krishnan RP. Critical appraisal of different triggering pathways for the pathobiology of pemphigus vulgaris-A review. Oral Diseases. Jun 21, 2021. DOI: 10.1111/odi.13937 [Online head of print]

[10] Tavakolpour S. Pemphigus trigger factors: Special focus on pem-phigus vulgaris and pemphigus foliaceus. Archives of Dermatological Research. 2018;**310**:95-106

[11] Juhasz MLW, Doan L, Rojek NW. Cocaine-induced pemphigus vulgaris. JAAD Case Reports. 2021;**9**:45-47

[12] Jamora MJJ, Jiao D, Bystryn JC. Antibodies to desmoglein 1 and 3, and the clinical phenotype of pemphigus vulgaris. Journal of the American Academy of Dermatology. 2003;**48**:976-977

[13] Hammers CM, Stanley JR. Mechanisms of disease: Pemphigus and Bullous Pemphigoid. Annual Review of Pathology. 2016;**11**:175-197

[14] Aktan Ş. The Etiopathogenesis of Autoimmune Bullous Diseases. Türkderm. 2011;**1**:8-15

[15] Femiano F. Pemphigus vulgaris: Recent advances in our understanding of its pathogenesis. Minerva Stomatologica. 2007;**56**(4):215-223

[16] Kaur B, Kerbrat J, Kho J, Kaler M, Stefanos K, Cirillo N. Mechanism-based therapeutic targets of pemphigus vulgaris: A scoping review of pathogenic molecular pathways. Experimental Dermatology. 2022;**31**(2):154-171

[17] DiMarco C. Pemphigus: Pathogenesis to treatment. Medical Journal. 2016;**99**:28-31

[18] Wojnarowska F, Venning VA, Burns T, Breathnach S, Cox N, Griffiths C. Rook's Textbook of Dermatology. 8th ed. Vol. 2. New York: Blackwell Science; 2010

[19] Amagai M, Bolognia JL, Jorizzo JL, Schaffer JV. Dermatoloji. 3. baskı. Cilt 1. Philadelphia: Elsevier; 2012. pp. 469-471. Pemfigus; s

[20] Porro AM, Seque CA, Ferreira MCC, Enokihara MMS. Pemphigus vulgaris. Anais brasileiros de dermatologia. 2019;**94**:264-278

[21] Sar-Pomian M, Rudnicka L, Olszewska M. The significance of scalp involvement in Pemphigus: A literature review. BioMed Research International. 2018;**2018**:6154397

[22] Smith MS, Moscarelli R, Panse G, Parkash V. Cervical Pemphigus Vulgaris presenting as postmenopausal bleeding. International Journal of Gynecological Pathology. 2021;**40**(5):477-481

[23] Montagnon CM, Lehman JS, Murrell DF, Camilleri MJ, Tolkachjov SN. Intraepithelial autoimmune bullous dermatoses disease activity assessment and therapy. Journal of the American Academy of Dermatology. 2021;**84**(6):1523-1537

[24] Chams-Davatchi C, Rahbar Z, Daneshpazhooh M, Mortazavizadeh SMA, Akhyani M, Esmaili N, et al. Pemphigus vulgaris activity score and assessment of convergent validity. Acta Medical Iran. 2013;**51**(4):224-230

[25] Payne AS, Stanley JR. Pemphigus. In: Goldsmith LA, Katz SI, Gilchrest BA, et al., editors. Fitzpatrick's Dermatology in General Medicine. 8th ed. Vol. 1. McGraw Hill; 2012. p. 586

[26] Hertl M, Jedlickova H, Karpati S, Marinovic B, Uzun S, Yayli S, et al. Pemphigus. S2 Guideline for diagnosis and treatment—Guided by the European Dermatology Forum (EDF) in cooperation with the European Academy of Dermatology and Venereology (EADV). Journal of the European Academy of Dermatology and Venereology. 2015;**29**(3):405-414

[27] Abasq C, Mouquet H, Gilbert D, et al. ELISA testing of anti-desmoglein 1 and 3 antibodies in the management of pemphigus. Archives of Dermatology. 2009;**145**:529

[28] Bystryn JC, Rudolph JL. Pemphigus. Lancet. 2005;**366**:61-73. DOI: 10.1016/S0140-6736(05)66829-8

[29] Yanovsky RL, McLeod M, Ahmed AR. Treatment of pemphigus vulgaris: Part 1—Current therapies. Expert Review of Clinical Immunology. 2019;**15**(10):1047-1060

[30] Baum S, Greenberger S, Samuelov L, et al. Methotrexate is an effective and safe adjuvant therapy for pemphigus vulgaris. European Journal of Dermatology. 2012;**22**:83-87

[31] Ioannides D, Chrysomallis F, Bystryn JC. Ineffectiveness of cyclosporine as an adjuvant to corticosteroids in the treatment of pemphigus. Archives of Dermatology. 2000;**136**(7):868-872

[32] Cummins DL, Mimouni D, Anhalt GJ, et al. Oral cyclophosphamide for treatment of pemphigus vulgaris and foliaceus. Journal of the American Academy of Dermatology. 2003;**49**(2):276-280

[33] Zhang W, Wei S, Peng X, Xie S, Zhang Z, Zeng K, et al. Short-term intravenous infusion of cyclophosphamide in the treatment of refractory Pemphigus Vulgaris: A Retrospective Study. Dermatology. 2021;**237**(2):185-190

[34] Sinha AA, Hoffman MB, Janicke EC. Pemphigus vulgaris: Approach to treatment. European Journal of Dermatology. 2015;**25**:103-113

[35] Werth VP, Fivenson D, Pandya AG, et al. Multicenter randomized, double-blind, placebo-controlled, clinical trial of dapsone as a glucocorticoid sparing agent in maintenance-phase pemphigus vulgaris. Archives of Dermatology. 2008;**144**:25-32

[36] Didona D, Maglie R, Eming R, Hertl M. Pemphigus: Current and future therapeutic strategies. Frontiers in Immunology. 2019;**10**:1418

[37] Harman KE, Brown D, Exton LS, Groves RW, Hampton PJ, Mohd Mustapa MF, et al. British Association of Dermatologists' guidelines for the management of pemphigus vulgaris 2017. The British Journal of Dermatology. 2017;**177**:1170-1201

[38] Langrish CL, Bradshaw JM, Francesco MR, Owens TD, Xing Y, Shu J, et al. Preclinical efficacy and anti-inflammatory mechanisms of action of the bruton tyrosine kinase inhibitor rilzabrutinib for immune-mediated disease. Journal of Immunology. 2021;**206**(7):1454-1468

[39] Murrell DF, Patsatsi A, Stavropoulos P, Baum S, Zeeli T, Kern JS, et al. Proof of concept for the clinical effects of oral rilzabrutinib, the first Bruton tyrosine kinase inhibitor for pemphigus vulgaris: The phase II BELIEVE study. The British Journal of Dermatology. 2021;**185**(4):745-755

[40] Egu DT, Sigmund AM, Schmidt E, Spindler V, Walter E, Waschke J. A new ex vivo human oral mucosa model reveals that p38MAPK inhibition is not effective to prevent autoantibody-induced mucosal blistering in pemphigus. The British Journal of Dermatology. 2020;**182**:987-994

[41] Murrell DF, Pena S, Joly P, Marinovic B, Hashimoto T, Diaz LA, et al. Diagnosis and management of pemphigus: Recommendations by an international panel of experts. Journal of the American Academy of Dermatology. 2018;**2**:21

[42] Joly P, Litrowski N. Pemphigus group (vulgaris, vegetans, foliaceus, herpetiformis, brasiliensis). Clinics in Dermatology. 2011;**29**(4):432-436

[43] De D, Kanwar AJ. Childhood pemphigus. Indian Journal of Dermatology. 2006;**51**:89-95

[44] Kincaid L, Weinstein M. Rituximab therapy for childhood pemphigus vulgaris. Pediatric Dermatology. 2016;**33**(2):e61-e64

[45] Gürcan H, Mabrouk D, Razzaque AA. Management of pemphigus in pediatric patients. Minerva Pediatrica. 2011;**63**(4):279-291

[46] Wananukul S, Pongprasit P. Childhood pemphigus. International Journal of Dermatology. 1999;**38**:29-35

[47] Kaufman AJ, Ahmed AR, Kaplan RP. Pemphigus, myasthenia gravis, and pregnancy. Journal of the American Academy of Dermatology. 1988;**19** (2 Pt 2):414-418

[48] Rangel J. Pregnancy-Associated "Cutaneous Type". Pemphigus Vulgaris Journal. 2016;**20**(1):e101

[49] Kalayciyan A, Engin B, Serdaroglu S, Mat C, Aydemir EH, Kotogyan A. A retrospective analysis of patients with pemphigus vulgaris associated with pregnancy. The British Journal of Dermatology. 2002;**147**(2):396-397

[50] Weinberg ED. Pregnancy-associated depression of cell-mediated immunity. Reviews of Infectious Diseases. 1984;**6**(6):814-831

[51] Gushi M, Yamamoto Y, Mine Y, Awazawa R, Nonaka K, Taira K, et al. Neonatal Pemphigus vulgaris. The Journal of Dermatology. 2008;**35**:529-535

[52] Lin L, Zeng X, Chen Q. Pemphigus and pregnancy. Analysis and summary of case reports over 49 years. Saudi Medical Journal. 2015;**36**(9):1033-1038

[53] Kanwar AJ, Thami GP. Pemphigus vulgaris and pregnancy—A reappraisal. The Australian & New Zealand Journal of Obstetrics & Gynaecology. 1999;**39**:372-373

[54] Braunstein I, Werth V. Treatment of dermatologic connective tissue disease and autoimmune blistering disorders in pregnancy. Dermatologic Therapy. 2013;**26**(4):354-363

[55] Hup JM, Bruinsma RA, Boersma ER, de Jong MC. Neonatal Pemphigus vulgaris: Transplacental transmission of antibodies. Pediatric Dermatology. 1986;**3**:468-472

[56] Daneshpazhooh M, Chams-Davatchi C, Valikhani M, Aghabagheri A, Mortazavizadeh SM, Barzegari M, et al. Pemphigus and pregnancy: A 23-year experience. Indian Journal of Dermatology, Venereology and Leprology. 2011;**77**:534

[57] Lehman JS, Mueller KK, Schraith DF. Do safe and effective treatment options exist for patients with active Pemphigus vulgaris who plan conception and pregnancy? Archives of Dermatology. 2008;**144**:783-785

[58] Cozzani E, Cacciapuoti M, Parodi A, Rebora A. Pemphigus following tetanus and diphtheria vaccination. The British Journal of Dermatology. 2002;**147**:188-189

[59] De Simone C, Caldarola G, D'agostino M, Zampetti A, Amerio P, Feliciani C. Exacerbation of pemphigus after influenza vaccination. Clinical and Experimental Dermatology. 2008;**33**(6):718-720

[60] Damiani G, Pacifico A, Pelloni F, Iorizzo M. The first dose of COVID-19 vaccine may trigger pemphigus and bullous pemphigoid flares: Is the second dose therefore contraindicated? Journal of the European Academy of Dermatology and Venereology. 2021;**35**:645-647

[61] Waldman RA, Creed M, Sharp K, et al. Letter in Reply: Toward a COVID-19 vaccine strategy for pemphigus patients on rituximab. Journal of the American Academy of Dermatology. 2020;**84**:197-E198

Chapter 8

Perspective Chapter: Diagnosis and Treatment of Venous Leg Ulcer

Vesna Karanikolic and Aleksandar Karanikolic

Abstract

Venous leg ulcer (VLU) represent a pathological tissue change in the form of a defect in the lower leg which occurs as a complication of chronic venous insufficiency. The prevalence of VLUs varies between 1.5–3% in the total population and 4–5% in persons over the age of 80. Venous ulcer is usually localized on the inner side of the lower third of the leg, oval, circular or irregular in shape. It is usually fibrous or covered with fresh granules that bleed heavily to the touch. It is very important to have a comprehensive clinical examination at the very beginning. Subsequent non-invasive and sometimes invasive tests may be indicated for diagnosis and treatment planning. Inadequate diagnosis results in inadequate therapy. The goal of therapy is complete restitution of the tissue defect and prevention of recurrence. The three basic elements of VLUs therapy are: local therapy, compression therapy and surgical treatment. If VLUs do not heal despite the application of standard therapeutic modalities, there are opportunities to apply new treatment technologies. The modern approach to the treatment of VLUs is based on the application of various biophysical interventions and medical devices.

Keywords: venous disease, venous leg ulcers, wound healing, diagnosis, venous leg ulcers treatment

1. Introduction

Venous leg ulcer (VLU) represent a pathological tissue change in the form of a defect in the lower leg which occurs as a complication of chronic venous insufficiency (CVI) [1]. Chronic ulceration is defined as ulceration on the lower leg that lasts (does not heal) within 6 weeks, and is caused by various etiopathogenetic factors [2].

Venous leg ulcers often heal slowly and result in long-term suffering and intensive use of health care resources [3, 4]. A VLUs represent a growing health problem, and they are a condition that is very expensive to treat for both the health system and patients.

A VLUs endangers the patient's normal life. Treatment of VLUs requires dedication and cooperation between the patient and the doctor. The health-related impact of VLUs is increasingly recognized as a valuable outcome measure for assessing interventions, especially when complete cure is unlikely [5]. Adults with VLUs often have multiple disabling symptoms, including pain, sleep disturbance, depression, swelling of the lower extremities, fatigue and symptoms associated with inflammation of lower leg (redness, localized heat, discomfort due to high exudate levels and itching) [6].

The prevalence of VLU varies between 1.5–3% in the total population and 4–5% in persons over the age of 80 [1]. Studies have shown that 1–2% of the adult population either has or has had venous ulceration [7]. The prevalence of VLU in Western European countries in the population over the age of 18 is 0.1–0.3% [1].

It is very important to point out that a certain number of VLUs heal very slowly or not at all. In a period of about 4 months with the application of adequate therapy, about 50% of VLUs heals [8, 9]. However, about 20% of VLUs do not heal even after 2 years from the beginning of treatment, and about 8% even after 5 years from the beginning of treatment [1]. At the annual level, the recurrence rate of VLUs ranges from 6–15% [1]. The risk of recurrence over a period of 1 year ranged from 30–57% [1].

Risk factors for VLUs are numerous, and most patients have more than one. Most of these factors are immutable and this group includes being female, elderly, having previous venous thrombosis of the legs, pulmonary embolism, multiparity, musculoskeletal and joint diseases [7, 10]. Obesity and sedentarianism are risk factors that can be influenced on [11]. The genetic traits of an individual can also be emphasized as a predisposing factor [7, 12], but the specific gene or set of genes responsible for the occurrence of this disease has not been determined so far. In people with varicose veins, Forkhead box C2, located on chromosome 16q24 [13], was isolated.

Despite the application of different standard treatment modalities for VLUs, a certain percentage of venous ulcers do not heal. Studies have shown that prolonged healing time or refractoriness to applied therapy may be due to an increase of T lymphocytes and granulocytes, lack of oxygen, growth factor and cytokine imbalance [10]. For this reason, we are working on the development of modern therapeutic modalities, while the number of new techniques for the VLUs care has increased in recent years and is constantly improving [14].

2. Symptomatology

Venous ulcer is usually localized on the inner side of the lower third of the leg, oval, circular or irregular in shape. The surface of the ulcer depends more on the degree of development than on the etiology. It is usually fibrous or covered with fresh granules that bleed heavily to the touch (**Figure 1**).

The ulcer area is thickened, pigmented and induced, together with subcutaneous adipose tissue. These changes correspond to lipodermatosclerosis, which is in fact a pre-ulcerative condition [15].

The absence of lipodermatosclerosis in the vicinity of the ulcer surface suggests that the ulcer may not be of venous origin. The presence of dilated venules, most often around the maleolus, below the ulcer surface, is also significant as a consequence of the transmission of increased venous tension through insufficient communicating veins. The presence of larger, dilated incompetent communicating veins is very significant for venous ulcers. An ulcer localized on the lateral side of the lower leg is often associated with an incompetent saphenous vein [16]. The presence of edema, lipodermatosclerosis and varicose superficial veins also supports the venous ulcer genesis. When examining ulcers, it is necessary to always examine the condition of the arterial circulation [17].

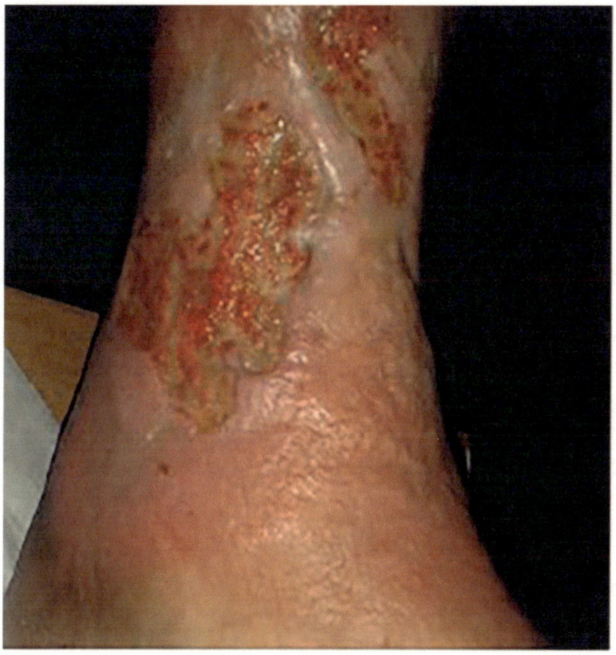

Figure 1.
Typical venous ulceration.

3. Diagnosis

Although simple at first glance, the diagnosis of venous disorders is essentially difficult due to specific hemodynamic conditions in the venous bloodstream.

A well-taken anamnesis can greatly help us in making an adequate diagnosis, and just the taking of anamnesis is considered to be a special skill, but for now there are no adequately conducted studies on the value of specific items for anamnesis. It is necessary to take data related to [18]: major symptoms exhibited and experienced, previous medical history, varicosity and treatment of varices, superficial and deep venous thrombosis, leg ulcer, peripheral arterial vascular disorder, diabetes mellitus, rheumatoid arthritis, extensive leg trauma, nutritional status, patient mobility, family anamnesis and specific leg ulcer aspects (duration, pain, previous treatment, symptoms of ulcer infection, the ankle joint mobility).

Today, the following diagnostic procedures are used to examine the venous system: Color-flow duplex ultrasound in the diagnosis of vascular diseases is widespread today, both because of its high sensitivity and accuracy, and the fact that it is a simple and safe diagnostic procedure. This method measures the diameter of the blood vessel, the duration of reflux, the presence of flow and the compressibility of the vein. The examination is performed in a standing position [19]. When examining the deep venous system up to the inferior vena cave, the patient is placed in a supine position [20]. The duration of reflux in normal proximal veins of the legs is <1 s while in distal veins <0.5 s.

Direct venous pressure measurement is an invasive diagnostic method where venous pressure is directly measured using a cannula in the superficial vein of the foot [21]. It was found that there is a direct correlation between the height of the pressure in the vein of the foot and the height of the pressure in the deep veins at the height of the ankle. Direct measurement of venous pressure is rarely used today because it is an invasive diagnostic technique and is not recommended as a routine diagnostic method in patients with venous ulcers.

Ankle-brachial pressure index (ABPI) is used to evaluate adequate arterial blood flow. A large number of studies have shown that about 30% of patients with VLUs also have a disease of the peripheral arterial system. Ulcers that occur in these patients may be due to diseases of the peripheral arterial system or occur in combination with venous insufficiency. Normal ABPI values range from 0.91–1.20. If ABPI is >0.8 arterial abnormality on the arteriogram is generally ruled out (chance >95%) [22].

Plethysmography, phlebodynamometry and phlebography, are less used methods due to inferior accuracy and associated risks [23, 24].

Application of bacteriological examination or biopsy of ulceration and pathohistological examination will be applied in case of suspicion of infection or malignant etiology of ulceration.

4. Differential diagnosis of VLU

The success of the treatment of venous ulcers of the lower extremities depends on the accuracy of the diagnosis. Infectious ulcers are mostly found in the tropics, while neoplastic ones are relatively rare. Ulcers associated with rheumatic disease or diabetes are also common in everyday clinical practice [7]. There is a whole range of etiological causes of ulcers on the lower extremities (**Table 1**).

Differential diagnosis of leg ulcers	
Vascular	venous, ischemic, mixed arterovenous, arteriovenous fistulas, venous malformations, vasculitis, diabetic ulcers, etc.
Traumatic	after sclerotherapy, after surgical interventions, accidental
Edema	lymphedema, renal, cardiac
Infection	tropical ulcers, cutaneous tuberculosis, syphilis, leprosy, parasitic and fungal infections
Malignant disease	Marjolin ulcer, primary squamous cell carcinoma, lymphoma, basal cell carcinoma, malignant melanoma
Other	immunodeficiency, contact dermatitis, nutrition disorder

Table 1.
Differential diagnosis of leg ulcers.

5. Principles of VLUs treatment

The therapy of VLUs is complex and is determined on the basis of: etiology, clinical picture, echosonographic findings, thrombotic status, laboratory findings, comorbidities, nutritional deficiencies, risk factors, economic and medical possibilities for diagnosis and therapy. The goal of therapy is complete restitution (reconstruction) of the tissue defect and prevention of recurrence [25]. Improvement of hemodynamic status (reduction of venous hypertension and venous stasis) is the primary therapeutic goal. The three basic elements of VLUs therapy are [26]:

1. local therapy

2. compression therapy

3. surgical treatment

Adequate VLUs therapy should reduce venous hypertension in the micro and macro circulation [26].

5.1 Local VLUs therapy

Local VLUs therapy is based on the application of the TIME treatment principle [27]:

- Tissue management

- Inflammation and infection control

- Moisture balance

- Epithelial (edge) advancement

Chronic wounds can traditionally be bandaged with gauze, antiseptics, topical antibiotics and adsorbents. This type of therapy requires daily bandaging, making the treatment expensive and ineffective [28].

By wound cleaning, we mean the removal of necrosis, fibrin or other deposits. Necrotic tissue can be removed surgically or treated with an enzymatic wound cleanser. The wound cleans itself by autolysis, if none of these methods is chosen. When performing surgical debridement of ulceration, debridement should be performed to avoid damage to healthy tissue [29]. Antiseptics such as povidone-iodine, chlorhexidine, acetic acid etc. are often used today in the VLUs treatment.

The use of dressings in the treatment of VLUs is efficient and pharmacoeconomically justified. The use of dressings in the treatment of VLUs has shown a significant advantage over the classic gauze bandage in a large number of studies. The advantages of dressing applying in the treatment of VLUs are reflected in [30]:

- faster wound healing (allow constant temperature and humidity, which allows faster cell migration).

- reducing the risk of infection (achieved by releasing silver ions or creating an impermeable barrier to bacteria and viruses).

- greater comfort and cost-effectiveness (do not require daily dressing, reduce painful sensitivity of the wound, and provide significantly better quality of life).

Dressings are divided into primary and secondary. Primary dressings are in direct contact with the wound surface, while secondary dressings have the role of fixing and holding the primary dressing, which also protects the wound surface from the external environment. Today, dressings have the role of both primary and secondary [31, 32].

Type of dressings	Mode of operation
Gels, alginate dressings with additives (Ringer, 0,9%Nacl)	Activation of autolysis
Hydrocolloids, foam, hydrocapillary or silicone coatings	Granulation, creating a moist environment and absorbing secretions
Membranes, acrylates, therapeutic dressings (non-resorbable / resorbable) collagen coatings, cellulose hydrobalanced dressings, nets, films	Reepithelialization
Dressings with the addition of silver, iodine, medical honey, polyhexanide	Anti-inflammatory action

Table 2.
Type and mode of dressings action.

The division of dressings according to the mode of action on wound healing is shown in **Table 2**.

5.2 Compression therapy in the treatment of VLUs

Compression therapy is the most effective form of VLUs conservative treatment. The advantage of this therapy is that it is used on an outpatient basis, patients are able to work during treatment and it is also cheaper compared to surgical treatment [33]. This method of treatment can be applied continuously or intermittently. Before applying the compression bandage, it is necessary to perform local treatment of the ulcer surface, cover the ulcer surface with sterile gauze, after which a compressive bandage is placed. The application of external compression reduces transmural pressure and improves skin changes. Compression bandage compresses the extremities, thus reducing the effect of venous hypertension. Depending on the stage of the vein disease, different degrees of compression therapy are applied.

Compression therapy can be achieved with short-elastic and long-elastic bandages, as well as various compression systems (compression gloves, socks and clothing) [34]. The materials used to make compressive agents have different extensibility, and create different pressures under the applied compressive agents both at rest and while walking.

In relation to the degree of compression, compression means are divided into four classes (**Table 3**) [35].

These compression values refer to in vivo measurements in the medial B_1 area (end of the Achilles tendon / calf muscle insertion) measured while lying down [36].

Compression systems may contain elastic and inelastic materials. Multilayer systems (two-layer and four-layer) function as inelastic systems even if they contain mainly elastic components. An inelastic bandage is known to have high stiffness compared to an elastic bandage. The stiffness of the compression therapy system can be determined by determining the static stiffness index (SSI). This index is determined by measuring the values of the pressure between the compression system and the patient's skin (subband pressure). Pressure is measured first when the patient is lying down and then in a standing position. The difference between these two measurements is SSI. If SSI is >10, the compression system is characterized as inelastic, while if SSI is <10, the compression system is marked as elastic [37].

Compression therapy systems in which SSI is high (inelastic or multilayer compression system) give higher pressure during standing and lower pressures when the patient is lying down compared to a system with lower SSI (elastic compression system).

Class	Levels of compression	Indications
Class 1	<25 mmHg	Prevention of DVT, Mild oedema, Tired-aching legs
Class 2	25–35 mmHg	Mild VV, Mild to moderate oedema, VV during and after pregnancy
Class 3	35–45 mmHg	Venous ulcers (including healed ulcers) DVT, Superficial thrombophlebitis, Following venous surgery and sclerotherapy, VV with severe oedema, Post-thrombotic syndrome, Mild lymphoedema
Class 4	45–60 mmHg	Severe lymphoedema, Severe CVI

Table 3.
Levels of compression and indications.

Contraindications	
Absolute	**Relative**
Advanced peripheral artery disease (critical ischemia)	Mild to moderate peripheral artery disease
Decompensated heart failure	Advanced peripheral polyneuropathy
Septic phlebitis	Chronic compensated heart failure
Phlegmasia cerulea dolens	Intolerance or allergy to the materials used
Advanced peripheral artery disease (critical ischemia)	Treatment-related pain
	Florid infectious diseases (initial phase of erysipelas/ cellulitis)

Table 4.
Absolute and relative contraindications for the application of compressive therapy.

Contraindications to the use of compression therapy are shown in **Table 4** [38]:

The use of compression therapy may be associated with the appearance of certain signs and symptoms that indicate the appearance of complications. The most common complications of compression therapy are necrosis, skin trauma, discoloration, pain, paresthesia, burning sensation, etc. [39].

5.3 Surgical treatment

Surgical treatment of VLUs is one of the types of treatment. Today, surgical procedures are performed on the superficial venous system, deep venous system and venous perforators. It should also be noted that surgical procedures on these three venous systems can be combined [40]. One of the ways of VLUs surgical treatment is the Vigoni-Schmeller procedure. This method involves excision of ulcers and surrounding altered tissue with removal of compartment syndrome of the lower leg by the Hach method [41].

6. New technologies applied in VLUs treatment

The modern approach to the treatment of VLUs today is based on the application of various biophysical interventions such as electromagnetic therapy, phototherapy, electrical stimulation and ultrasound therapy. The modern method of treatment today includes the use of stem cell therapies, biological skin equivalents (such as bilayered living cellular construct (BLCC), or 3D-printed hydrogel dressing [42, 43].

In addition to the application of standard methods of treating VLUs, the following are also used: oxygen therapies, negative pressure wound therapy and platelet-rich plasma therapy. The use of a muscle pump activator or device with occasional pneumatic compression in a number of patients with VLUs has been shown to be very successful [44, 45].

Electromagnetic therapy (EMT) also has a significant place in VLUs therapy. EMT devices generate a pulsed electromagnetic field (PEMF). PEMF increases the number of fibroblasts and macrophages in the wound, which results in rapid wound healing. Studies have shown that PEMF increases the deposition of fibrin and collagen and reduces the inflammatory process [46].

Low-level light therapy (LLLT) as a variant of phototherapy has a prominent place in the treatment of VLUs [47, 48]. The use of LLLT devices activates cells through a photochemical effect. There is an increase in cellular activity [43] resulting in accelerated tissue healing, granulation tissue formation, increased protein synthesis, increased cell proliferation, anti-inflammatory modulation and pain reduction [43, 49]. This method is a non-contact method of treating VLUs, and LLLT devices usually direct a beam of light around the entire surface of the wound [48].

Electrical stimulation (ES) stimulates angiogenesis by activating mitogen-activated protein kinase (MAPK) and increasing vascular endothelial growth factor (VEGF). The application of ES leads to increased fibroblast proliferation by stimulating the production of fibroblast growth factors (FGF). The application of ES has been shown to be effective in reducing the inflammatory process and regulating bacterial growth [50].

Ultrasound therapy (UT) has found a significant place in the treatment of VLUs as one of the auxiliary therapeutic modalities [51, 52]. The effect of ultrasound on tissues is reflected in the increase of blood flow in the tissue and the induction of physical changes in the structure of collagen. This type of therapy promotes cell proliferation, angiogenesis and protein synthesis. UT also accelerates the formation of granulation tissue, has anti-inflammatory and anti-edematous effects [51, 52]. However, previous research on the application of UT has not given a clear answer on the in vivo healing process [51].

Clinical studies have shown that stem cell therapy (SCT) promotes wound healing in each wound repair phase. The application of SCT accelerates the healing process of VLUs, with a significant reduction in wound area and quality tissue regeneration [53, 54].

Oxygen therapy has a prominent place in the treatment of VLUs. Chronic wound tissues have a very small amount of oxygen, and due to hypoxia, the wound healing process is slowed down. This is particularly pronounced if a transcutaneous oxygen partial pressure (pO_2) is lower than 40 mmHg [55]. Oxygen therapy accelerates wound healing and does not reveal relevant cell damage risk [55, 56]. Today, the following methods of oxygen therapy are used: hyperbaric oxygen therapy and topical oxygen therapy.

Negative pressure wound therapy (NPWT) accelerates the healing process of VLUs. This is achieved through several mechanisms: reduction of local edema as well as reduction of the number of bacteria, inflammatory mediators and wound exudates. NPWT promotes angiogenesis, promotes tissue perfusion, stimulates tissue granulation, causes wound shrinking, and contraction of its edges [47, 57].

Platelet-rich plasma (PRP) or autologous platelet-rich plasma is a suspension of platelets obtained from whole blood [58]. The concentration of platelets in PRP is two to six times higher than that in the blood [59]. To form a liquid or gel that contains multiple growth factors, PRP is most commonly mixed with thrombin. PRP supplies not only a number of growth factors but also signaling cytokines that also play a key role in new tissue synthesis, angiogenesis, or inflammation regulation [58].

The role of growth factors in wound healing is very complex. Certain growth factors (e.g. TGF-beta) play different roles in different phases of healing. To date, in spite of many years of research, only one growth factor (Becaplermin, PDGF) is registered for the treatment of diabetic foot ulcers and not for venous ulcers [60].

7. Discussion

Venous leg ulcers occur as a complication of CVI. With the aging of the world's population, an increase in the number of obese people with various chronic diseases, the number of patients with VLUs will increase. These patients' performance will be a significant burden on the health care system [61].

Venous leg ulcers are significantly more common in the elderly. In 13% of people, VLUs first appears before the age of 30, and 22% before the age of 40. For this reason, patients with VLUs have a reduced quality of life and varying degrees of physical disabilities. These patients suffer varying degrees of acute and chronic pain [62].

The application of modern diagnostic and therapeutic modalities in the treatment of VLUs in combination with available evidence-based data will reduce the number of patients who will not heal VLUs and who will relapse. Therefore, the use of standard methods of treatment and the use of expensive advanced therapeutic agents is of particular importance.

It is very important to have a comprehensive clinical examination at the very beginning. Subsequent non-invasive and sometimes invasive tests may be indicated for diagnosis and treatment planning. Inadequate diagnosis results in inadequate therapy.

The application of objective tests aims to confirm the diagnosis, determine the etiology of the disease, locate the anatomical site of the venous disease (superficial, deep, and perforating venous system) and the severity of the disease, or identify coexisting peripheral arterial disease [63].

Taking a good medical history is imperative of a good clinical examination. Patients with VLUs have a rich medical history and a number of concomitant comorbidities. Unfortunately, there are not enough studies that have shown the value of specific items for the anamnesis [25]. In practice, it has been shown to be very important to take all data related to the previous medical history as well as the family history and the specific aspects of the ulcer [18].

In order to monitor the healing rate of ulcers, it is very important to perform an accurate and consistent wound measurement. Wound location, area, and characteristics should be documented. Traditionally, length and width are measured in perpendicular distances of wound borders (the longest length with the greatest width at right angles). This measurement can be done manually or via digital photography. These wound measurement methods are inconsistent and sometimes inaccurate. The use of digital software is recommended. The study of Cardinal et al. showed that oval or circular ulcers initially heal better than wounds with large indentations, multiple segments and skin swellings at the edges. VLUs documentation is important for estimating the healing rates. If in the period from 4 weeks there is no reduction in wound area by 30%, it is unlikely that VLUs will heal by week 12 [64]. Patients with VLUs that heal slowly are ideal candidates for advanced therapy.

In order to make a diagnosis, the following diagnostic procedures are recommended: ABPI and duplex venous mapping. If duplex venous mapping cannot be used to make a valid diagnosis, phlebography, venous angiotomography, and venous angioresonance are recommended [64].

The success and sensitivity of the color-flow duplex ultrasound depend on the researchers and the coefficient of variation of reflux measurements ranges from 30–45% [65]. Studies have shown that duplex diagnostics has high sensitivity and specificity in the diagnosis of superficial and deep venous leg systems [65, 66]. Today, this method represents the gold standard in the diagnosis of venous diseases, enables further classification of chronic venous insufficiency and selection of the optimal treatment of venous diseases.

ABPI test is widely applied in the diagnosis of peripheral occlusive artery disease, because of its accessibility, affordable price, lack of risk, a sensitivity of 95% and a specificity of 99% [64]. Determination of ABPI is not the most reliable in patients with diabetes mellitus because compression of the arteries may not be possible due to medial sclerosis.

Taking an ulcer biopsy is a quick, easy, and effective way to identify less common etiologies in ulcers that are unusual in appearance and where there is a reasonable suspicion of a malignant etiology. Sometimes it is necessary to take multiple biopsy specimens to get an accurate diagnosis [67].

Standard sampling for bacterial colonization has no therapeutic consequence and thus is meaningless. Wound swabs should only be taken if there are signs of infection, prior to initiating therapy, and for MSRA detection. Cultivation and eventual use of antibiotics is only indicated if there are signs of VLUs infection [68].

Successful treatment of VLUs requires a multidisciplinary team to make an adequate diagnosis, assess the condition of the vascular system and determine other factors that affect the healing of ulceration.

The basis of VLUs treatment is to reduce or eliminate the effect of venous hypertension. This is achieved through the use of compression therapy, surgical treatment of venous abnormalities, local ulcer treatment, systemic medications that aid healing and complementary measures [64].

There is relatively little data in the medical literature regarding the cleansing of venous ulcers. The results of a number of prospective and retrospective studies related to surgical debridement of VLUs have shown that this method has a certain place in treatment. The results of a prospective study showed that the presence of dense fibrosis and high levels of mature collagen in ulcer tissue samples directly positively correlates with the speed and success of VLUs healing [26].

Extensive and deep debridement of VLUs that were refractory to therapy until the absence of dense fibrosis and mature collagen in the ulceration is recommended.

The results of a number of studies have shown that there are no justifiable reasons for the use of antiseptics, in principle, cytotoxic agents. Cleaning with ordinary clean water has the same result as cleaning with isotonic sodium solution [26].

The use of dressings in the treatment of VLUs has shown a significant advantage over the classic gauze bandage in a large number of studies. Proper use of dressings is based on clinical protocols containing the etiology of ulceration, clinical assessment of ulceration (depth, size, degree of purity, contamination, surrounding skin condition, amount of exudate), presence of infection, and general patient condition [30].

Modern dressings today provide optimal physio-chemical conditions necessary for normal wound healing, preventing the development of infection, controlling exudates, reducing the number of debridements and reducing the need for more painful dressings [69, 70].

Effective compression is achieved by precise application of the bend system, which should provide mild compression at rest, but also effective compression during all types of activities. All compression therapy systems achieve this to some extent, and the choice of a bandage or socks requires selection on an individual basis.

The two main principles on which compression therapy is based are [71]:

- creating a closed system that allows internal pressures to be evenly distributed in the leg.

- variation of subbandage pressure according to limb shape and bend tension.

Understanding the principles of compression therapy allows us to define the ideal compression system. The characteristics of an ideal compression system are: includes inelastic component, provides good anatomical grip, enables smooth operation and mobility, provides comfort at rest, easy to apply and adapts to the size and shape of the limbs and does not cause an allergic reaction and shows endurance.

Compression therapy systems must be compatible so that they can be effectively applied in different limb sizes and shapes, while providing therapeutic levels of compression without the risk of damage. The use of multicomponent compression systems has shown significantly better efficiency in the healing of venous ulcers compared to the use of one-component compression systems. Multicomponent compression greater than 30 mm/Hg showed, in addition to high efficiency in wound healing, a reduction in the recurrence of venous ulcerations [72, 73].

After the ulcer has healed, elastic stockings with graduated compression of the appropriate size are used, with a pressure of 30–40 mmHg. In most patients, knee pads are sufficient. In fact, socks above the knee or other compression devices that exceed the height of the knee are uncomfortable to wear and occlude the popliteal vein during knee flexion. Ankle compression >40 mmHg is rarely required. If the patient is associated with arterial insufficiency, socks that produce less pressure around the ankle joint are needed, so as not to lead to skin necrosis [71].

It should be noted that it is very important to apply surgical therapy in order to treat the underlying venous disease whenever possible. The use of surgery can improve and accelerate healing, as well as reduce the risk of recurrence [64].

Unfortunately, up to this date, no randomized studies have been performed on the use of this treatment for VLUs. The problem with the application of surgical therapy in the treatment of VLUs is the lack of valid randomized, controlled studies. Previous studies have had an uneven number of patients and different surgical techniques have been applied. None of the previous studies has shown the advantage of surgical therapy over VLUs conservative treatment.

Based on the recommendations of the Scottish guidelines, surgical therapy should not be the method of choice in the VLUs treatment (an active ulcer). Surgical therapy is also not recommended as a secondary prevention after VLUs healing [74]. The data obtained from the ESHAR study showed that there is no advantage of surgery over compression therapy in the treatment of patients with varicose veins of the lower extremities. However, this study showed that in relation to the occurrence of disease recurrence, surgical therapy proved to be more successful [75].

The number of new technologies and use of grafting techniques used in the treatment of VLUs has increased in recent years. The future may hold micro- and pixel-grafts, spray on cells and the use of 3D printing to prefabricate vascularized grafts to assist in wound coverage.

Some of the new technologies used in the treatment of VLUs require broader evidence of clinical efficacy and can be considered as experimental therapies [76].

8. Conclusion

Venous leg ulcers occur as a complication of CVI. Venous leg ulcers are significantly more common in the elderly. A VLUs represent a growing health problem, and they are a condition that is very expensive to treat for both the health system and patients. The application of modern diagnostic and therapeutic modalities in the treatment of VLUs in combination with available evidence-based data will reduce the number of patients who will not heal and who will relapse. Therefore, the use of standard treatment methods and the use of expensive advanced therapeutic agents is of particular importance.

Author details

Vesna Karanikolic* and Aleksandar Karanikolic
Faculty of Medicine, University of Niš, Serbia

*Address all correspondence to: vkaranikolic@gmail.com

References

[1] The Venous Forum of the Royal Society of Medicine and Societas Phlebologica Scandinavica. The management of chronic venous disorders of the leg: An evidence based report of an international task force. Phlebology. 1999;**14**(1):23-25

[2] Nelson EA, Adderley U. Venous leg ulcers. BMJ Clinical Evidence. 2016;**2016**(15):1902

[3] Anand S, Dean C, Nettleton R, Praburaj D. Health related quality of life tools for venous-ulcerated patients. The British Journal of Nursing. 2003;**12**:48-59

[4] Abbade LPF, Lastoria S. Venous ulcer: Epidemiology, physiopathology, diagnosis and treatment. International Journal of Dermatology. 2005;**44**:449-456

[5] Howard A, Davies AH. Health-related quality of life in patients with venous ulceration. Phlebology. 2001;**16**(1):12-16

[6] Jones J, Barr W, Robinson I, Carlisle C. Depression in patients with chronic venous ulceration. The British Journal of Nursing. 2006;**15**:S17eS23

[7] Bonkemeyer S, Gan R, Townsend P. Venous ulcers: Diagnosis and treatment. American Family Physician. 2019;**100**(5):298-305

[8] Rabe E, Pannier-Fischer F, Bromen K, et al. Bonner Venenstudie der Deutschen Gesellschaft fur Phlebologie. Epidemiologische Untersuchung zur Frage der Haufigkeit und Ausspagung von chronischen Venenkrankheiten in der stadtischen und landlichen Wohnbevolkerung. Phlebologie. 2003;**32**:1-14

[9] Amsler F, Willenberg T, Blattler W. In search of optimal compression therapy for venous leg ulcers: A meta-analysis of studies comparing diverse bandages with specifically designed stockings. Journal of Vascular Surgery. 2009;**50**:668-674

[10] Santler B, Goerge T. Chronic venous insufficiency—A review of pathophysiology, diagnosis, and treatment. Journal der Deutschen Dermatologischen Gesellschaft. 2017;**15**(5):538-556

[11] Rahmani J, Haghighian Roudsari A, Bawadi H, et al. Relationship between body mass index, risk of venous thromboembolism and pulmonary embolism: A systematic review and dose-response meta-analysis of cohort studies among four million participants. Thrombosis Research. 2020;**192**:64-72

[12] Crawford JM, Lal BK, Durán WN, et al. Pathophysiology of venous ulceration. Journal of Vascular Surgery: Venous and Lymphatic Disorders. 2017;**5**(4):596-605

[13] Serra R, Buffone G, de Franciscis A, et al. A genetic study of chronic venous insufficiency. Annals of Vascular Surgery. 2012;**26**(5):636-642

[14] Kranke P, Bennett MH, Martyn-St James M, et al. Hyperbaric oxygen therapy for chronic wounds. Cochrane Database of Systematic Reviews. 2015;**6**:CD004123

[15] Korting HC, Callies R, Reusch M, et al. Dermatologische Leitlinienarbeit 2007 in der Perspektive. Journal der Deutschen Dermatologischen Gesellschaft. 2007;**5**:1-3

[16] Mali JWH, Kuiper JP, Hamers A. Acro-angiodermatitis van de voet.

Op acrosarcoma Kaposi gelijkende afwijkingen bij chronische veneuze insufficientie. Nederlands Tijdschrift voor Geneeskunde. 1966;**110**:790-796

[17] Situm M, Kolić M. Atypical wounds: Definition and classification. Acta Medica Croatica. 2012;**66**(1):5-11

[18] Chaby G, Senet P, Ganry O, et al. Angio-dermatology group of the french society of dermatology. Prognostic factors associated with healing of venous leg ulcers: A multicenter, prospective, cohort study. The British Journal of Dermatology. 2013;**169**:1106-1113

[19] Coleridge-Smith P, Labropoulos N, Partsch H, et al. Duplex ultrasound investigation of the veins in chronic venous disease of the lower limbs–UIP consensus document. Part I. Basic principles. European Journal of Vascular and Endovascular Surgery. 2006;**31**:83-92

[20] De Maeseneer M, Pichot O, Cavezzi A, et al. Union Internationale de Phlebologie. European Journal of Vascular and Endovascular Surgery. 2011;**42**:89-102

[21] Payne SPK, London NJM, Newland DJ, et al. Ambulatory venous pressure: Correlation with skin condition and role in identifying surgically correctable disease. European Journal of Vascular and Endovascular Surgery. 1996;**11**:195-200

[22] Bernatchez SF, Eysaman-Walker J, Weir D. Venous leg ulcers: A review of published assessment and treatment algorithms. Advanced Wound Care (New Rochelle). 2022;**11**(1):28-41

[23] van Bemmelen PS, van Ramshorst B, Eikelboom BC. Photoplethysmography reexamined: Lack of correlation with duplex scanning. Surgery. 1992;**112**(3):544-548

[24] Neglén P, Raju S. Intravascular ultrasound scan evaluation of the obstructed vein. Journal of Vascular Surgery. 2002;**35**(4):694-700

[25] Colenci R, Abbade LPF. Fundamental aspects of the local approach to cutaneous ulcers. Anais Brasileiros de Dermatologia. 2018;**93**(6):859-870

[26] Powers JG, Higham C, Broussard K, et al. Wound healing and treating wounds: Chronic wound care and management. Journal of the American Academy of Dermatology. 2016;**74**(4):607-625

[27] Dowsett C, Ayello E. TIME principles of chronic wound bed preparation and treatment. The British Journal of Nursing. 2004;**13**(15):16-23

[28] Ligresti C, Bo F. Wound bed preparation of difficult wounds: An evolution of the principles of TIME. International Wound Journal. 2007;**4**(1):21-29

[29] Frykberg RG, Banks J. Challenges in the treatment of chronic wounds. Advanced Wound Care (New Rochelle). 2015;**4**(9):560-582

[30] Norman G, Westby MJ, Rithalia AD, et al. Dressings and topical agents for treating venous leg ulcers. Cochrane Database of Systematic Reviews. 2018;**6**(6):CD012583

[31] McLain NE, Moore ZE, Avsar P. Wound cleansing for treating venous leg ulcers. Cochrane Database of Systematic Reviews. 2021;**10**(3):CD011675

[32] Karrer S. Topische Ulkustherapie. Der Hautarzt. 2005;**56**(12):1165-1178

[33] Stücker M, Link K, Reich-Schupke S, et al. Compression and venous ulcers. Phlebology. 2013;**28**(1):68-72

[34] Woo KY, Alavi A, Evans R, et al. New advances in compression therapy for venous leg ulcers. Surgical Technology International. 2013;**23**:61-68

[35] Vicaretti M. Compression therapy for venous disease. Australian Prescriber. 2010;**33**:186-190

[36] Weller CD, Buchbinder R, Johnston RV. Interventions for helping people adhere to compression treatments for venous leg ulceration. Cochrane Database of Systematic Reviews. 2013;**9**:CD008378

[37] Partsch H. The static stiffness index: A simple method to assess the elastic property of compression material in vivo. Dermatologic Surgery. 2005;**31**:625-630

[38] Dissemond J, Assenheimer B, Bültemann A, et al. Compression therapy in patients with venous leg ulcers. JDDG. 2016;**14**(11):1072-1087

[39] Rabe E, Partsch H, Morrison N, et al. Risks and contraindications of medical compression treatment—A critical reappraisal. An international consensus statement. Phlebology. 2020;**35**(7):447-460

[40] Juntermanns B, Kröger K, Waldhausen P, et al. Ulcus cruris venosum – chirurgische Therapie [Venous ulcus cruris-Surgical treatment]. Hautarzt. 2022;**73**(6):491-500

[41] Hach W, Prave F, Hach-Wunderle V, et al. The chronic venous compartment syndrome. VASA. 2000;**29**:127-132

[42] Cereceres S, Lan Z, Bryan L, et al. Bactericidal activity of 3D-printed hydrogel dressing loaded with gallium maltolate. APL Bioengineering. 2019;**3**:026102

[43] Bavaresco T, Pires AUB, Moraes VM, et al. Low-level laser therapy for treatment of venous ulcers evaluated with the Nursing Outcome Classification: Study protocol for a randomized controlled trial. Trials. 2018;**19**:372

[44] Harris C, Duong R, Vanderheyden G, et al. Evaluation of a muscle pump-activating device for non-healing venous leg ulcers. International Wound Journal. 2017;**14**:1189-1198

[45] Alvarez OM, Markowitz L, Parker R, et al. Faster healing and a lower rate of recurrence of venous ulcers treated with intermittent pneumatic compression: Results of a Randomized Controlled Trial. Eplasty. 2020;**20**:e6

[46] Aleksandrowicz H, Owczarczyk-Saczonek A, Placek W. Venous leg ulcers: Advanced therapies and new technologies. Biomedicines. 2021;**9**:1569. DOI: 10.3390/biomedicines9111569

[47] Cuomo R, Nisi G, Grimaldi L, et al. Use of ultraportable vacuum therapy systems in the treatment of venous leg ulcer. Acta Bio-Medica. 2017;**88**:297-301

[48] Illescas-Montes R, Atkinson RA, Cullum N. Low-level light therapy for treating venous leg ulcers. Cochrane Database of Systematic Reviews. 2018;**2018**:CD013061

[49] Romanelli M, Piaggesi A, Scapagnini G, et al. EUREKA study-the evaluation of real-life use of a biophotonic system in chronic wound management: An interim analysis. Drug Design, Development and Therapy. 2017;**11**:3551-3558

[50] Rajendran SB, Challen K, Wright KL, et al. Electrical Stimulation to Enhance Wound Healing. Journal of Functional Biomaterials. 2021;**12**:40-44

[51] Beheshti A, Shafigh Y, Parsa H, et al. Comparison of high-frequency and MIST ultrasound therapy for the healing of venous leg ulcers. Advances

in Clinical and Experimental Medicine. 2014;**23**:969-975

[52] Cullum N, Liu Z. Therapeutic ultrasound for venous leg ulcers. Cochrane Database of Systematic Reviews. 2017;**5**:CD001180

[53] Coalson E, Bishop E, Liu W, et al. Stem cell therapy for chronic skin wounds in the era of personalized medicine: From bench to bedside. Genes Diseases. 2019;**6**:342-358

[54] Raghuram AC, Yu RP, Lo AY, et al. Role of stem cell therapies in treating chronic wounds: A systematic review. World Journal of Stem Cells. 2020;**12**:659-675

[55] Harries RL, Bosanquet DC, Harding KG. Wound bed preparation: TIME for an update. International Wound Journal. 2016;**13**(3):8-14

[56] Ren SY, Liu YS, Zhu GJ, et al. Strategies and challenges in the treatment of chronic venous leg ulcers. World Journal of Clinical Cases. 2020;**8**:5070-5085

[57] Alkhateep Y, Zaid N, Fareed A. Negative pressure wound therapy for chronic venous ulcer: A randomized-controlled study. Egypt Journal of Surgery. 2018;**37**:196-199

[58] Huber SC, de Moraes MB, Quintero M, et al. A case series of platelet rich plasma in chronic venous ulcers. Regeneration Therapy. 2021;**18**:51-58

[59] Suthar M, Gupta S, Bukhari S, et al. Treatment of chronic non-healing ulcers using autologous platelet rich plasma: A case series. Journal of Biomedical Science. 2017;**24**:16-20

[60] Neumann HAM, Cornu-Thenard A, Junger M, et al. S3-guideline on venous leg ulcer. JEADV. 2016;**30**:1843-1875

[61] Woo K, Lo C, Alavi A, et al. An audit of leg and foot ulcer care in an Ontario community care access centre. Wound Care Canada. 2007;**5**(1):19-S27

[62] Hopman WM, Buchanan M, Van Den Kerkhof EG, Harrison MB. Pain and health-related quality of life in people with chronic leg ulcers. Chronic Diseases Injection. 2013;**33**:167-174

[63] Vivas A, Lev-Tov H, Kirsner RS. Venous leg ulcers. Annals of Internal Medicine. 2016;**165**:ITC17-32

[64] Abbade LPF, Frade MAC, Pegas JRP, et al. Consensus on the diagnosis and management of chronic leg ulcers: Brazilian Society of Dermatology. Anais Brasileiros de Dermatologia. 2020;**95**(1):1-18

[65] Baker SR, Burnand KG, Sommerville KM, et al. Comparison of venous reflux assessed by duplex scanning and descending phlebography in chronic venous disease. Lancet. 1993;**341**:400-403

[66] Lurie F, Comerota A, Eklof B, et al. Multicenter assessment of venous reflux by duplex ultrasound. Journal of Vascular Surgery. 2012;**55**:437-445

[67] Romanelli M, Miteva M, Romanelli P, Barbanera S, Dini V. Use of diagnostics in wound management. Current Opinion in Supportive and Palliative Care. 2013;**7**:106-110

[68] Moore K, Hall V, Paull A, et al. Surface bacteriology of venous leg ulcers and healing outcome. Journal of Clinical Pathology. 2010;**63**:830-834

[69] Blumberg SN, Maggi J, Melamed J, et al. A histopathologic basis for surgical debridement to promote healing of venous ulcers. Journal of the American College of Surgeons. 2012;**215**:751-757

[70] Dogra S, Rai R. Venous leg ulcer: Topical treatment, dressings and surgical debridement. Indian Dermatology Online Journal. 2014;**5**(3):371-373

[71] Mościcka P, Szewczyk MT, Cwajda-Białasik J, Jawień A. The role of compression therapy in the treatment of venous leg ulcers. Advances in Clinical and Experimental Medicine. 2019;**28**(6):847-852

[72] Karanikolic V, Binic I, Jovanovic D, et al. The effect of age and compression strength on venous leg ulcer healing. Phlebology. 2018;**33**(9):618-626

[73] Karanikolic V, Golubovic M, Stevanovic G, et al. The influence of compression strength, patient and wound variables on venous leg ulcers healing. Dermatologica Sinica. 2019;**37**(4):194-198

[74] Taylor E. Guidelines for the assessment & management of patients suffering from venous leg ulcers. NHS Herefordshire CCG. 2014:14-22

[75] Barwell JR, Davies CE, Deacon J, et al. Comparison of surgery and compression with compression alone in chronic venous ulceration (ESCHAR study): Randomized controlled trial. Lancet. 2004;**363**:1854-1859

[76] Eriksson E, Liu PY, Schultz GS, et al. Chronic wounds: Treatment consensus. Wound Repair and Regeneration. 2022;**30**(2):156-171

Section 3

Innovative Technologies and Therapies for Wound Healing

Chapter 9

Role of Skin Substitutes in Burn Wound Reconstruction

Elizabeth Concannon, Lindsay Damkat-Thomas, Patrick Coghlan and John E. Greenwood

Abstract

Skin substitutes have modernised burn wound reconstruction since their use was first pioneered by Burke and Yannas in the 1980s. Skin substitutes offer a solution to the problem of insufficient autologous skin graft availability in major burn wound closure. A growing body of evidence supports the role of skin substitutes in both acute major burns and secondary burn scar resurfacing. Classification of skin substitutes has become increasingly complex given the large variety of synthetic and biologic dermal matrices now available as the result of ongoing advances in regenerative medicine techniques. Classification systems are required to assist clinicians with selection and comparison of outcomes across a wide diversity of skin substitutes. Professor John Greenwood, invented, designed and developed one such dermal substitute, 'Biodegradable Temporising Matrix', which is approved for use across the globe for reconstruction of major burns and complex wounds. This chapter provides a review of available classification systems for skin substitutes with a summary of the latest evidence in relation to their role and impact on burn wound outcomes. Future developments toward the elusive 'ideal' skin substitute may be possible through ongoing research efforts focused on clinical translation of modern skin tissue engineering techniques for burn wound reconstruction.

Keywords: dermal substitutes, skin substitutes, burn reconstruction, biodegradable temporizing matrix, skin graft, tissue engineering

1. Introduction

The skin is the largest organ of the body and is responsible for many essential functions that no skin substitute has been able to fully replicate to date. Skin substitutes can be defined as any material used to provide biologic wound coverage on a temporary or permanent basis. Skin substitutes may be differentiated from simple, inert, wound dressings in that they possess properties that allow them to enhance repair of skin after injury, expedite regeneration and improve scar quality [1–3].

Epidermal and superficial partial thickness burns have the potential to heal by epidermal regeneration from adnexal nests of epidermal stem cells with minimal scarring, provided the burn wound remains protected and free from infection. Conventional management of debrided deep dermal and full thickness burns has been to achieve wound closure with autologous skin grafts since they were first introduced in the nineteenth century. Early wound closure minimises the severity of scarring and functional impairment caused by permanent dermal loss. However, autologous skin graft donor site availability is frequently limited in major burn patients, particularly when the total body surface area of burn (TBSA) exceeds 25%. Donor site morbidity from skin autograft harvest includes acute physiological insult to the burn patient, blood loss, pain and additional wounding and scarring. Allograft and xenografts are less desirable than autograft due to inherent issues with delayed graft rejection and risk of infection.

A vast array of skin substitutes have been developed through advances in tissue engineering and biomaterials. Skin substitutes have not yet eliminated the requirement for autologous skin grafting in deep or full thickness burns. However, they have the potential to circumvent some issues associated with autologous graft in terms of availability or lack thereof, donor site morbidity and failure to adequately replace dermal elements in deeper injuries. Skin substitutes can provide clinical benefits in terms of wound healing that have been outlined, as follows [4]:

- Protect the wound from infection and loss of fluid
- Provide a stable and biodegradable template for the synthesis of neodermal tissue
- Either host or enable the influx of cells that will function as dermal cells, producing dermal tissue rather than scar tissue
- Allow ease of handling and resist tear forces

Simplified classification systems can aid clinicians in selection of appropriate skin substitutes for burn wound reconstruction. Robust classifications can also benefit research efforts by allowing comparison of outcomes across a growing range of available skin substitutes, categorised based on their properties.

2. Classification of skin substitutes

Skin substitutes encompass a diverse group of materials and may be classified based on five main properties [5–7], as outlined with examples in **Table 1**.

Permanence: Temporary or permanent
Material source: Biological (either natural biological or constructed biological dermal substitutes), synthetic or mixed (biosynthetic) dermal substitutes
Layering: Single layer, bilayer, multilayer
Replaced region: Epidermal component only, dermal component only, composite (dermal and epidermal components)
Cellularity: Acellular or cellular

This classification system inspired by factorial design reported by Davison-Kotler et al. (**Figure 1**) [7]. borrows elements from four earlier classification systems which have been summarised in **Table 2** [8–11]. Classification systems can be helpful to both researchers in comparing outcomes of different skin substitutes and to clinicians who need to understand their composition in order to make an appropriate selection based on the clinical scenario faced.

Skin substitute properties	Subgroups	Examples of materials used in burn wounds
Permanence	Temporary	Allograft, Amniotic membrane, Biobrane, Suprathel, Alloderm, Apligraf
	Permanent	Biodegradable Temporising Matrix (BTM), Integra, Matriderm
Material source	Biological	Allograft, Amniotic membrane, Alloderm, Apligraf, Matriderm
	Biosynthetic	Integra, Biobrane, Dermagraft
	Synthetic	Biodegradable Temporising Matrix (BTM), Suprathel
Layering	Single layer	Alloderm, Matriderm, Suprathel, Cultured Epithelial autograft
	Bilayer	Biobrane, Integra, BTM
Replaced region	Epidermal	Epicel, Recell, Suprathel, Cultured Epithelial autograft, Biobrane
	Dermal only	Alloderm, Dermagraft, Matriderm
	Composite	Allograft, Apligraf, Integra, BTM
Cellularity	Acellular	Integra, BTM, Matriderm, Biobrane, Suprathel
	Cellular	Allograft, Amniotic membrane, Epicel, Recell, Apligraf, Dermagraft

Table 1.
Classification of skin substitutes by various properties.

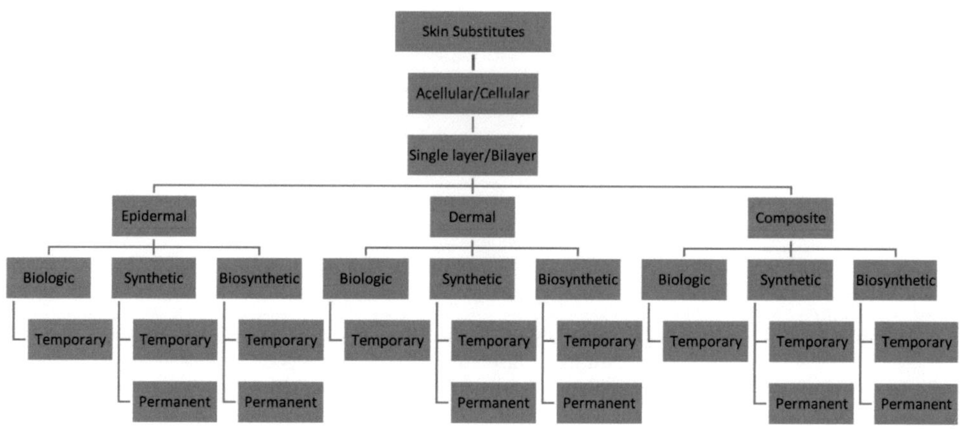

Figure 1.
Skin substitute classification adapted from Davison-Kotler et al. [7].

Classifications have evolved over time in parallel with advancements in skin substitute design. A commonality to all classification systems was an emphasis placed on the tissue layer replaced by the skin substitute in question, be it epidermal, dermal or composite skin replacement. This concept marries well with standard categorisation of burns and other wounds by the depth of injury when planning reconstructive requirements. Earlier classification systems failed to differentiate between products based on permanence [8], material source [8] and cellularity [8–10]. The omission

Classification system author	Description	Categories
Balasubramani [8]	Categorised by the tissue layer the produce replaces	Class I: Substitutes consisting of cultured epidermal equivalent only (e.g., Epicel) Class II: Substitutes consisting of dermal components from processed skin or manufactured with extracellular matrix proteins such as collagen (e.g., Dermagraft) Class III: Composite skin substitutes including both dermal and epidermal components (e.g., Integra)
Kumar [9]	Categorised by the tissue layer the product replaces, layering and material source	Class I: Temporary, impervious, materials that replace epidermal function (e.g., Suprathel) Class II: Epidermal (e.g., Epicel or dermal skin substitutes (e.g., Matriderm or Alloderm) Class III: Composite skin substitutes replacing both layers (e.g., Integra, BTM)
Ferreira [10]	Categorised by location, permanence, and material source with lettering system	Permanence: *Permanent (P)* assigned to materials which lack degradation *Temporary (T)* assigned to materials which degrade over time Origin: *Biological (b)* assigned to materials that are autologous, allogeneic, or from another species *Biosynthetic (bs)* assigned to materials that are derived from a biological source, however, also contain synthetic, nondegradable materials such as silicone or nylon Location: *Composite (C)* indicates the skin substitute replaces both dermal and epidermal components of skin *Dermal (D)* indicates the skin substitute replacesthe dermal component of the skin *Epidermal (E)* indicates the skin substitutereplaces the epidermal component of the skin
Vyas and Vasconez [11]	Categorised by cellularity, the tissue layer the product replaces and permanence	This review suggested categorisation of skin substitutes based on cellularity in addition to the tissue layer the product is replacing and the permanence of the skin substitute
Davison-Kotler [7]	Incorporated elements from all four above classifications	Algorithmic system fully outlined in **Figure 1**. Five properties used to categorise skin substitutes: Permanence: Temporary (biodegradable)/ Permanent (nonbiodegradable) Material Source: Natural (i.e., Biological)/ Synthetic/Both Layering: Single layer/Bilayer Replaced region: Epidermis/Dermis/Both Cellularity: Acellular/Cellular

Table 2.
Chronological development of skin substitute classification systems.

of these integral features created classification systems that were non-intuitive and confusing, whereby some dissimilar products could be placed in the same category or qualify for multiple categories.

The system outlined by Davison-Kotler et al. [7] allows multiple key properties to be simultaneously incorporated, since all skin substitutes possess a variety of characteristics. This multifactorial classification system allows for clear and comprehensive descriptive categorisation of commercially available skin substitutes with potential to expand to include novel skin substitutes still under development. A glossary to further expand

Skin substitute (manufacturer)	Structure	Mechanism of action and limitations
Allograft (N/A)	Human cadaveric split-thickness skin grafts. Available cryopreserved or glycerol preserved.	Vascularises temporarily as per autograft but is a passive temporizer with eventual rejection after 3–4 weeks. Fresh allograft confers risk of disease transmission due to retention of residual DNA.
Amniotic membrane (N/A)	Innermost layer of placenta consisting of epithelial layer, basement layer and avascular stroma, hyaluronan and decorin. Available cryopreserved or glycerol-preserved.	Promotes epithelial cell migration and adhesion with anti-inflammatory and anti-scarring properties. Efficacious in protecting the wound bed and reducing bacterial load but has poor mechanical stability.
Alloderm (Lifecel corporation)	Acellular cadaveric human dermis, processed to remove epidermis and cells	Provides a scaffold for fibroblast and vascular ingrowth, single stage reconstruction with autologous graft. Limitations include antigenicity, availability and shelf life.
Apligraf (Organogenesis Inc.)	Cultured human foreskin-derived neonatal fibroblasts in a bovine type I collagen matrix with stratified keratinocytes	Provides a scaffold for host cell migration and population with barrier function provided by keratinocyte layer. Inconsistent cell survival, collagen composition and vascularisation.
Biobrane (Smith & Nephew)	Silicone membrane bonded to porous nylon mesh impregnated with cross linked T1 porcine collagen peptides	Dermal collagen peptides allow adherence to the wound, semipermeable outer membrane allows exudate drainage and evaporative water loss control, e.g., partial thickness burns/donor sites.
Biodegradable Temporising Matrix (BTM) (Novosorb Polynovo®)	Completely synthetic dermal scaffold composed of impermeable polyurethane seal overlying layer of biodegradable polyurethane foam	Bi-layered dermal matrix widely used in acute and delayed burn wound reconstruction. Robust integration and neo-vascularisation reported even in application to infected or avascular wounds such as exposed tendon.
Cultured Epidermal Autograft (N/A)	Keratinocytes cultured from biopsy of autologous skin. 3-week turnaround for 10,000-fold keratinocyte expansion. Culture process which may use murine fibroblasts and foetal calf serum.	Variable graft take and poor long term graft stability in large and deep burn wounds due to poor regeneration of basement membrane proteins which have key role in epidermal adhesion and skin homeostasis. Processing times long and costly. Culture using animal derived cells carries risk of immunogenicity and prion disease transmission.

Skin substitute (manufacturer)	Structure	Mechanism of action and limitations
Dermagraft (Intercytex Ltd.)	Cryopreserved cultured neonatal dermal fibroblasts on a bioresorbable polyglactin mesh	Provides scaffold of extracellular matrix consisting of growth factors and collagens, tenascin, vitronectin, and GAGs.
Epicel (Vericel Corporation)	Petroleum gauze and autologous keratinocyte sheets co-cultured with murine cells	2–8 mm cell layers thick, indicated for deep dermal and full-thickness burns
Integra (Integra LifeSciences)	Biosynthetic dermal scaffold composed of polysiloxane polymer overlying cross-linked T1 bovine collagen and shark glycosaminoglycan (chondroitin-6-sulphate)	Bi-layered dermal matrix widely used in two-stage acute and delayed burn wound reconstruction. Available in single layer of collagen only for single stage reconstruction. Infection during integration phase generally requires removal or replacement.
Matriderm (Medskin Solutions)	Single layer of non-crosslinked bovine collagen and tendon derived elastin hydrolysate. 1 or 2 mm thick matrices available.	Dermal matrix which provides neodermis for autograft application either as one stage (1 mm construct) or two staged (2 mm construct) procedure.
ReCell (Avita Medical)	Autologous keratinocytes obtained from cultured autologous skin biopsy, suspended in solution that can be sprayed onto wound bed	Accelerated epithelialisation from in vivo wound models but human application and long term wound stability remains controversial and further independent clinical studies ongoing. Fibroblasts and melanocytes also delivered to wound
Suprathel (Polymedics Innovations)	Microporous, absorbable synthetic copolymers, mostly polylactic acid	Similar indications for use as Biobrane with no biologic component.

Table 3.
Glossary with description of skin substitutes in alphabetical order.

on the examples skin substitutes provided in this chapter is found in **Table 3**. This list is not exhaustive and many additional commercially products are available but it serves to illustrate the classification systems outlined, with a particular focus on materials utilised commonly in contemporary management of burns and other extensive wounds.

2.1 Skin substitute properties

2.1.1 Permanence

Skin substitutes can be subdivided into two groups with distinct objectives and indications in burn care with regards to their permanence: namely temporary and permanent skin substitutes. Permanence may be defined by biodegradability as described in the classification reported by Davison-Kotler et al. [7]. However, many bilayered skin substitutes such as Integra and Biodegradable Temporising Matrix, (BTM), have a non-biodegradable outer component that requires removal before autografting of a slowly biodegradable scaffold following ingrowth of host cellular material (no polyurethane residues present by 18 months in the case of BTM) [12]. A more intuitive definition preferred by the authors of this chapter has been provided by Ferreira et al. [10] who describes the distinction as follows: Temporary skin substitutes 'refer to those that remain in the wound for the period of time necessary to modulate and improve the characteristics of the lesion and are replaced by autogenous grafts. Permanent materials are those that restore part or the total structure of the skin and remain on the wound bed even after a possible grafting of autogenous skin for complete coverage of the lesion.' Similarly, permanence is defined by the FDA as any material persisting more than 30 days in a wound, therefore permanence does not imply infinite presence in a wound.

Temporary skin substitutes do not generally achieve full integration with the wound bed. However, they may temporarily adhere while they promote healing by protecting, reducing water loss and accelerating epithelialisation.

The *objective* of temporary skin substitutes is to provide a moist environment, protect the wound from water loss and bacterial invasion while limiting the number of dressing changes.

Indications include definitive dressing of superficial or partial thickness burns until epithelialisation, temporary excised burn wound closure while awaiting autografting, protection of widely meshed autografts, 'test' graft in questionable wound beds while awaiting burn depth demarcation, donor site dressing to facilitate epithelialisation and pain control.

Examples: Cadaveric allograft, Amniotic membrane, Biobrane, Suprathel

Permanent skin substitutes are generally composed of constructs or scaffolds that become integrated with the wound architecture by hosting or allow ingrowth of dermal cells, before eventual scaffold reabsorption.

The *objective* of permanent skin substitutes is to provide a stable but biodegradable template for the synthesis of neo-dermis by enabling the influx of cells that produce dermal tissue rather than scar tissue [13, 14]. Epidermal constructs alone have proven to be problematic in the absence of viable dermis due to inadequate long term wound stability. Scar fragility with propensity to mechanical damage and shear demonstrated following cultured epithelial autografting [15] highlighted the challenge of dermal-epidermal junction regeneration. Dermal and dermal-epidermal constructs have been developed in response to these issues, to improve the quality of healing and reduce scarring.

Indications include excised deep partial or full thickness burn wounds.

Examples: Biodegradable Temporising Matrix (BTM), Integra.

2.1.2 Material source

As the name suggests, biologic skin substitutes are made using biological materials from human or animal sources. Synthetic material refer to non-biological materials engineered in a laboratory to replace or support regeneration of one or more components of normal skin structure. Biosynthetic skin substitutes are those made using a combination of biological and synthetic materials. Skin substitutes with biological components may allow replication of a more natural neodermal structure generated by native extracellular matrix and can allow excellent re-epithelialisation, although staged procedures are often necessary due to slow vascularisation. Synthetic skin substitutes offer increased control over scaffold composition and less propensity to loss due to cross-species antigenicity or infective complications [16] as compared with materials with biological origins, following integration with the burn wounds to which they applied.

2.1.3 Layering

Single layered skin substitutes replace either the epidermal (e.g., Suprathel) or dermal (e.g., Matriderm) component of skin, the latter of which requires autologous skin grafting to complete the epidermal reconstruction. Bilayered dermal substitutes are designed to replace or replicate both dermal and epidermal layers during their application whether this is on a temporary basis (e.g., Biobrane) or a permanent basis (e.g., Integra, BTM). In the latter case a two-stage approach is required whereby the impermeable pseudo-epidermal layer is removed or 'delaminated' prior to autologous skin graft application for definitive wound closure. A two staged strategy is particularly advantageous in major burn patients by allowing autologous skin harvest to be deferred until such time as the patient has reached a point of physiological stabilisation, resolution of inhalational injury or other concomitant traumatic injury [12] and optimisation of cardiac or other medical comorbidities [17]. This approach also facilitates re-epithelialisation of donor site harvest for repeated harvest in major burn patients who may have a paucity of donor site due to their total body surface area of burn, while permitting mobilisation during the integration phase [18].

2.1.4 Replaced region

Skin substitutes can be categorised based on their ability to replace the epidermal, dermal or composite (epidermal and dermal) layers of skin. Epidermal replacement should, in theory, be sufficient for reconstruction of burn wounds and other wound with intact dermal elements. However, deeper dermal and full thickness injuries ultimately require epidermal and dermal reconstruction in order to achieve robust wound healing while minimising scar formation and loss of function. Replication of basement membrane and dermal-epidermal junction are one of several scientific challenges that has yet to be overcome by advanced skin substitute design (discussed in further detail in Section 2.5), in order to attain stable skin coverage for deep tissue injuries [19, 20].

2.1.5 Cellularity

Cellular skin substitutes contain viable cells such as keratinocytes or fibroblasts and as such they may incite an immunogenic host response due to antigenicity. These materials are bioengineered from human sources such as Dermagraft (source material: neonatal foreskin). The inclusion of cellularity as a property of skin substitutes was necessary given its implications for wound indications, risk of rejection, cost and regulatory issues.

2.2 Clinical applications of skin substitutes in acute burn care

To appreciate the use of skin substitutes in acute burn care an understanding of the pathophysiology of burn injury is essential. A burn is a defined an injury to tissues induced by heat, cold, friction, chemical, radiation or electrical energy. With regards to the utilisation of dermal substitutes for cutaneous burn wounds, the three most important factors are depth, size and anatomical location of the cutaneous burn.

2.2.1 Burn depth

Burn depth can be epidermal only, dermal (ranging from superficial to deep dermal) or full thickness. In real terms there are only two burn depths. In the first group the burns are superficial enough to heal spontaneously with acceptable functional and aesthetic outcome. These burns are classified as epidermal, superficial partial thickness and mid-dermal. The treatment is supportive and the corner stay is prevention of infection, which can deepen the burn and the control of pain. Pain control facilitates dressing changes and improves compliance with therapy and mobilisation. These burns heal spontaneously as there is an adequate volume of undamaged residual dermal tissue in the burn bed, as well as nests of epidermal cells located in the invaginated sheaths of adnexal structures. This results in re-epithelisation.

The second group (deep dermal to full thickness burns) undergo prolonged healing with granulation tissue and wound contracture, resulting in secondary intention healing. The treatment priorities for this group of burns is to abort the process of secondary intention healing replace it as closely as possible with primary intention healing. The surgical methods for doing this include excision and direct closure of small burns and burn wound excision with split thickness skin grafting for larger burns.

2.2.2 Burn size

As burn size increases the treatment options become more complex. Small burns of any depth can generally be managed with dressings or relatively minor procedures. For the more superficial burns increasing burns size results in increasing the frequency and volume of dressings, restricting mobility and more likely to cause pain. For deeper burns that require skin grafting the larger the burn the smaller the area of "donor" site for skin graft harvesting. The skin grafts are subsequently "meshed" to allow a greater surface area to be covered. The larger the size of the burn the smaller the donor site area becomes resulting in thinner grafts with wider mesh patterns and subsequent poorer scarring outcomes. Additionally, for burns of over 50% TBSA there may not be enough skin donor site to close the debrided burn wounds. Skin grafts can be harvested from the same donor site, but the area must be healed first, and temporising options are required to cover the debrided wounds.

2.2.3 Anatomical locations

Burns over joints can be challenging to manage. Superficial burns require early mobilisation to prevent stiffness and deeper burns require meticulous debridement and skin grafting and intensive mobilisation. Debrided full thickness burns may result in the exposure of deeper structures such as tendon and bone. This results in unfavourable reconstruction if skin graft is used alone and often skin graft failure.

2.2.4 Skin substitutes replacing the epidermis: treatment of superficial dermal burns

For superficial partial thickness burns where the epidermis and a variable amount of dermis is damaged skin substitutes designed to replace the epidermal layer are of value, particularly in larger burns and burns of the hands and joints. Examples of materials that are commonly used as epidermal substitutes in acute burns include:

- Biobrane

- Suprathel

To be of benefit epidermal substitutes must be applied shortly after the burn injury, preferably within 24–48 hours. The burn wound must be meticulously cleaned and residual debris including particulate matter and detached epidermis removed.

Shaving the skin is also recommended as is a through wash with iodine solution. Application under general anaesthetic or sedation is recommended as the preparation may be painful. Mobilisation can begin at 48 hours and once the substitute has adhered. Dressing changes will only require the outer layers to be removed at the substitute should remain intact and undisturbed. Within 2–3 weeks it is expected that the substitute will detach as the skin beneath re-epithelialises. It is imperative to monitor for infection and if this occurs the substitute must be removed and conventional dressings applied. The risk of infection can be reduced with meticulous burn wound preparation and consideration of antibiotics.

Epidermal substitutes play an important role in the management of burns that are destined to heal themselves by preventing infection (which may convert the burn into a deep dermal/full thickness injury that will not heal by itself) and treating pain (allowing patients to tolerate dressing changes, early mobilisation and expediting hospital discharge).

2.2.5 Skin substitutes replacing the dermis: treatment of full thickness burns

The early definitive closure of burn wounds is problematic when the total body surface area exceeds 50% as burn are begins to exceed the available skin donor site area. Dermal substitutes in this setting are used to actively temporise the wound bed until split skin grafting can be performed. Examples of dermal substitutes commonly used in acute burns include:

- Integra

- Biodegradable Temporising Matrix (BTM)

The dermal matrix strategy was developed to combat these issues. Pioneered by Burke and Yannis [1, 2], the strategy involved producing a scaffold to allow autologous tissue in growth and establish a neo-dermis. The material developed, Integra, is a cross-linked type 1 collagen scaffold supported by shark chondroitin-6-suplahte glycosaminoglycan. It is physiologically closed with a bonded pseudo-epidermis of silicone. The expense of the product and issues arising from placing non-vascularised biological material on the surface of a wound in an immune compromised patient and anticipating neovascularisation without infection has resulted in variable usability and success in acute burns. The cost of this product often limits its use to very large burn wounds or as a 'patch-up' to cover persistent wounds that remain following primary auto-grafting procedures.

The development of biodegradable polymers and, at the start of this millennium, a completely synthetic, biodegradable polyurethane dermal matrix was designed and developed in Adelaide, Australia, using biodegradable polymer developed in Melbourne, Australia; this is known as the NovoSorb Biodegradable Temporising Matrix (BTM; Polynovo). The synthetic composition means that is not prone to infection by micro-organisms and if it does occur it is localised, not requiring removal or replacement [16]. The loss of skin graft over integrated BTM is uncommon and as also observed with Integra, the appearance of the meshed graft is considerably improved compared to autografting alone. The presence of a 'neo-dermis' provides a bed across which interstitial epithelialisation can occur without needing granulation tissue and so the cosmetic appearance is improved. In fact, the thinner the graft, the better the appearance and the less obvious the mesh pattern. The presence of a 'neo-dermis' provides a bed across which interstitial epithelialisation can occur without needing granulation tissue and so the cosmetic appearance is improved. In fact, the thinner the graft, the better the appearance and the less obvious the mesh pattern

2.3 Clinical applications of skin substitutes in secondary burn wound resurfacing

The long-term outcome of scarring for survivors of large burn injuries is unpredictable. Skin grafted areas can form unstable pathological scars resulting in itch, pain and reduced function, particularly if the burn scar cross joints. Additionally, the aesthetic appearance is less than ideal.

A method to treat this involves scar excision and re-surfacing using dermal substitutes and split skin grafting. The introduction of skin substitute is beneficial in two ways. Firstly, the secondary contracture associated with using split skin grafts is reduced when using a dermal interface. Secondly the scar quality and pliability is improved when split skin grafting is used in conjunction with skin grafting. Frequently used skin substitutes in secondary burn wound reconstruction include:

- Matriderm
- Integra
- Biodegradable temporizing matrix

The surgical technique for scar excision remains constant but the choice of dermal substitute is dependent upon surgeon preference, size of defect and patient choice.

2.3.1 Matriderm

The application of Matriderm involves a single stage procedure, which may be preferable to the staged reconstruction required for both Integra and BTM. The wound bed requires meticulous preparation and application of Matriderm. It can be challenging to use over large defects and is sheet split skin grafting rather than meshed is generally required and therefore requires available and good quality donor sites [5, 8].

2.3.2 Integra

Integra requires a two-stage application, firstly the excision of the scar application of the dermal substitute. Then, once integrated, delamination and application of split skin grafting. Timing between the two procedures varies dependent upon integration. As burn resurfacing is an elective surgery the risk of infection with Integra is somewhat mitigated in comparison to its use in acute burn wound care. The functional and aesthetic outcome of Integra has been observed to be reliable [1–3, 5, 8].

2.3.3 Biodegradable Temporising Matrix

Similar to Integra BTM is a two-stage procedure. The patient can be managed in an outpatient setting until integration is completed. The risk of infection in an elective setting is minimal due to the synthetic nature of the product and the aesthetic and functional outcomes are comparable with the more established dermal substitutes [12, 16–18].

2.4 Future advances toward an ideal dermal substitute

2.4.1 Ideal skin substitute

The ideal skin substitute does not yet exist. The following features have been proposed as desirable properties to consider in the development of novel skin substitutes [5, 6].

- Inexpensive and cost-effective
- Easy to store with long shelf life
- Non-antigenic or low antigenicity
- Durable and resistant to shear but flexible
- Prevents evaporative water loss
- Tolerant of hypoxia
- Presence of dermal and epidermal components
- Provides a bacterial barrier and resist infection
- Rheology comparable to skin—drapes and conforms well
- Easy to prepare, secure and store
- Grows with patient growth (suitable for paediatric wounds)
- Avoids scar hypertrophy/contracture
- Single stage application

2.4.2 Scientific challenges and future advances

Several scientific and regulatory challenges must be overcome in the development of the aspirational ideal skin substitute. Creating an anatomical and physiological substitute for normal skin is a challenge faced by burns and trauma patients that has involved tissue bioengineers, polymer chemists, cellular and molecular biologists, surgeons, nurses, and therapists. A critical challenge in skin substitute design has been replication or regeneration of basement membrane the undulating dermal-epidermal junction which it produces through a process of paracrine dialogue between fibroblasts and keratinocytes. This specialised junction is responsible for limiting shear by establishing a molecular bond that anchors the cellular epidermis to the extracellular matrix of the dermis [19, 20].

As such, epidermal-only substitutes may offer a clinical adjunct to expedite reepithelialisation in conjunction with other wound reconstruction strategies but are insufficient in replication of autologous skin graft due to their limited expansion rate, mechanical fragility on handling, tendency to blister in vivo and vulnerability to shear after application. Reconstructive strategies using novel composite epidermal-dermal constructs [21–23], although challenging to engineer, offer theoretically increased wound stability compared with combining separate dermal and epidermal substitutes which lack the critical component of a functional dermal-epidermal junction required for long term graft stability. A randomised comparison of an engineered skin substitute with autograft [22] (autologous keratinocytes and fibroblasts attached to a collagen-based scaffold) in 15 paediatric patients demonstrated reduced mortality and requirements for donor skin harvesting, for autografting of full- thickness burns of greater than 50% TBSA. A pre-clinical study of a fibrin-based human skin substitute [23] with epidermal and dermal components (fibroblasts cultured in fibrin gel with keratinocytes seeded on top) carried out on in vitro deep burn necrotic tissue showed similar outcomes compare with split-thickness skin graft, concluding that this could potentially represent a viable management option for deep burn injuries, without the need for autologous skin graft. The challenge of further clinical research efforts will be to evaluate and compare between the ever-growing variety of reconstructive strategies that have been made possible due to the wide array of skin substitute products now commercially available.

New frontiers of research are being forged through clinical translation of advanced tissue bio-engineering techniques combined with 3D printing technology [24–26] to produce novel bi-layered and even tri-layered constructs with hypodermis [25]. Positive clinical results obtained with autologous and allogeneic TESSs based on human adult skin cells and human mesenchymal stem cells regarding successful engraftment (60–90% in the majority of studies [24]) safety, re-epithelialization and wound healing rates, are promising. Takami et al. has developed a TESS composed of autologous cultured keratinocytes, fibroblasts, and cadaveric de-cellularised allogenic dermal matrix.

This skin substitute demonstrated at 96% graft survival rate in four patients with debrided full thickness burn wounds with no delayed graft loss [27]. Although many tissue engineered skin substitutes (TESS) remain at pre-clinical development stage, they offer hope that the ultimate goal of developing an ideal skin substitute is attainable through further clinical research efforts.

3. Conclusion

This chapter outlines classification systems for skin substitutes and their evolution over time in line with advances in skin engineering technology, evidence supporting their clinical applications with regards to acute and secondary burn wound reconstruction and future advances toward the aspirational goal of developing an ideal dermal substitute.

Conflict of interest

Professor John Greenwood designed and developed the skin substitute known as Novosorb Biodegradable Temporising Matrix (BTM) and has a small residual shareholding with the company that manufactures this product, Polynovo.

Dr. Elizabeth Concannon and Dr. Lindsay Damkat-Thomas have no conflicts of interest to declare.

Author details

Elizabeth Concannon[1*], Lindsay Damkat-Thomas[2], Patrick Coghlan[1] and John E. Greenwood[1]

1 Adult Burn Service, Royal Adelaide Hospital, Adelaide, Australia

2 Middlemore Hospital, Auckland, New Zealand

*Address all correspondence to: lizconcannon@gmail.com

References

[1] Yannas IV, Burke JF. Design of an artificial skin. I. Basic design principles. Journal of Biomedical Materials Research. 1960;**14**(65):81

[2] Burke JF, Yannas IV, et al. Successful use of a physiologically acceptable artificial skin in the treatment of extensive burn injury. Annals of Surgery. 1981;**194**(4):413-428

[3] Dai C, Shih S, Khachemoune A. Skin substitutes for acute and chronic wound healing: An updated review. The Journal of Dermatological Treatment. 2020;**31**(6):639-648

[4] van der Veen V, van der Wal M, van Leeuwen M, Ulrich M, Middelkoop E. Biological background of dermal substitutes. Burns. 2010;**36**:305

[5] Sheridan RL, Tompkins RG. Skin substitutes in burns. Burns. 1999;**25**:97-103

[6] Sheridan RL. Skin substitutes in burns—Letter to the Editor. Burns. 2001;**27**:92

[7] Davison-Kotler E, Sharma V, Kang NV, Garcia-Gareta E. A new and universal classification system of skin substitutes inspired by factorial design. Tissue Engineering, Part B: Reviews. 2018;**24**(4):1-8

[8] Balasubramani M, Kumar TR, Babu M. Skin substitute: A review. Burns. 2001;**27**:534

[9] Kumar P. Classification of skin substitutes. Burns. 2008;**34**:148

[10] Ferreira M, Paggiaro A, Isaac C, Neto N, Santos G. Skin substitutes: Current concepts and a new classification system. Revista Brasileira de Cirurgia Plástica. 2011;**2001**(26):696

[11] Vyas K, Vasconez H. Wound healing: Biologics, skin substitutes, biomembranes and scaffolds. Healthcare. 2014;**2**(3):356-400

[12] Greenwood JE, Schmitt B, Wagstaff MJ. Experience with a synthetic bilayer Biodegradable Temporising Matrix in significant burn injury. Burns Open. 2018;**2**(1):17-34

[13] Bloemen MC, Van der Wal MB, Verhaegen PD, et al. Clinical effectiveness of dermal substitution in burns by topical negative pressure: A multicenter randomized controlled trial. Wound Repair and Regeneration. 2012;**20**(6):797-805

[14] Bloemen MC, Van Leeuwan MC, Van Vucht NE, et al. Dermal substitution in acute burns and reconstructive surgery: A 12-year follow-up. Plastic and Reconstructive Surgery. 2010;**125**(5):1450-1459

[15] Compton CC, Press W, Gill JM, et al. The generation of anchoring fibrils by epidermal keratinocytes: A quantitative long-term study. Epithelial Cell Biology. 1995;**4**(3):93-103

[16] Cheshire PA, Herson MR, Cleland H, Akbarzadeh S. Artificial dermal templates: A comparative study of NovoSorb™ Biodegradable Temporising Matrix (BTM) and Integra® Dermal Regeneration Template (DRT). Burns. 2016;**42**(5):1088-1096

[17] Marriott R, Concannon E, Solanki NS, Greenwood JE. Sternotomy through anterior chest wall burns temporised with an implanted

synthetic dermal matrix. Burns Open. 2021;**5**(4):1-5

[18] Schmitt B, Heath K, Kurmis R, Klotz T, Wagstaff MJD, Greenwood J. Early physiotherapy experience with a biodegradable polyurethane dermal substitute: Therapy guidelines for use. Burns. 2021;**47**(5):1074-1083

[19] Dearman BL, Boyce ST, Greenwood JE. Advances in skin tissue bioengineering and the challenges of clinical translation. Frontiers in Surgery. 2021;**8**:640879

[20] Aleemardani M, Triki MZ, Green NH, Claeyssens F. The importance of mimicking dermal-epidermal junction for skin tissue engineering: A review. Bioengineering. 2021;**8**:148

[21] Kelly C, Wallace D, Moulin V, et al. Surviving an extensive burn injury using advanced skin replacement technologies. Journal of Burn Care & Research. 2021;**42**(6):1288-1291

[22] Boyce S, Simpson P, Rieman M, et al. Randomized, paired-site comparison of autologous engineered skin substitutes and split-thickness skin graft for closure of extensive, full-thickness burns. Journal of Burn Care & Research. 2017;**38**:61-70

[23] Kljenak A, Tominac Trcin M, Buji M, et al. Fibrin gel as a scaffold for skin substitute—Production and clinical experience. Acta Clinica Croatica. 2016;**55**:279-289

[24] Sierra-Sanchez A, Kim KH, Blasco Morente G, Arias-Santiago S. Cellular human tissue-engineered skin substitutes investigated for deep and difficult to heal injuries. npj Regenerative Medicine. 2021;**6**:35

[25] Zimoch J, Zielinska D, Michalak-Micka K, et al. Bio-engineering a pre-vascularised human tri-layererd skin substitute containing a hypodermis. Acta Biomaterialia. 2021;**134**:215-227

[26] Choi WS, Kim JH, Ahn CB, Lee JH, Kim YJ, Son KH, et al. Development of a multi-layer skin substitute using human hair keratinic extract-based hybrid 3D printing. Polymers. 2021;**13**:2584

[27] Takami Y, Yamaguchi R, Ono S, et al. Clinical application and histological properties of autologous tissue-engineered skin equivalents using an a cellular dermal matrix. Journal of Nippon Medical School. 2014;**81**:356-363

Chapter 10

Nanotechnological Interventions and Mechanistic Insights into Wound-Healing Events

Sourabh Soni, Rubbel Singla and Yogendra S. Padwad

Abstract

Wound-healing cascade is highly dynamic and composed of four continuous but overlapping phases that are precisely programmed. Successful healing occurs when these phases occur sequentially in a specific time frame and thus require multipotent wound-healing material. Nanotechnology has revolutionized the field of wound dressings by the development of various types of nanotechnology-based drug delivery systems and materials to treat hard-to-heal wounds. In this chapter, the advantages and the limitations associated with nanoparticle-based wound-healing materials as well as recent trends and applications of nanotechnology-based approaches in advanced wound therapy for healing of cutaneous, chronic, and burn wounds will be detailed along with the molecular interventions involved. Efforts are targeted herein to address the most significant factors affecting cutaneous wound healing and the molecular mechanisms involved. This chapter describes several nanoparticle (NP)-based drug delivery systems to improve the healing potential of antimicrobial, anti-fungal, growth factors, and other bioactive agents. While much remains to be learned, a better understanding of the factors influencing wound repair and nanotechnological interventions therein may lead to therapeutics that improve the healing process.

Keywords: nanomaterials, wound-healing process, therapeutics, delivery systems, wound dressings, molecular mechanisms, wound-healing events

1. Introduction

Wound occurs mainly because of an injury, burn, surgery, infectious disease, or a pathological condition that leads to a compromise in the overall integrity of the tissue. Wounds are considered as major healthcare challenge affecting several million people globally due to the underlying complications resulting from infections and comorbidities such as diabetes. Lifestyle disorders enhance the risk of complications and lead to improper/delayed wound-healing processes. Despite of thousands of marketed products available to treat wounds, it is still considered as a burden to the individual and to the society at large [1].

Managing wounds is not at all easy, especially due to the various steps involved in the healing process. Most of the healing methods rely on the “tried and tested” approach, but off-late, there has been a high influx of new products in the market, as well as the latest technologies, to increase the wound repair armamentarium. A vast majority of the new products in the market are refurbished and updated versions of the older ones. Most of the newer wound management products are the result of newer fields of research and investigation. Older wound-healing products, such as plain gauze, are still being extensively used as dressing in hospitals, but better and advanced understanding and novel technologies have resulted in certain products that aid in achieving the ideal moist, protected, and warm wound-healing microenvironment. The bioactive properties such as antimicrobial action and immune modulation create a microenvironment favorable for healing. The current wound care products in the market include alginate, cellulose, chitosan, collagen, and hyaluronic acid.

Nobel laureate Richard Feynman in 1959 first predicted the emergence of a new field of study that deals with structures ranging in the nanoscale. Sixty years later, the impact that nanotechnology has in our lives these days is huge, it is playing a role in important fields such as diagnostics and therapeutics *via* its role in the development of various medical devices [2]. With the rapid growth of nanotechnology as a research field worldwide, a plethora of nanomaterials has garnered importance in the biomedical and healthcare sectors. Several nanotechnology-based products are currently being investigated to aid in wound healing. Owing to their interesting properties at both chemical and physical levels, nanomaterials have gained a lot of attention in research [3]. Nanodevices being innovative provide us with a wide range of benefits such as entry across cellular barriers, nonantigenic, anti-shear stress, and gas-exchange permeability, modulation of biocompatibility, and bioavailability of drugs as well as nanodelivery option [4–7]. Nanotherapies lead to improvement of the healthcare sector by enhancement of currently available medical prognosis and treatments for challenges such as impaired wound healing. Despite the development of potential biomaterials and nanotechnology-based applications for wound healing, this scientific knowledge is not translated into an increase of commercially available wound-healing products containing nanomaterials [8].

2. Wounds and wound types

A wound is generally described as a tissue disruption from the normal anatomic structure leading to a subsequent loss of function [9]. The classical way to define a wound is to say that it is a disruption in the anatomic and cellular continuity of a tissue. Wounds tend to rupture the skin's epithelial integrity and may occur with or without microbial infection [10]. Wound may take place on many occasions during an individual's lifetime due to chemical, physical, and microbial factors influencing it. The physiological response by an individual to an injury is termed as wound healing, which involves integrated sbiochemical and cellular events leading to the regaining of functional and structural integrity at the injury site [11]. Healing of a wound starts right from the time of injury and carries on throughout the wound repair with the duration and extent varying according to the wound. Wound healing involves the action of many cells, soluble mediators and growth factors, and cell-extracellular matrix interactions. The coordinated action of all these events leads to the healing of wound *via* the process of hemostasis, inflammation, and epithelization, followed by fibroplasia and angiogenesis, finally resulting in wound contraction and remodeling [10, 12].

Humans possess an *in situ* property of wound healing, that is, self-regeneration, which depends on a person's age, gender, living habits, environment, microbial infection, and types of wounds [13]. This leads to various criteria for wound classification: etiology, level of microbial infection, and morphology. Firstly, based on etiology, the wounds could be classified into abrasions, burns, cuts, lacerations, and stab wounds. Based on microbial infections, wounds have been categorized mainly into three groups: aseptic, contaminated, and septic wounds. There is one more characterization: closed and open wounds. Wounds are termed as closed when the skin shows no damage, but the underlying layer is injured while in open wounds the skin injury leads to exposure of the underlying tissue [14]. Finally, the duration of healing is a prime factor in wound management that leads to other criteria of wound categorization: acute and chronic wounds, which are discussed here in detail.

2.1 Acute wounds

A wound that follows an orderly and timely process of healing is termed as acute wound. These wounds tend to repair themselves following the normal stages of healing and results in timely restoration of anatomical and functional trait. They are generally caused by traumatic injury or surgery with healing time ranging from a week to a maximum of a month [10].

2.2 Chronic wounds

The wounds that fail to follow the normal procedure of the healing process thus leading to impairment in timely repair are called chronic wounds, which include diabetic and pressure wounds as well as venous and arterial ulcers. Generally, one or more than one stages of the wound-healing cascade are prolonged due to various factors leading to incomplete and disrupted healing [10]. Ulcers tend to remain in the chronic inflammation stage in pathological conditions and are characterized by an abundant infiltration of neutrophils and reactive oxygen species that release enzymes such as collagenase and elastase, leading to the destruction of cells, connective tissue, and growth factors [15]. These nonhealing wounds have a perpetual inflammation state, and they frequently relapse due to disrupted and dis-coordinated healing events [10, 16].

Millions of people globally suffer from chronic wounds affect, accounting for massive healthcare costs with estimates suggesting an annual burden of about $30 billion in the USA alone [17]. Bacterial infection is the most frequent complication of chronic wounds, hence the search for effective treatment options that evade infections has been a continuous process over centuries with antibiotic-resistant strains emerging as a major concern [18]. The imbalances in various signaling networks coordinating cellular interactions lead to nonhealing, chronic wounds characterized by prolonged inflammation, decreased angiogenesis, impaired cellular function, and bacterial infection [19–21]. The rate of chronic wound healing differs from acute wounds and shows dependence on the patient's immunological status [22]. Despite extensive efforts to develop therapeutic strategies for the effective treatment of chronic wounds, so far, limited clinical success has been achieved [23].

3. Wound-healing cascade

Wound healing, the normal response in mammals to injury, is a complex and dynamic biological process that is evolutionarily conserved, highly coordinated, and spatiotemporally regulated. The wound-healing cascade has three sequential yet overlapping but distinct phases: inflammation, new tissue formation, and remodeling [12, 16, 24]. These coordinated phases of healing involve the interaction of immune and nonimmune cells, as well as soluble mediators and extracellular matrix components [16, 25]. Additionally, the dynamic link between skin and the microbial population also contributes to the process outcome. Under normal circumstances, wounds heal by themselves, but depending on the extent of tissue damage, the process varies [26, 27]. Wound healing is a very interesting research field, with many mechanisms still not fully understood.

The process of wound healing initiates immediately after injury with the hemostasis phase. The fibrin clot formed here acts like a barrier and leads to moisture retention [10]. Traditional gauze-based dressings target this healing phase by retaining moisture and preventing excessive bleeding [28]. This is followed by inflammation (beginning soon after injury), which may continue for a week with the release of pro-inflammatory cytokines from injured tissue leading to the attraction of circulating leucocytes at the site [29]. Subsequently, the proliferation phase starts, which involves angiogenesis, granulation, epithelialization, and wound contraction. Finally, after around 3 weeks of injury begins the maturation phase, which might take as long as 2 years for completion [30]. The cascade of wound-healing events along with the signaling and the cellular changes involved is further discussed in detail and diagrammatically explained in **Figure 1**.

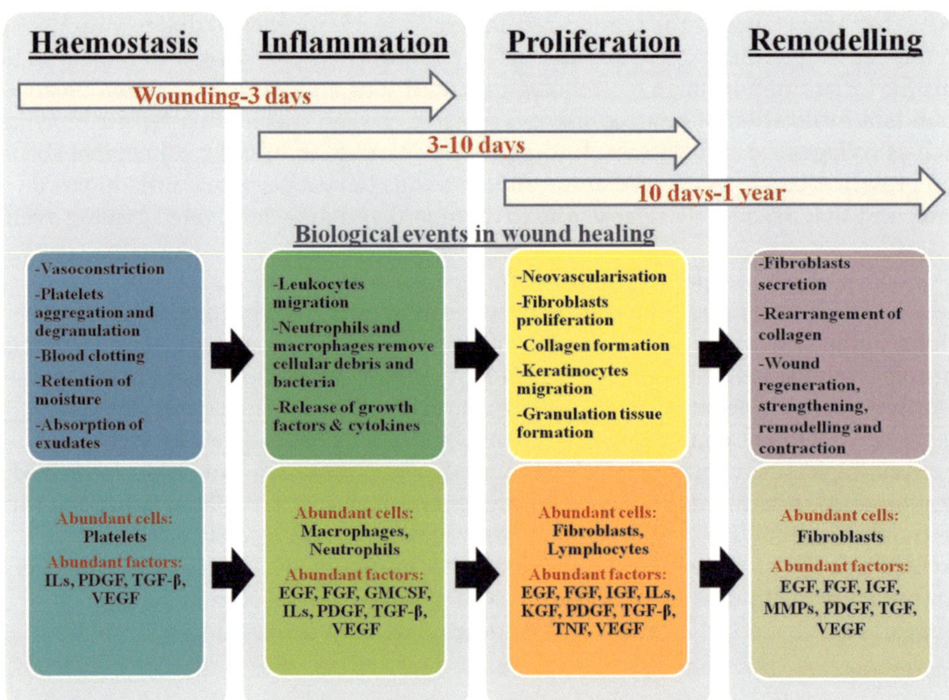

Figure 1.
Diagrammatic representation of various nanotechnology-based therapies used in different stages of wound healing. The currently employed nanostrategies for wound management are presented in this figure. The list provided here is intended to be just an illustration and is not comprehensive.

DOI: http://dx.doi.org/10.5772/intechopen.106481

3.1 Hemostasis and inflammation phase (begins soon after injury and continues for 3 days)

Hemostasis and inflammation occur soon after tissue injury and constitute the first and the foundation phase of wound repair. It leads to the formation of a platelet plug to prevent blood loss, removal of dead tissues and to prevent infection, and employs the components of the coagulation, inflammatory, and immune cascade to accomplish these tasks (**Figure 1**) [31, 32]. Further, the fibrin matrix acts as a scaffold for the infiltrating cells that are essential for later phases of wound healing. The clot consists of collagen, fibrin molecules, fibronectin, platelets, and thrombin. The fibrin clot operates as a scaffold hence aiding the migration of neutrophils, monocytes, leukocytes, keratinocytes, fibroblasts, and endothelial cells, and simultaneously forms a matrix for concentrating cytokines and growth factors [31, 33, 34]. The soluble factors released by these initiate the inflammatory phase aimed at establishing an immune barrier against infections [10].

In response to complement system activation, the next step is the recruitment of neutrophils to the wound site [35]. Following the formation of the clot, a stress signal is transmitted with neutrophils being the first cells to respond. This causes nearby vessels to vasodilate and accumulation of inflammatory mediators to facilitate the sudden rise in cellular traffic. Neutrophils release proteolytic enzymes such as proteases, which clean up the wounded area by removing cellular debris and invading bacteria [18, 31]. Neutrophils lead to the creation of reactive oxygen species that in combination with chlorine lead to wound sterilization [31]. *In vitro* studies have indicated the possibility that neutrophils could change the cytokine expression and phenotype of macrophages, leading to an innate immune response during wound healing [36]. This phase is sometimes called as the "lag phase," where in the absence of tensile strength in the wound, the recruitment of the migrating cells and various factors must be managed for the healing process [33].

Approximately 2–3 days post-injury, the monocytes from the neighboring tissue migrate to the wound site and finally differentiate into macrophages, which are seemingly crucial for the healing cascade. They cause phagocytosis of cell debris, apoptotic cells, and pathogens and lead to the secretion of various soluble factors [37, 38]. Despite their importance, the role of neutrophils and macrophages has not been well elucidated in wound repair. Reports have suggested that deficiency of one of these cells can be compensated *via* redundancy in the inflammation phase [39], whereas when cells of both types are absent, wound repair still takes place, with a lesser scarring response [40]. Macrophages synthesize various enzymes such as collagenases, cytokines, and growth factors like epidermal growth factor (EGF), basic fibroblast growth factor (bFGF), interleukins (ILs), platelet-derived growth factor (PDGF), transforming growth factor-β (TGF-β), tumor necrosis factor-α (TNF-α), and vascular endothelial growth factor (VEGF), leading to the promotion of cell proliferation and extracellular matrix (ECM) synthesis (**Figure 1**) [31, 41]. The inflammatory phase essentially supplies growth factors and cytokines that keep the wound-healing process intact and are quite crucial in the later stages of wound repair [25, 42]. Past evidence suggests that the extent of scarring depends on the amount of inflammation. This is validated by reports that show that the hypothesis behind scarless healing of fetus wounds is the lack of intrauterine inflammation [43].

3.2 Proliferative phase (Day 3–10)

Proliferation is the second phase of wound healing, which takes place from 3 to 10 days post-injury. This stage is characterized by new tissue formation, cellular migration, and proliferation (**Figure 1**). In this phase, the focus is on covering the injured surface, the synthesis of granulation tissue, and the reformation of the vascular network [33, 44, 45]. It indicates the start of angiogenesis and the synthesis of the ECM components. In the first step, keratinocytes migrate to the injured dermis and angiogenesis occurs. New capillaries sprout replacing the fibrin clot with granulation tissue, resulting in a new substrate for migration of keratinocytes during later stages of the healing (**Figure 1**). Capillaries help in nutrient supply during the granulation and tissue deposition phase, in absence of which a chronic wound will develop [31]. The keratinocytes proliferate and mature to restore the epithelial barrier. There is also secretion of cytokines such as ILs, TNF-α, enzymes like matrix metalloproteinase (MMPs), and growth factors like EGF, PDGF, TGF-β, and VEGF by the activated macrophages and de-granulated platelets (**Figure 1**) [46]. The concentrations of these factors vary and are dependent on the immunological state of the individual [42]. Excessive synthesis of granulation tissue and collagen causes scar formation [47]. Several pathways play an important role in restoring the normal anatomy, physiology, and functional status of the injured tissue with mitogen-activated protein kinases (MAPK), phosphoinositide 3-kinase (PI3K)/Akt, TGF-β, and Wnt/β-catenin being the major ones [48].

Vascular system restoration is a complex cascade in the injured tissue involving various cellular and molecular events. The most important angiogenesis upregulators are VEGF and FGF [49]. In a study, VEGF application to diabetic animal wounds normalized the healing process [50]. Later in this phase of repair, fibroblasts differentiate into myofibroblasts upon stimulation by macrophages [51]. Myofibroblasts being contractile in nature bring the wound edges together over time. Further, in combination with myofibroblasts, they produce extracellular matrix and lead to collagen and scar formation [52]. Fibroblasts secrete IL-6 and keratinocyte growth factors (KGFs) that act as stimuli causing migration of neighboring keratinocytes to the injury site, leading to their proliferation and differentiation into the epidermis [31]. Keratinocytes present at the wound edges cause re-epithelialization of the wound [53, 54].

Proliferative phase ends with the formation of acute granulation tissue [31]. During this phase, the proliferating endothelial cells get activated by VEGF, leading to the formation of new capillaries. By this time, the remodeling phase has already been initiated. The fibrin-based wound matrix is replaced with scar tissue characterized by high-cellular density due to fibroblasts, granulocytes, and macrophages, as well as capillaries and collagen bundles, hence termed granulation tissue [25, 33, 44, 53, 55]. This tissue is highly vascular because angiogenesis is still incomplete. By the end of this phase, myofibroblasts differentiation reduces the population of maturing fibroblasts, which are further terminated *via* apoptosis [56].

3.3 Maturation and remodeling phase (Day 10–1 year)

Remodeling is the third and the last phase of wound repair that begins around 2 weeks post-injury and may last up to 1 year or longer, based on various factors [10]. During this stage, all the cellular processes activated post-injury wind down and come to an end, the new epithelium is formed, and the final scar tissue develops. The granulation tissue formation ceases *via* cellular apoptosis, leading to an acellular and avascular mature wound [57]. Majority of the cellular components exit from the wound site or undergo apoptosis, and the resulting mass consists of collagen and other ECM proteins. During wound maturation, the ECM components undergo various changes characterized by collagen deposition in a well-arranged network form (**Figure 1**). 4–5 weeks post-injury, collagen continues to be synthesized. Stronger collagen I replace the previously predominant collagen III produced during the proliferative phase [58]. Normally, around 90% of collagen present in skin is type I, but during the granulation phase in the wounded skin type III, levels reach up to 30% [31]. In cases with excessive collagen formation, generation of hypertrophic scar occurs [31]. The regulation of skin integrity and homeostasis occurs through the epithelial–mesenchymal interactions [59].

Further, myofibroblasts lead to wound contractions thereby decreasing the scar surface [38, 60]. The angiogenesis processes now diminish causing the blood flow in the wound to decline, and the acute metabolic activity in the wound now slows down and finally diminishes. However, the injured tissue never tends to regain the properties of healthy skin. Certain skin components never recover completely such as the hair follicles and sweat glands that possess no potential to heal potential post-injury [61]. The epidermal layer of the scar formed differs from surrounding healthy skin post-healing [33]. Even years after the injury, the collagen in the scar never gets the fully organized structure seen in healthy skin. Furthermore, the wound strength never returns to 100% [31].

4. Management of wounds through nanotherapeutic approaches

As described above, wound healing is a dynamic and highly regulated process. Wound closure can be realized by either regeneration or repair. The process of healing has been described as a playing orchestra where an organized interplay of various factors, such as cells, cytokines, and growth factors, leads to tissue repair [55]. However, when this intricate balance gets disrupted, the healing process is affected with recent reports suggesting that the absence of a particular cell or a mediator gets compensated so that the tissue repair process goes on [42]. The currently used wound management strategies have certain limitations in fulfilling the needs of comprehensive care [62]. Hence, wound healing remains a challenge and a burden [63]. The treatment modalities in practice are specifically based on the type of wounds, with inadequate management leading to complications such as chronic wounds, fibrosis, compromised tissue functioning, or even amputation [64]. The best prevention technique against undesirable outcomes during healing is the effective management during the early stages of the process to prevent wounds to progress to chronic conditions.

Recent advances in interdisciplinary research have brought bioactive materials to the forefront as smart wound care materials [8, 65]. Bioactive materials can potentially be exploited to target any phase of the healing process by their direct cellular interactions or indirectly through ECM. Biopolymers are one of the most widely exploited bioactive materials used for wound care because they possess useful properties such as ability to support cell growth, biocompatibility, biodegradability, durability, and regenerative potential [66]. Dermal substitutes and human skin equivalents are the two food and drug administration (FDA)-approved biomaterial therapies promoting healthy healing *via* their interaction with the wound microenvironment [67–70]. Due to the increased understanding of the healing process, there has been an emergence of dressing-based wound-healing materials [71]. Modern dressings have been designed for successful healing by providing a beneficial wound microenvironment with control on moisture and absorbance of excess exudates. Active dressings have been known to alter the wound microenvironment *via* targeting microbial load and excessive proteases or aiding tissue growth by alginate, chitosan, hyaluronan, and collagen matrices acting as scaffolds [72–74]. There have been plenty of reports that demonstrate the advantages of modern dressings harboring cells and recombinant growth factors, but still, the majority of the clinical modalities are based on safety evaluation rather than efficacy [75].

Chronic wounds demand very robust and efficacious therapies that address the various challenges of a deregulated healing process. Many of the novel approaches have failed in delivering specific healing outcomes, which have further made way for the introduction of several nanotechnology-based wound-healing therapies [7]. The chronic nature and associated complications of nonhealing wounds have led to the emergence of nanotechnology-based therapies for ultimately repairing the injured tissue [65]. Multitudes of nanotherapeutic approaches have been introduced to efficiently manage the wounds and remove any related possible complications (**Figures 2** and **3**) [76]. The advantage of using nanomaterials over other wound dressings is their tenability, low cytotoxicity, good biocompatibility, drug delivery ability, and versatility of physicochemical properties endowing them with many unique features [71, 76, 77]. Furthermore, nanoscale helps them in enhanced penetration to the injury site and a high interaction probability with the biological target [78]. Consequently, NPs possess the ability of controlled and sustained the release of therapeutics, resulting in accelerated wound repair [72].

5. Nanoparticles used as therapeutic materials for wound repair

A range of metallic NPs, polymeric NPs, peptide-loaded nanostructures, and carbon-based nanomaterials have been investigated for applicability in wound repair due to the astonishing physical, chemical, and biological characteristics, such as their ease of fabrication, biodegradability, and biocompatibility [79, 80]. The aim of any injury due to burns or accidents is to achieve healing and epithelialization as soon as possible without any side effects [81]. A variety of nanomaterials used for the treatment of wounds and their brief mechanistic action are given in detail in the following sections (**Figures 2** and **3**).

5.1 Metallic nanoparticles

In the past literature, different varieties of metal or metal oxide NPs were reported for their wound-healing application. Metal NPs, such as silver, gold, and zinc, are frequently used for dermal wound treatment due to their ease of use and large surface-area-to-volume ratio. These metal NPs provide a moist wound environment and possess strong antimicrobial activity [82]. Silver NPs (AgNPs) are among the ones used in most of the dressings available in the market. AgNPs as well as silver are known to show great antimicrobial action against wide spectra of microbes that include bacteria, fungi, yeast, and even viruses [83]. A nanogel prepared from biologically synthesized AgNPs from cell-free extract of *Saccharomyces boulardii* resulted in superior healing of burn wounds in rats as compared to marketed formulations [81]. AgNPs successfully interrupt the quorum sensing mechanism, resulting in decreased biofilm formation and detoxification of the bacterial toxins [84]. AgNPs carry the silver ions (Ag^+) that are solely responsible for antimicrobial activity by interfering with the respiratory chains at the cytochrome, damaging cell wall, binding with DNA,

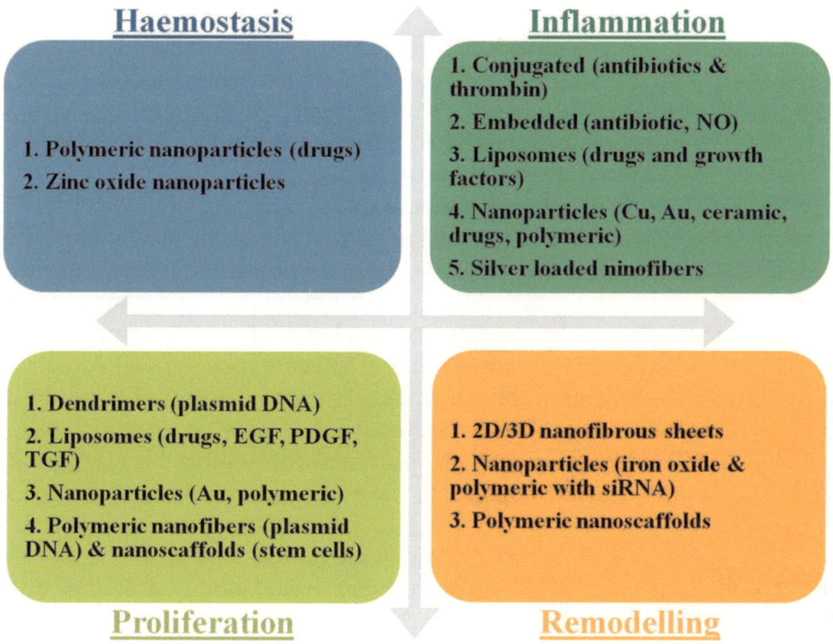

Figure 2.
Schematic representation of the main biological phases and events in the wound healing cascade along with the most abundant cells and soluble factors present in each phase, which is responsible for wound repair. The arrows at the top indicate the timeline of healing phases suggesting the overlapping nature of the wound healing cascade.

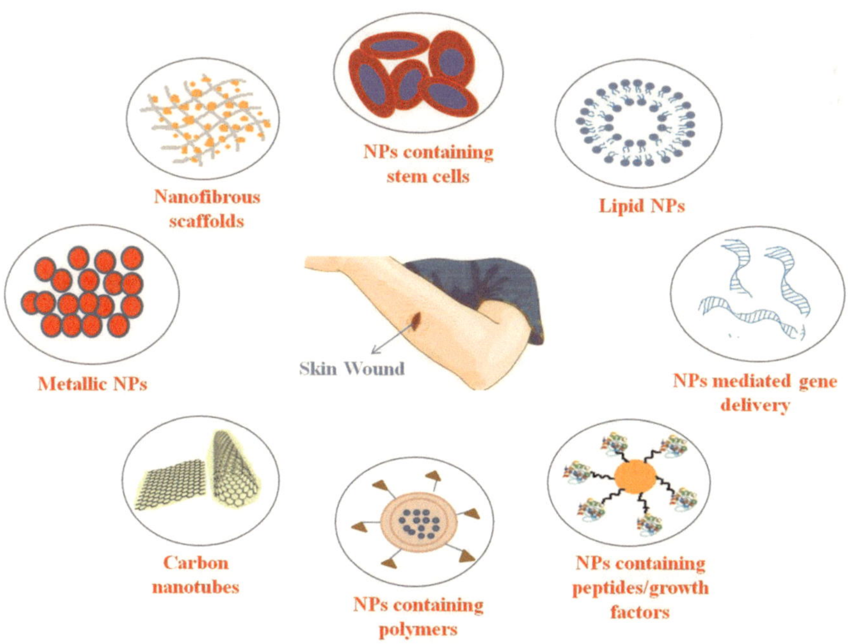

Figure 3.
Pictorial representation of the various types of nanotechnology-driven wound repair materials currently under research/available in the market.

and inhibiting its replication [85, 86]. In a recent *in vitro* study, it was demonstrated that the use of AgNPs led to a significant decrease in levels of inflammatory cytokines, oxidative stress in human keratinocytes and dermal fibroblasts that ultimately accelerated the rate of healing [87]. In a burn wound model, topical application of AgNPs tends to reduce the neutrophil count and IL-3 levels along with an increase in levels of IL-10, TGF-β, VEGF, and interferon-gamma (IFN-γ) [88].

Gold NPs (AuNPs) are way more biocompatible than other metallic NPs. It is very exciting to describe that AuNPs alone or along with other drugs have also been examined for their wound-healing efficacy [71]. The proteasome inhibitory activity, antibacterial, and antioxidant potential of AuNPs synthesized using aqueous extract of the rind of *Citrullus lanatus* may serve as potential candidates for wound healing [89]. Electrospun scaffold containing pharmaceutical intermediate-capped AuNPs provided a remedy for the treatment of full-thickness wounds infected by multi-drug resistant (MDR) bacteria [90]. The antibacterial mechanism of action of AuNPs illustrates that AuNPs alter the membrane potential and inhibit the ATP synthase enzyme that ultimately causes a collapse in the energy metabolism of the cell and cell death [91].

The inherent antibacterial nature of zinc oxide (ZnO) NPs promotes the applicability of such nanomaterials in numerous hydrogel-based wound dressings. In a study, cotton wound dressings impregnated with AgNPs, ZnO NPs, and mixed Ag/ZnO NPs resulted in high antibacterial action of wound dressings (**Figure 3**). Bandages impregnated with a liquid solution of AgNPs showed more antibacterial activity as compared to ZnO and mixed Ag/ZnO NPs [92]. ZnO-NPs successfully prepared from aqueous leaf extract of the plant *Barleria gibsoni* exhibited a remarkable wound-healing potential in rats and acted as an effective and better topical antimicrobial formulation to treat burn wounds [93]. In another study, the authors explored the healing potential of Ag-ZnO composite NPs in Wistar rats and showed comparatively faster healing in 10 days as compared to pure AgNPs and dermazin (the standard drug) [94]. Topical administration of antibacterial ZnO NPs also decreased bacterial skin infections in mice model by the induction of disintegration of the cell membrane and oxidative stress response in macrophages [95]. Iron oxide NPs were also evaluated for wound healing purposes. Fe_2O_3 NPs conjugated with thrombin significantly stimulated incisional wound healing by improving the tensile strength of the skin and reducing scar formation [96].

5.2 Nanoparticles containing polymers

Wound dressing materials are often based on polymeric nanostructures that include either synthetic or natural polymers. Mainly, poly(lactic-co-glycolic acid) (PLGA), poly(ethylene glycol) (PEG), poly(lactic acid) (PLA), and polycaprolactone (PCL) are the mostly used synthetic polymers to engineer biomaterials for wound care applications [97]. Natural biodegradable polymers are chitosan, cellulose, alginates, and hyaluronic acids, which have played a well-versed role in the healing of wounds. In a study, electrospun nanofibers prepared from the blend of PLA and hyperbranched polyglycerol and loaded with curcumin showed wound-healing potential. *In vitro* scratch assay results indicated that the curcumin-loaded electrospun nanofibers were able to completely cover the wound within 36 h [98]. In another study, curcumin-PLGA nanostructures resulted in two-fold increase in wound-healing potential when compared to either PLGA or curcumin. Curcumin-loaded PLGA NPs reduced reactive oxidative species (ROS) and downregulated expression of anti-oxidative molecules (glutathione peroxidase and NFκβ) that are responsible for reducing the inflammatory responses (**Figures 2** and **3**) [99]. A hybrid alginate hydrogel cross-linked by calcium gluconate crystals deposited in PCL-PEG-PCL was shown to promote wound regeneration in a full-thickness skin defect model of rats that suggested their great potential in skin tissue engineering [100].

Another important biopolymer, collagen is structural component of the extracellular matrix and is known for providing excellent strength to tissues [101]. Collagen nanofibers mat incorporated with AgNPs resulted in accelerated re-epithelialization, collagen production, and better wound contraction compared with plain collagen nanofibers. Due to its excellent biocompatibility and bioadhesive nature, collagen nanofibers mat promotes cell adhesion and interacts with cells and regulates cell migration, proliferation, and survival. Collagen dressings also result in accelerated fibroblast production and promote wound healing [102]. Another collagen-derived biopolymer, that is, gelatin has been used mainly in the establishment of biocompatible and biodegradable wound dressings. The porosity and interfiber distance of gelatin structure tend to promote healing. In a report, topical administration of gelatin wound scaffolds resulted in rapid wound closure and faster wound repair in a rat model [103]. Chitosan is another natural polymer that acts as an optimum wound-healing material as it bears film-forming capacity, gel-forming characteristics, positive charge, and a strong tissue adhesive trait in response to increased coagulation of blood [104]. Its analogous structure with glycosaminoglycan (main component of extracellular matrix) plays a great role in its utility in tissue engineering biomaterials [105]. In a study, chitosan-Ag-ZnO nanocomposite dressing enhanced the wound healing and promoted re-epithelialization and collagen deposition [106]. Similarly, a spongy bilayer wound dressing material composed of chitosan-Ag NPs and chitosan-*Bletilla striata* polysaccharide also showed hastened healing of skin wounds of mice, and the bilayer displayed improved mature epidermization and less inflammation on day 7 [107]. In another report, insulin-delivering chitosan NPs coated onto the electrospun PCL/collagen demonstrated nearly full wound closure when compared to the sterile gauze, which showed approximately 45% of wound closure [108].

Cellulose, another important biopolymer occurring abundantly, has been used widely in wound dressing applications due to its biodegradability, biocompatibility, and high tensile strength. Methylcellulose-containing AgNPs showed excellent antibacterial action and burn wound healing [109]. Nanocomposites containing cellulose nanocrystals (CNCs) incorporated with silver NPs have also been used for acute and diabetic wound healing in mice. The nanocellulose in these nanocomposites possessed good water-absorbing capacity and porous nature that assisted in the rapid healing of acute and diabetic wounds [110–112].

5.3 Peptide encapsulated nanostructures

Peptides of various types possess astonishing functions for wound-healing applications. But the controlled and prolonged delivery of peptides to the wound site is quite challenging. The use of NPs for encapsulation of peptides serves as a platform to provide sustained and controlled delivery of peptides and protect the peptides from degradation, thus promoting rapid healing of wounds [113]. In a study, solid lipid nanoparticle (SLN) encapsulating simultaneously LL37 and serpin A1 was used to deliver the agent at specific ratios. The developed nanostructures resulted in faster wound repair by promoting wound closure in fibroblasts and keratinocytes and increasing antibacterial action against bacteria *S. aureus* and *E. coli* as compared to bare LL37 or serpin A1 alone. LL37 is well-known endogenous host defense peptide possessing the antimicrobial trait and takes part in the regulation of the healing process. Further, Serpin A1, an elastase inhibitor has been reported to demonstrate healing properties [114]. In another report, a recombinant fusion protein comprised of stromal cell-derived growth factor-1 (SDF1) and elastin-like peptide (ELPs) was developed, which possess the tendency to self-assemble into NPs. SDF1 is known to promote neovascularization for early re-epithelialization of cutaneous wounds in diabetic mice. ELPs are non-immunogenic, non-pyrogenic, and biologically compatible derivatives of tropoelastin. The topical application of wounds treated with SDF1-ELP NPs resulted in 95% closure of full-thickness wounds by day 21, and complete closure by day 28. On the other hand, only 80% of wound closure was achieved by treatment with free SDF1, ELP alone, or vehicle control by day 21, and the wounds took 42 days for complete closure [115]. In another study, heparin mimetic peptide nanofibers angiogenic scaffolds were developed for slow release of growth factors and protection from degradation. Heparin mimetic peptide nanofibers have the potential to bind and enhance the activity and production of major angiogenic growth factors, such as VEGF, and thus provided a therapeutic way to accelerate the healing of diabetic wounds [116]. Another similar study demonstrated the use of heparin-mimetic peptide nanofiber gel for increasing the rate of healing of burn injuries [117].

A different study reported the simple one-step cross-linking strategy for the preparation of collagen peptide with recombinant human collagen (RHC)-chitosan nanofibers for wound healing. The results showed rapid epidermalization and angiogenesis in Sprague–Dawley (SD) rat scalding model after treatment with *in situ* cross-linked nanofibers (**Figure 3**). The *in situ* cross-linked nanofibers behaved well as a scaffold showing better cell attachment and proliferation. The breakdown products of RHC played a role as chemotactic agents for the faster synthesis of granulation tissue for showing better healing performance [118]. A different type of hybrid multifunctional nanofibrous matrix composed of poly(citrate)-ε-poly-lysine and PCL was designed to inhibit MDR bacteria and enhance full-thickness wound healing [119].

5.4 Carbon-based nanomaterials

Carbon nanomaterials, such as graphene oxide (GO)-NPs, carbon dots, and fullerenes, possess the potential to be used as skin repair agents (**Figure 3**). The application of carbon nanotubes (CNTs) to wound healing provides enhanced functionality for dressing, delivery of antiseptics in a controlled manner, and real-time monitoring of healing events. Polyvinyl alcohol (PVA) functionalized multi-walled CNTs further conjugated with glucose oxidase enzyme showed antibacterial activity against bacterial pathogens due to the generation of hydrogen peroxide. The antibacterial activity of the developed nanomaterials opened innovative ways for the potential of such materials in wound-healing applications [120]. In a study, GO nanosheets incorporated in ultrafine biopolymer fibers were tested for skin wound-healing potential in adult male rats. From the *in vivo* studies, it was found that a large open wound ($1.5 \times 1.5\ cm^2$) was completely regenerated after 14-day of injury. Pathological studies confirmed the formation of thick dermal tissue and complete epithelialization in the presence of 1.5wt% GO nanosheets [121]. In a different study, a novel 3D collagen scaffold containing carbon-based 2D layered material, GO was characterized for periodontal healing of dogs. GO scaffold was implanted into dog class II furcation defects, and periodontal healing was examined after 4 weeks of surgery. The outcomes suggested that GO scaffold was biocompatible and possessed excellent bone and periodontal tissue formation ability [122]. Onion-derived carbon nanodots that comprised hydrophilic group-decorated amorphous nanodots exhibited accelerated healing in a full-thickness wound model of rat model attributed to its radical scavenging action [123]. Carbon C_{60} fullerenes exhibited fascinating properties that balance several pathological mechanisms accountable for hampering the wound repair pathway [124]. In a different study, C_{60} fullerene functionalized with cationic three dimethyl pyrrolidinium groups was examined to rescue mice from fatal wound infections of Gram-negative species, *Proteus mirabilis* and *Pseudomonas aeruginosa.* The study results successfully revealed that mice infected with *P. mirabilis* showed 82% survival due to the photodynamic therapy of fullerenes as compared to only 8% survival of mice without treatment [125].

5.5 Solid lipid nanomaterials

Various kinds of lipid nanomaterials, such as SLN, liposomes, micelles, nanostructured lipid carriers (NLC), or vesicles, have been used as therapies for wound healing (**Figure 3**). SLNPs encapsulated with morphine were reported to increase keratinocyte migration, proliferation, and differentiation responsible for accelerated wound repair [126]. In this context, liposome with silk fibroin hydrogel core was designed to stabilize bFGF. The study indicated that the skin permeability of bFGF was significantly enhanced by the developed liposomal system, and a major part of the encapsulated growth factor penetrated the skin dermis. Application of bFGF encapsulated liposomes resulted in improvement in the morphology of hair follicles at the wound site with hair regrowth shown on a deep second scald mice model. The healing action was mainly found to be associated with inhibiting scar formation and promoting vascular growth in dermis, which may serve as a potential candidate to improve wound healing [127]. In another study, liposomes were loaded with dexamethasone-phosphate. The liposomes were further surface modified with either PEG or phosphatidylserine. Both formulations resulted in decreased IL-6 and TNF-α release and increased efferocytosis activity. A faster uptake and a higher potency were induced by phosphatidylserine-modified liposomes as compared to PEG-modified liposomes. Liposomes after shell modification with phosphatidylserine promoted dexamethasone delivery to macrophages and induced a phenotype favorable for chronic wound healing [128]. The topical administration of recombinant human EGF loaded into lipid nanocarriers showed accelerated healing of full-thickness cutaneous wounds in a porcine model. The administration of 20 μg of nanoencapsulated lipid carriers twice a week increased the wound closure rate, as well as improved the wound quality in *in vivo* experiments [129].

Micelles were also proposed as suitable candidates for the delivery of hydrophobic molecules to the wound site for the healing of chronic wounds. In this respect, a biodegradable hydrogel system cutaneous wound dressing was developed containing curcumin encapsulated in micelles. Curcumin suffers from problems such as low water solubility, poor oral bioavailability, and rapid first-pass metabolism. The application of developed micelles in both incision and excision wound models showed higher collagen level, better granulation, remarkable reduction in superoxide dismutase content, and small increase in catalase activity causing an enhancement in the healing of cutaneous wounds [130]. Another study demonstrated that clarithromycin-loaded micelles were prepared *via* self-assembly of chitosan with a mixture of linoleic and oleic acids. These micelles exhibited good biocompatibility, induced cell proliferation, and showed 20-times greater clarithromycin loading capacity in comparison to its water-saturated solution, suggesting the potential of micelles in wound-healing applications [131].

6. Nanomaterials as delivery agents carrying therapeutic molecules

Many therapeutic molecules such as nitric oxide, various antibiotics and anti-oxidative compounds, bioactive molecules, and vitamins possess great potential for wound healing. But each of these has few problems associated with solubility, stability, degradation by enzymes, temperature sensitivity, and so on. Because of these problems, the topical applicability of these compounds decreases to a large extent. Therefore, a need was felt to develop nanotechnology-based carriers to encapsulate these compounds for enhancing their efficacy.

6.1 Nanoparticles containing bioactive molecules for healing

Nanoencapsulated bioactive molecules also served as promising approach for skin tissue engineering. NPs encapsulated with bioactive ingredients help in slow and sustained release of the active moiety to the target site and increase the stability of molecules [132]. As an important natural molecule, curcumin suffers from limitations of poor solubility and fast degradation rate that hinder its applicability as an anti-oxidative and antimicrobial agent. To overcome these limitations, curcumin-loaded NPs have been synthesized, which enhanced the wound healing in the murine model as compared to pure curcumin [133]. In another report, efforts have been made to prepare curcumin-loaded chitosan NPs that were then impregnated into collagen-alginate scaffolds. Such prepared nanoscaffolds resulted in complete epithelization and granulation tissue formation for rapid healing of wounds in diabetic mice (**Figures 2** and **3**) [134]. An important study demonstrated the effect of guanidinylated chitosan NPs loaded with five different bioactive molecules (EGF, ascorbic acid, hydrocortisone, insulin, and 1,25-dihydroxyvitamin D_3). These biomolecules are beneficial for stimulating skin fibroblasts and keratinocyte proliferation but have limited applicability as they are unstable in wound dressing fabrication and storage. The prepared wound dressings resulted in stable delivery of bioactive factors and enhancement of skin wound healing in Wistar rats [135]. In a similar study, curcumin NPs were embedded in gelation microsphere hydrogels. These thermosensitive and MMP-9 responsive hydrogels induced drug release at the wound bed and resulted in acceleration of diabetic skin wound healing due to their ability to promote cell migration and antioxidant nature [136].

Another important flavonoid, quercetin, is also known for its antioxidant nature. But its topical application is limited due to low solubility, low stability, and less release after application. To overcome these limitations, quercetin was encapsulated into mesoporous silica NPs carrying a copolymer. These NPs showed thermoresponsive behavior that acts to provide the potential of such particles in dermal delivery [137]. In another study, topical application of chitosan-fibrin scaffolds impregnated with quercetin significantly accelerated the process of wound healing [138]. Similarly, baicalin-loaded nanohydrogels comprised of a dispersion of cholesterol-derivatized gellan in phosphate buffer. Baicalin (a flavone glycoside)-loaded nanohydrogels demonstrated complete skin restoration and inhibition of specific inflammatory markers causing rapid skin wound healing in *in vivo* mice [139].

6.2 Nanoparticles for nitric oxide delivery

Nitric oxide is an important diatomic molecule that is synthesized by three different isoforms of enzyme nitric oxide synthases by the conversion of amino acid L-arginine. In the skin, different forms of nitric oxide are produced and released by various cells involved, such as macrophages, keratinocytes, melanocytes, and fibroblasts. In wound healing, nitric oxide is synthesized in the early inflammatory phase by inflammatory macrophage cells, whereas many cells secrete nitric oxide in the proliferative phase during wound healing. Nitric oxide being lipophilic in nature possesses the tendency to interact with various biomolecules. It can cross various biological barriers to reach the target site and diffuse along a concentration gradient to rapidly move from cell to cell. Nitric oxide is antibacterial in nature, modulates the immune response, maintains homeostasis and regulates wound healing, and helps in collagen deposition, cell proliferation, and wound contraction [140]. In this context, topical application of nitric oxide for acute and chronic wound healing always remained a challenge. To meet this challenge, engineering NPs mediated nitric oxide release to the wound bed served as a novel approach to allow its free radicals to exert antibacterial action [141].

In this respect for nitric oxide delivery, nitric oxide released from NPs system constituted of composite of polymer/glass hydrogel was tested for its efficacy in methicillin-resistant *Staphylococcus aureus* (MRSA) abscesses in mice. The study results documented that antibacterial nitric oxide-NPs treatment of abscesses reduced the involved area and bacterial load, and ultimately improved the skin architecture [142]. In a recent study, a novel wound-healing material was formulated by combining chitosan with electrospun PCL nonwoven mat for the loading of nitric oxide. Nitric oxide was released in a sustained fashion from the developed wound dressing under the physiological conditions. *In vivo* wound healing evaluated in full-thickness cutaneous wounds of mice resulted in accelerated wound healing through re-epithelialization and granulation formation due to immunomodulation and enhanced collagen synthesis provided by the sustained release of nitric oxide [143]. Nitric oxide released from silica NPs has been demonstrated to exert a bactericidal activity against *P. aeruginosa*, which is one of the important pathogens causing wound infections in hospitals [144]. In a different report, nitric oxide donor precursor glutathione was encapsulated chitosan NPs with an encapsulation efficiency of 99.60% (**Figure 2**). Small size and positive zeta of chitosan NPs led to the delivery of nitric oxide through the skin for topical applications due to the affinity of positively charged chitosan NPs with negatively charged phospholipids that further result in changing the permeability of the skin membrane and reducing the skin barriers [145].

6.3 Antibiotics-loaded nanoparticles for wound repair

There are many types of wounds that fail to heal and turn into chronic wounds [146]. The major cause of delayed healing of such wounds is the persistence of infectious agents or microbial growth around the wound bed [147]. The major goal of any wound-healing treatment is to control the microbial infections to allow normal healing to proceed. Conventional therapies to treat microbial infections are based on either the systemic administration of antibiotics or the topical application of antibiotic formulations [146]. The systemic administration of antibiotics causes toxicity along with kidney and liver complications, but topical application of antibiotics provides high local concentration with a short residence time on the wound surface [148].

Therefore, an appropriate antimicrobial therapy of the wound to control microbial colonization is still required for optimum wound care. The delivery of antibiotic therapy *via* NPs offers great potential advantages, such as slow and sustained delivery, targeted delivery, and decrease in toxicity and improvement in antimicrobial and pharmacokinetic properties (**Figure 2**) [149].

In this respect, a novel wound dressing based on the Spanish Broom fibers impregnated with vancomycin-loaded chitosan NPs was designed, which showed an increased antibacterial action against *S. aureus* and was not toxic to HaCaT keratinocytes as compared to the fibers containing vancomycin without NPs [150]. In another study, chitosan nanofibers mat was functionalized with thiol groups, and gentamicin-loaded liposomes (17% loading efficiency) were immobilized covalently. Liposomes showed sustained and controlled release of gentamicin during 16 h, achieving a steady state at 24 h [151]. Nanofibers of small diameter exhibit unique properties such as excellent mechanical properties, flexibility in surface functionalities, and high specific surface area for wound healing [152]. Chitosan is used in such dressings because its biodegradable, cell adhesive, and possesses hemostatic activity and high mechanic strength [153]. In another study, ZnO NPs were coated with gentamicin and integrated into the chitosan matrix to yield a ZnO/gentamicin-chitosan gel (**Figure 2**). The resulting gel showed 91% of gentamicin release after 8 h and evidenced a four-fold minimum inhibitory concentration (MIC) reduction for *S. aureus* and 2-fold reduction of MIC for *P. aeruginosa*. The resulting antibacterial gels could serve as potential candidates for wound healing [154]. Few other reports well-documented the loading of antibiotics in NPs or nanofibers matrix for the sustained release of antibiotic drugs to prepare wound dressings. Ampicillin-incorporated electrospun polyurethane scaffolds [155], PVA films containing tetracycline hydrochloride-loaded quaternized chitosan NPs [156], tetracycline hydrochloride-loaded electrospun nanofibers mats based on chitosan, and PVA NPs [157] wound dressings have shown biocompatibility and strong antibacterial activity against different strains of bacteria.

7. Engineered scaffolds and nanocomposites for wound healing

One most important feature of the modern dressings used for the therapeutic purpose for skin tissue repair involves the designing of engineered biocompatible nanoscaffolds to mimic the structure of ECM (**Figures 2** and **3**). Such nanoscaffolds should possess the properties such as porous nature, biocompatibility, tendency to incorporate and release various growth factors/antibiotics in a controlled manner, and support for the attachment of cells and their proliferation [158]. Scaffold-based tissue-engineered nanocomposites have been known to accelerate chronic wound healing by improvement in angiogenesis [159]. Various nanotechnology-based methods such as electrospinning, phase separation, and self-assembly have been devised for the formation of such scaffolds [65]. Electrospinning is the most favored method among all these methods for the preparation of nanofibrous scaffolds for skin tissue engineering [160]. For promoting diabetic wound healing and increasing collagen content, nanofibrous glucophage-loaded collagen/PLGA scaffolds were fabricated by electrospinning [161]. In another study, electrospun PCL scaffolds resulted in fibroblast attachment and proliferation. Full-thickness skin wounds of guinea pigs healed within 35 days after treatment with these membranes [162]. Similarly, electrospun membrane of PCL/chitosan nanofibers/aloe vera was fabricated to mimic both the layers of skin. Top dense layer was composed of PCL to provide mechanical strength to the wounded site, and bottom layer of the dressing consisted of chitosan nanofibers and aloe vera to provide bactericidal activity for promoting skin wound healing [163]. Electrospun chitosan-poly(ethylene oxide) (PEO) nanofibrous scaffold-incorporated PLGA NPs were studied for *in vivo* wound healing [164]. In another report, chitosan NPs and TiO_2 NPs were incorporated in polyurethane nanocomposites membranes, which showed 71.5% improvement in swelling when compared to neat polyurethane membrane and resulted in increase in tensile strength and antibacterial activity suitable for wound healing [165]. Multilayer wound dressing prepared by electrospun polyurethane nanofibers loaded with Semellil extract and other layer chitosan nanofiber resulted in 94% wound closure after 14 days [166].

Another material, that is, nanocomposites have also been proved beneficial for wound healing due to the properties possessed by its dispersed phase and reinforcing fillers. The nanocomposites serve as optimum wound dressing materials as they provide better mechanical strength due to the synergistic action of both the components. In a study, nanocomposites of collagen sponges and AuNPs showed greater tensile strength and indicated a faster wound healing [167]. In a different report, cerium nanocrystals were immobilized onto mesoporous silica NPs to develop ROS scavenging nanocomposites for wound healing. Ceria nanocrystals are known to reduce ROS and to protect the cell from oxidative damage. Silica NPs act as nanobridge between nanomaterial and tissue matrix for rapid wound closure. The nanocomposite prepared from both the components resulted in accelerated wound healing due to their synergistic action [168]. Another type of nanocomposites was prepared by using bacterial cellulose and hyaluronic acid. Bacterial cellulose has high-water-absorbing capacity and porous nature responsible for enhancing the wound-healing rate, whereas hyaluronic acid is biocompatible and possesses gel-forming capacity. The developed nanocomposites facilitated the growth of fibroblast cells and promoted the tissue repair [169]. Nanocomposites wound dressing for chronic wounds prepared from halloysite and chitosan oligosaccharides showed better skin re-epithelization and reorganization as compared to halloysite or chitosan alone [170].

8. Nanomaterials incorporated with growth factors for healing

Healing occurs as a cellular response to wounding/injury, and it involves a variety of cells such as macrophages, fibroblasts, keratinocytes, and neutrophils. In general, the wound-healing process is regulated by various factors, such as microbial infections, wound type, patient conditions, lesser growth factors, and cytokine release. Impaired or delayed wound healing is very much affected by the decreased production of different growth factors by the cells that will ultimately cause the lengthening of healing time and leads to various other complications [171]. Various growth factors such as VEGF, EGF, PDGF, FGF, and TGF-β play a great role in promoting the wound-healing process *via* decreasing inflammation, promoting cell proliferation of fibroblasts and epithelial cells, increasing angiogenesis and ultimately re-epithelialization [158]. Topical administration of growth factors as wound dressings is quite unsatisfactory due to their low biodegradability, instability of protein structure under certain physiological conditions, and enzymatic degradation [172]. In this regard, new drug delivery systems to deliver growth factors at the target wound site in a controlled fashion were developed using nanotechnology (**Figures 2** and **3**) [173].

In this context, gold NPs have been used to conjugate the keratinocyte growth factor. The gold NPs effectively promoted the proliferation of keratinocytes in contrast to unloaded gold NPs or keratinocyte growth factor. *In vivo* full-thickness wound model resulted in enhanced of healing by promoting re-epithelialization by the application of growth factor conjugated NPs. In this study, gold NPs were favored for use due to their biocompatibility and versatile nature for surface functionalization [174]. In another study, recombinant human EGF-loaded nanostructured lipid carriers (NLCs) were checked for their wound-healing efficacy in full-thickness excisional wound porcine model. *In vivo* healing experiments showed that topical application of 20 μg of recombinant human epidermal growth factor (rhEGF)-NLC enhanced the percentage rate of wound closure by day 25 as compared to administration of 75 μg of free rhEGF and NLC by migration and proliferation of fibroblast cells and deposition of collagen in the newly healed wound [129]. Human EGF was loaded into thiolated heparin and diacrylated PEG hydrogels *via* photopolymerization for wound healing. *In vivo* full-thickness wounds in mice showed accelerated wound closure as compared to EGF solution due to sustained release of EGF from biocompatible hydrogel [175]. In a similar manner, wound dressing composed of chitosan-hyaluronic acid composite sponge containing VEGF encapsulated fibrin NPs was designed for diabetic wounds. From the released studies, it was found that 64% of the encapsulated VEGF in NPs was released in 72 h with an initial burst release of 29% in 2 h, which was supposed for the initial sprouting of blood vessels. *In vitro* studies showed that endothelial cells seeded on these hydrogels showed capillary-like tube formation beneficial in wound-healing angiogenesis [176]. From all these studies, it can be inferred that NPs enhance the release of growth factors and thus accelerate the wound-healing process.

9. Gene (RNAi and siRNA) delivery by nanotherapeutic agents for wound repair

It is a well-known fact that miRNAs can be critical regulators of wound repair [177], but the miRNAs involved and their specific role in wound healing remains unclear. Recently, a new method for the identification of functional miRNAs, which get elevated during skin injury, has been described. This group has identified miR-223 as a new potential therapeutic target influencing acute inflammation in wounds that are *S. aureus* infected [178].

RNAi therapy has been used to specifically silence gene expression of overexpressed targets in chronic wounds [179]. NP-based approach has been implemented to protect the effector molecule in siRNA from degradation *via* intracellular RNases leading to targeted delivery [180]. Of late, gold NP conjugates with spherical nucleic acid (SNA) have also been employed for efficient *in vivo* siRNA delivery [181]. The importance of SNA nanotechnology lies in its ability to cross the epidermal barrier, thereby permitting its use in topical therapeutics (**Figures 2** and **3**). Nevertheless, a pertinent demand for more efficacious and refined novel RNAi-based therapeutics for tissue repair. Such products should overcome the drawbacks of presently available materials in use and provide for better retention, bioavailability, effectiveness, safety, and selective targeting [180].

A combination of gene therapy and tissue engineering commonly called as gene-activated matrix therapy has come to the fore as a method to enhance or knockdown a specific target gene playing a role in bone, cartilage, or skin regeneration [182]. The major advantage of this approach is the higher stability of DNA in comparison to the growth factor therapy [182, 183]. However, the major flaw of this technique is the need for repeated injections of colloidal and naked DNA to the wound site and the short-term and inconsistent gene expression [183]. To overcome these issues, nucleic acids have been impregnated into electrospun nanofibrous meshes to increase tissue regeneration and to decrease scarring [183]. More recently, polyester scaffolds have been used for the management of cutaneous wounds [179, 184]. Furthermore, electrospun scaffolds having a mixture of PLA and PCL were employed for the delivery of plasmid that encodes keratinocytes' growth factor [184].

10. Nanomaterials incorporated with stem cells to prompt healing

Therapeutic approaches for wound healing that involves stem cells have been studied extensively in the past, and they have shown great promise in promoting angiogenesis and facilitating re-epithelialization [185]. Adipose-derived stromal cells (ASCs), bone marrow (BM)-derived endothelial progenitor cells, BM-derived mesenchymal stem cells (BM-MSCs), BM-derived mononuclear cells (BM-MNCs), placenta-derived SCs, and umbilical cord-derived MSCs have been shown to have a therapeutic role in wound repair [185, 186]. The probable mechanism of action is, however, not well elucidated, but the hypothesis says that SC therapy tends to provide a dynamic wound microenvironment *via* their paracrine effect, hence, hastening the healing cascade [187]. In a recent study, it was shown that when MSCs are directly delivered to the wound site, they induce cell death; this effect was then attenuated by using bioengineered delivery platform for therapies [188].

Currently, SCs are used for local administration to wounds by the way of dressings, injections, sprays, and systemic administration. Recently, nanotechnology-driven approaches were employed to synthesize nanomatrices possessing customized biophysical properties, leading to controlled differentiation of SCs. BM-MSCs attached to collagen/PLGA nanofiber scaffold showcased faster closure of wounds [189]. The BM-MSC/nanoscaffold composite approach was explored for wound healing and regeneration (**Figures 2** and **3**). Subsequently, a mixture of MSCs, growth factors, and the matrix was used in the production of nanoscaffolds to mimic human skin characteristics [187, 190]. Polymeric nanofibers having biomimetic potential can simulate the native tissue thereby forming an ideal SC niche. Despite significant advancements in this field in the past, no SC therapy for chronic wound management has yet been FDA approved [185]. It is highly likely that in the future, viable treatments will use SCs in combination with other local/systemic therapies.

11. Nanotechnology-driven targeted delivery achieves cell-type specificity

The field of targeted/site-specific delivery of nanomaterials is still in its young days in comparison to various other nanotechnologies used for wound-healing applications. Targeted delivery of therapeutics is highly recommended and significant to reduce side effects, improve efficacy, and reduce therapy costs [180]. This also overcomes the limitation of a low viable cell number homing the target tissue that has often been associated with systemic stem cell therapy. This platform is highly versatile and can be customized for the targeted delivery of cells, DNA, proteins siRNA, and small drugs, to any target tissue. This is achieved by complexing the NP with the therapeutic agent and with the aid of a molecular recognition molecule integrated within the NP.

Recently, SDF1 was used for targeted delivery to the injury site employing ROS stimulus-responsive polymeric NPs as delivery vehicles [191]. The nanocarrier-targeted delivery platform demonstrated high efficiency and biocompatibility to direct SCs to the injured tissues, resulting in enhanced angiogenesis and repair of injury with no toxicity or immunogenicity involved.

12. Advantages of nanotechnology over conventional methods for healing

Nanotechnology offers several advantages to nanomaterial dressings as compared to dressings prepared by conventional methods for wound healing applications. The various advantages of nanomaterials considered for skin tissue engineering include: (i) nano-dimensions impart proper structure to cells/tissues for their adhesion, differentiation, and proliferation, (ii) due to particular chemical composition and physical structure, nanomaterials serve as analogous structures to extracellular matrix [192], (iii) nanomaterials have high mechanical strength due to which these can act to reinforce various organic/synthetic scaffolds for tissue engineering [193], (iv) high conductivity of carbon-based nanomaterials provides electrical stimulation to scaffolds for skin tissue repair [194, 195], (v) micro/nanoencapsulation of important growth factors/bioactive agents help them to release these molecules in a slow and sustained manner at the target wound site [196, 197], (vi) NPs impart better biocompatibility, bioactivity and enhance interactions of scaffolds to cells or proteins [198], and (vii) NPs possess astonishing properties that are far better in terms of high Young's modulus, high tensile strength, and high surface-area-to-volume ratio as compared to the bulk materials from which nanomaterials are being prepared. All these advantages of NPs make them successful candidates for tissue repair and wound healing applicability.

13. Conclusions and future perspectives

Millions of people around the globe are being affected by chronic wounds, with current research showing limited success in producing FDA-approved efficacious therapeutic agents. This may be attributed to the fact that chronic wound pathology is highly complex as is the tissue repair process. Hence, researchers are in dire need to develop alternative therapeutic approaches for the management of nonhealing wounds that would be viable and efficient as per the FDA norms. The factors that are known to impede the development of therapeutics for chronic wounds include variability of patients and comorbidities, limited understanding of patient pathophysiology, complexity and costs associated with clinical trials, and the general lack of awareness in the public.

Despite a multitude of previously existing materials, healing in chronic conditions is still compromised. Hence, the future wound repair materials should possess a plethora of functions and properties such as antimicrobial, biomimetic, bioresponsive, and hemostasis to provide a suitable microenvironment for wound repair. Therefore, developing an appropriate combinational therapy that targets dysfunctional cellular processes remains the major challenge. Future advances in the understanding of the complex wound healing process will surely aid in this front. The emergence of multifunctional nanotechnologies, in the wound healing arena, showcases the high expectations toward this field. However, gaining in-depth information about their physicochemical properties and their possible toxicity remains a huge hurdle in promoting these nanotechnologies for human use. Recent developments in the nano-field have led to the development of matrices, scaffolds, skin substitutes, embedded/loaded dressings, etc., which mimic the integrity of the skin. Soon unique phenotype–genotype characteristics will lead way to tailored therapies. This will provide a platform to create new nanotechnology-driven approaches, hence, streamlining and facilitating personalized treatment plans.

For the clinical translation of nanotechnology-based products, there is an urgent need for improved tools and better analytical methods. Comprehensive efforts are necessary to develop chronic wound care products with target and site-specificity to negate the undesirable effects of the nanosystems in humans. In due course of time and with the ever-increasing reports about exciting new nanotechnology platforms, the day is not far when the international standards on biocompatibility and toxicity of various nanotherapies are met with. In a nutshell, our current knowledge about the development of nanotherapeutics, together with our understanding of phenotype–genotype characteristics and chronic wound pathology, will be instrumental in promoting and conceptualizing next-generation wound repair nanotechnologies.

Acknowledgements

The authors acknowledge the Director, CSIR-IHBT for his valuable guidance and support. RS and SS thank UGC and CSIR, respectively, for providing research fellowships and AcSIR for Ph.D. registration. YSP thanks the financial assistance from the Council of Scientific and Industrial Research (CSIR), Government of India in the form of project MLP0204. The CSIR-IHBT publication number of this article is 4347.

List of abbreviations

Ag^+	silver ions
AgNP	silver nanoparticle(s)
ASCs	adipose-derived stromal cells
AuNP	gold nanoparticle(s)
bFGF	basic fibroblast growth factor
BM-MNCs	bone marrow-derived mononuclear cells
BM-MSCs	bone marrow-derived mesenchymal stem cells
BM	bone marrow
CNCs	cellulose nanocrystals
CNT	carbon nanotubes
ECM	extracellular matrix
EGF	epidermal growth factor
ELPF	elastin-like peptide
FDAF	food and drug administration
FGF	fibroblast growth factor
GO	graphene oxide
IFN-γ	interferon-gamma
ILs	interleukins
KGF	keratinocyte growth factor
MAPK	mitogen-activated protein kinases

MDR	multi-drug resistant
MIC	minimum inhibitory concentration
MMPs	metalloproteinase
MRSA	methicillin-resistant *S. aureus*
NLC	nanostructured lipid carriers
NP	nanoparticle(s)
PCL	polycaprolactone
PDGF	platelet-derived growth factor
PEG	poly(ethylene glycol)
PEO	poly(ethylene oxide)
PI3K	phosphoinositide 3-kinase
PLA	poly(lactic acid)
PLGA	poly(lactic-co-glycolic acid)
PVA	poly(vinyl alcohol)
RHC	recombinant human collagen
rhEGF	recombinant human epidermal growth factor
ROS	reactive oxidative species
SC	stem cell(s)
SD	sprague dawley
SDF1	stromal cell-derived growth factor-1
SLN	solid lipid nanoparticle
SNA	spherical nucleic acid
TGF-β	transforming growth factor-β
TNF-α	tumor necrosis factor-α
VEGF	vascular endothelial growth factor
ZnO	zinc oxide

Author details

Sourabh Soni[1,2†$], Rubbel Singla[2,3†] and Yogendra S. Padwad[1,2*]

1 Pharmacology and Toxicology Laboratory, Dietetics and Nutrition Technology Division, CSIR—Institute of Himalayan Bioresource Technology (CSIR-IHBT), Palampur, Himachal Pradesh, India

2 Academy of Scientific and Innovative Research (AcSIR), Ghaziabad, India

3 Nanobiology Laboratory, Biotechnology Division, CSIR—Institute of Himalayan Bioresource Technology (CSIR-IHBT), Palampur, Himachal Pradesh, India

*Address all correspondence to: yogendra@ihbt.res.in

† These authors contributed equally.

$Current address: Division of Pulmonary and Critical Care Medicine, Brigham and Women's Hospital, Department of Medicine, Harvard Medical School, Boston, MA, USA.

References

[1] Dhivya S, Padma VV, Santhini E. Wound dressings—A review. BioMedicine. 2015;**5**(4):24-28

[2] Seetharam RN. Nanomedicine—Emerging area of nanobiotechnology research. Current Science. 2006;**91**(3): 260

[3] Nandhini J, Neeraja P, Rajkumar SRJ, Umapathy V, Suresh S. Comparative studies of microwave and sol–gel-assisted combustion methods of $NiFe_2O_4$ nanostructures: synthesis, structural, morphological, opto-magnetic, and antimicrobial activity. Journal of Superconductivity and Novel Magnetism. 2017;**30**(5): 1213-1220

[4] Suri SS, Fenniri H, Singh B. Nanotechnology-based drug delivery systems. Journal of Occupational Medicine and Toxicology. 2007;**2**(1): 16-21

[5] Medintz IL, Mattoussi H, Clapp AR. Potential clinical applications of quantum dots. International Journal of Nanomedicine. 2008;**3**(2):151

[6] Sandhiya S, Dkhar SA, Surendiran A. Emerging trends of nanomedicine—An overview. Fundamental & Clinical Pharmacology. 2009;**23**(3):263-269

[7] Shalaby MA, Anwar MM, Saeed H. Nanomaterials for application in wound healing: Current state-of-the-art and future perspectives. Journal of Polymer Research. 2022;**29**(3):1-37

[8] Blanco-Fernandez B, Castaño O, Mateos-Timoneda MÁ, Engel E, Pérez-Amodio S. Nanotechnology approaches in chronic wound healing. Advances in Wound Care. 2021;**10**(5):234-256

[9] Lazarus GS, Cooper DM, Knighton DR, Margolis DJ, Percoraro RE, Rodeheaver G, et al. Definitions and guidelines for assessment of wounds and evaluation of healing. Wound Repair and Regeneration. 1994;**2**(3):165-170

[10] Velnar T, Bailey T, Smrkolj V. The wound healing process: An overview of the cellular and molecular mechanisms. Journal of International Medical Research. 2009;**37**(5):1528-1542

[11] Mittal A, Sardana S, Pandey A. Herbal boon for wounds. International Journal of Pharmacy and Pharmaceutical Sciences. 2013;**5**:1-12

[12] Rodrigues M, Kosaric N, Bonham CA, Gurtner GC. Wound healing: A cellular perspective. Physiological Reviews. 2019;**99**(1):665-706

[13] Ghosh PK, Gaba A. Phyto-extracts in wound healing. Journal of Pharmacy & Pharmaceutical Sciences. 2013;**16**(5): 760-820

[14] Chhabra S, Chhabra N, Kaur A, Gupta N. Wound healing concepts in clinical practice of OMFS. Journal of Maxillofacial and Oral Surgery. 2017; **16**(4):403-423

[15] Diegelmann RF, Evans MC. Wound healing: An overview of acute, fibrotic and delayed healing. Frontiers in Bioscience. 2004;**9**(1):283-289

[16] Eming SA, Martin P, Tomic-Canic M. Wound repair and regeneration: Mechanisms, signaling, and translation. Science Translational Medicine. 2014;**6** (265):265sr6

[17] Nussbaum SR, Carter MJ, Fife CE, DaVanzo J, Haught R, Nusgart M, et al.

An economic evaluation of the impact, cost, and medicare policy implications of chronic nonhealing wounds. Value in Health. 2018;**21**(1):27-32

[18] Han G, Ceilley R. Chronic wound healing: A review of current management and treatments. Advances in Therapy. 2017;**34**(3):599-610

[19] Liang L, Stone RC, Stojadinovic O, Ramirez H, Pastar I, Maione AG, et al. Integrative analysis of miRNA and mRNA paired expression profiling of primary fibroblast derived from diabetic foot ulcers reveals multiple impaired cellular functions. Wound Repair and Regeneration. 2016;**24**(6):943-953

[20] Lindley LE, Stojadinovic O, Pastar I, Tomic-Canic M. Biology and biomarkers for wound healing. Plastic and Reconstructive Surgery. 2016;**138**(3): 18S-28S

[21] Loesche M, Gardner SE, Kalan L, Horwinski J, Zheng Q, Hodkinson BP, et al. Temporal stability in chronic wound microbiota is associated with poor healing. Journal of Investigative Dermatology. 2017;**137**(1):237-244

[22] Demidova-Rice TN, Hamblin MR, Herman IM. Acute and impaired wound healing: Pathophysiology and current methods for drug delivery, part 1: Normal and chronic wounds: Biology, causes, and approaches to care. Advances in Skin & Wound Care. 2012; **25**(7):304-315

[23] Mahmoudi M, Gould LJ. Opportunities and challenges of the management of chronic wounds: A multidisciplinary viewpoint. Chronic Wound Care Management and Research. 2020;7:27

[24] Garraud O, Hozzein WN, Badr G. Wound healing: Time to look for intelligent,'natural'immunological approaches? BMC Immunology. 2017; **18**(1):23-30

[25] Gurtner GC, Werner S, Barrandon Y, Longaker MT. Wound repair and regeneration. Nature. 2008;**453**(7193): 314-321

[26] Kirsner RS, Eaglstein WH. The wound healing process. Dermatologic Clinics. 1993;**11**(4):629-640

[27] Regan MC, Barbul A. The cellular biology of wound healing. Wound Healing. 1994;**1**:3-17

[28] Sezer AD, Cevher E. Biopolymers as wound healing materials: Challenges and new strategies. In: Biomaterials Applications for Nanomedicine. London, UK: InTech; 2011

[29] Steed DL. The role of growth factors in wound healing. Surgical Clinics of North America. 1997;**77**(3):575-586

[30] Cooper DM. Optimizing wound healing. A practice within nursing's domain. The Nursing Clinics of North America. 1990;**25**(1):165-180

[31] Broughton G, Janis JE, Attinger CE. Wound healing: An overview. Plastic and Reconstructive Surgery. 2006;**117** (7eS):1eS-32eS

[32] Stoica AE, Chircov C, Grumezescu AM. Nanomaterials for wound dressings: An up-to-date overview. Molecules. 2020;**25**(11):2699

[33] Robson MC, Steed DL, Franz MG. Wound healing: Biologic features and approaches to maximize healing trajectories. Current Problems in Surgery. 2001;**38**(2):72-140

[34] Woo YC, Park SS, Subieta AR, Brennan TJ. Changes in tissue pH and

temperature after incision indicate acidosis may contribute to postoperative pain. Anesthesiology: The Journal of the American Society of Anesthesiologists. 2004;**101**(2):468-475

[35] De Oliveira S, Rosowski EE, Huttenlocher A. Neutrophil migration in infection and wound repair: Going forward in reverse. Nature Reviews Immunology. 2016;**16**(6):378-391

[36] Daley JM, Reichner JS, Mahoney EJ, Manfield L, Henry WL, Mastrofrancesco B, et al. Modulation of macrophage phenotype by soluble product (s) released from neutrophils. The Journal of Immunology. 2005;**174**(4):2265-2272

[37] Koh TJ, DiPietro LA. Inflammation and wound healing: The role of the macrophage. Expert Reviews in Molecular Medicine. 2011;**13**:e23-e34

[38] Profyris C, Tziotzios C, Do Vale I. Cutaneous scarring: Pathophysiology, molecular mechanisms, and scar reduction therapeutics: Part I. The molecular basis of scar formation. Journal of the American Academy of Dermatology. 2012;**66**(1):1-10

[39] DiPietro LA, Wilgus TA, Koh TJ. Macrophages in healing wounds: Paradoxes and paradigms. International Journal of Molecular Sciences. 2021; **22**(2):950

[40] Martin P, D'Souza D, Martin J, Grose R, Cooper L, Maki R, et al. Wound healing in the PU. 1 Null mouse—Tissue repair is not dependent on inflammatory cells. Current Biology. 2003;**13**(13): 1122-1128

[41] DiPietro LA, Polverini PJ. Role of the macrophage in the positive and negative regulation of wound neovascularization. Behring Institute Mitteilungen. 1993; **92**:238-247

[42] Eming SA, Krieg T, Davidson JM. Inflammation in wound repair: Molecular and cellular mechanisms. Journal of Investigative Dermatology. 2007;**127**(3):514-525

[43] Redd MJ, Cooper L, Wood W, Stramer B, Martin P. Wound healing and inflammation: Embryos reveal the way to perfect repair. Philosophical Transactions of the Royal Society of London B: Biological Sciences. 2004;**359** (1445):777-784

[44] Strodtbeck F. Physiology of wound healing. Newborn and Infant Nursing Reviews. 2001;**1**(1):43-52

[45] Bauer SM, Bauer RJ, Velazquez OC. Angiogenesis, vasculogenesis, and induction of healing in chronic wounds. Vascular and Endovascular Surgery. 2005;**39**(4):293-306

[46] Golebiewska EM, Poole AW. Platelet secretion: From haemostasis to wound healing and beyond. Blood Reviews. 2015;**29**(3):153-162

[47] Potekaev NN, Borzykh OB, Medvedev GV, Pushkin DV, Petrova MM, Petrov AV, et al. The role of extracellular matrix in skin wound healing. Journal of Clinical Medicine. 2021;**10**(24):5947

[48] Bielefeld KA, Amini-Nik S, Alman BA. Cutaneous wound healing: Recruiting developmental pathways for regeneration. Cellular and Molecular Life Sciences. 2013;**70**(12):2059-2081

[49] Veith AP, Henderson K, Spencer A, Sligar AD, Baker AB. Therapeutic strategies for enhancing angiogenesis in wound healing. Advanced Drug Delivery Reviews. 2019;**146**:97-125

[50] Galiano RD, Tepper OM, Pelo CR, Bhatt KA, Callaghan M, Bastidas N, et al.

Topical vascular endothelial growth factor accelerates diabetic wound healing through increased angiogenesis and by mobilizing and recruiting bone marrow-derived cells. The American Journal of Pathology. 2004;**164**(6): 1935-1947

[51] Opalenik SR, Davidson JM. Fibroblast differentiation of bone marrow-derived cells during wound repair. The FASEB Journal. 2005;**19**(11): 1561-1563

[52] Werner S, Krieg T, Smola H. Keratinocyte–fibroblast interactions in wound healing. Journal of Investigative Dermatology. 2007;**127**(5):998-1008

[53] Martin P. Wound healing—Aiming for perfect skin regeneration. Science. 1997;**276**(5309):75-81

[54] Lau K, Paus R, Tiede S, Day P, Bayat A. Exploring the role of stem cells in cutaneous wound healing. Experimental Dermatology. 2009;**18**(11):921-933

[55] Krafts KP. Tissue repair: The hidden drama. Organogenesis. 2010;**6**(4): 225-233

[56] Darby IA, Desmoulière A. Scar formation: Cellular mechanisms. In: Textbook on Scar Management. Cham: Springer; 2020. pp. 19-26

[57] Lux CN. Wound healing in animals: A review of physiology and clinical evaluation. Veterinary Dermatology. 2022;**33**(1):91-e27

[58] Mathew-Steiner SS, Roy S, Sen CK. Collagen in wound healing. Bioengineering. 2021;**8**(5):63

[59] Szabowski A, Maas-Szabowski N, Andrecht S, Kolbus A, Schorpp-Kistner M, Fusenig NE, et al. c-Jun and JunB antagonistically control cytokine-regulated mesenchymal–epidermal interaction in skin. Cell. 2000;**103**(5): 745-755

[60] Gurtner GC, Evans GR. Advances in head and neck reconstruction. Plastic and Reconstructive Surgery. 2000; **106**(3):672-682

[61] Levenson SM, Geever EF, Crowley LV, Oates JF III, Berard CW, Rosen H. Healing of rat skin wounds. Annals of Surgery. 1965;**161**(2):293-308

[62] Sarabahi S. Recent advances in topical wound care. Indian Journal of Plastic Surgery: Official Publication of the Association of Plastic Surgeons of India. 2012;**45**(2):379-387

[63] Jarbrink K, Ni G, Sönnergren H, Schmidtchen A, Pang C, Bajpai R, et al. The humanistic and economic burden of chronic wounds: a protocol for a systematic review. Systematic Reviews. 2017;**6**(1):15-21

[64] Sen CK. Human wound and its burden: Updated 2020 compendium of estimates. Advances in Wound Care. 2021;**10**(5):281-292

[65] Hamdan S, Pastar I, Drakulich S, Dikici E, Tomic-Canic M, Deo S, et al. Nanotechnology-driven therapeutic interventions in wound healing: Potential uses and applications. ACS Central Science. 2017;**3**(3):163-175

[66] Baranwal J, Barse B, Fais A, Delogu GL, Kumar A. Biopolymer: A sustainable material for food and medical applications. Polymers. 2022;**14**(5):983

[67] Veves A, Falanga V, Armstrong DG, Sabolinski ML. Graftskin, a human skin equivalent, is effective in the management of noninfected neuropathic diabetic foot ulcers: A prospective

randomized multicenter clinical trial. Diabetes Care. 2001;**24**(2): 290-295

[68] Marston WA, Hanft J, Norwood P, Pollak R. The efficacy and safety of dermagraft in improving the healing of chronic diabetic foot ulcers: Results of a prospective randomized trial. Diabetes Care. 2003;**26**(6):1701-1705

[69] Driver VR, Lavery LA, Reyzelman AM, Dutra TG, Dove CR, Kotsis SV, et al. A clinical trial of Integra Template for diabetic foot ulcer treatment. Wound Repair and Regeneration. 2015;**23**(6): 891-900

[70] Wei EX, Kirsner RS, Eaglstein WH. End points in dermatologic clinical trials: A review for clinicians. Journal of the American Academy of Dermatology. 2016;**75**(1):203-209

[71] Kalashnikova I, Das S, Seal S. Nanomaterials for wound healing: Scope and advancement. Nanomedicine. 2015; **10**(16):2593-2612

[72] Parani M, Lokhande G, Singh A, Gaharwar AK. Engineered nanomaterials for infection control and healing acute and chronic wounds. ACS Applied Materials & Interfaces. 2016;**8**(16): 10049-10069

[73] Tamer TM, Valachová K, Hassan MA, Omer AM, El-Shafeey M, Eldin MSM, et al. Chitosan/hyaluronan/edaravone membranes for anti-inflammatory wound dressing: In vitro and in vivo evaluation studies. Materials Science and Engineering: C. 2018;**90**: 227-235

[74] Zeng HY, Huang YC. Basic fibroblast growth factor released from fucoidan-modified chitosan/alginate scaffolds for promoting fibroblasts migration. Journal of Polymer Research. 2018;**25**(3):1-9

[75] Pastar I, Stojadinovic O, Yin NC, Ramirez H, Nusbaum AG, Sawaya A, et al. Epithelialization in wound healing: A comprehensive review. Advances in Wound Care. 2014;**3**(7):445-464

[76] Korrapati PS, Karthikeyan K, Satish A, Krishnaswamy VR, Venugopal JR, Ramakrishna S. Recent advancements in nanotechnological strategies in selection, design and delivery of biomolecules for skin regeneration. Materials Science and Engineering: C. 2016;**67**:747-765

[77] Wang F, Zhang W, Li H, Chen X, Feng S, Mei Z. How effective are nano-based dressings in diabetic wound healing? A comprehensive review of literature. International Journal of Nanomedicine. 2022;**17**:2097

[78] Mordorski B, Rosen J, Friedman A. Nanotechnology as an innovative approach for accelerating wound healing in diabetes. Diabetes Management. 2015; **5**(5):329-332

[79] Gaharwar AK, Peppas NA, Khademhosseini A. Nanocomposite hydrogels for biomedical applications. Biotechnology and Bioengineering. 2014; **111**(3):441-453

[80] Kumar N, Chamoli P, Misra M, Manoj MK, Sharma A. Advanced metal and carbon nanostructures for medical, drug delivery and bio-imaging applications. Nanoscale. 2022;**14**: 3987-4017

[81] Kaler A, Mittal AK, Katariya M, Harde H, Agrawal AK, Jain S, et al. An investigation of in vivo wound healing activity of biologically synthesized silver nanoparticles. Journal of Nanoparticle Research. 2014;**16**(9):2605-2614

[82] Mihai MM, Dima MB, Dima B, Holban AM. Nanomaterials for wound

healing and infection control. Materials. 2019;**12**(13):2176

[83] Lara HH, Garza-Treviño EN, Ixtepan-Turrent L, Singh DK. Silver nanoparticles are broad-spectrum bactericidal and virucidal compounds. Journal of Nanobiotechnology. 2011; **9**(1):30-37

[84] Singh BR, Singh BN, Singh A, Khan W, Naqvi AH, Singh HB. Mycofabricated biosilver nanoparticles interrupt *Pseudomonas aeruginosa* quorum sensing systems. Scientific Reports. 2015;**5**:13719

[85] Bragg PD, Rainnie DJ. The effect of silver ions on the respiratory chain of *Escherichia coli*. Canadian Journal of Microbiology. 1974;**20**(6):883-889

[86] Xiu ZM, Zhang QB, Puppala HL, Colvin VL, Alvarez PJ. Negligible particle-specific antibacterial activity of silver nanoparticles. Nano Letters. 2012; **12**(8):4271-4275

[87] Frankova J, Pivodova V, Vágnerová H, Juráňová J, Ulrichová J. Effects of silver nanoparticles on primary cell cultures of fibroblasts and keratinocytes in a wound-healing model. Journal of Applied Biomaterials & Functional Materials. 2016;**14**(2):137-142

[88] Tian J, Wong KK, Ho CM, Lok CN, Yu WY, Che CM, et al. Topical delivery of silver nanoparticles promotes wound healing. ChemMedChem: Chemistry Enabling Drug Discovery. 2007;**2**(1): 129-136

[89] Patra JK, Baek KH. Novel green synthesis of gold nanoparticles using Citrullus lanatus rind and investigation of proteasome inhibitory activity, antibacterial, and antioxidant potential. International journal of nanomedicine. 2015;**10**:7253-7264

[90] Yang X, Yang J, Wang L, Ran B, Jia Y, Zhang L, et al. Pharmaceutical intermediate-modified gold nanoparticles: Against multidrug-resistant bacteria and wound-healing application via an electrospun scaffold. ACS Nano. 2017;**11**(6):5737-5745

[91] Gobin AM, O'Neal DP, Watkins DM, Halas NJ, Drezek RA, West JL. Near infrared laser-tissue welding using nanoshells as an exogenous absorber. Lasers in Surgery and Medicine. 2005;**37** (2):123-129

[92] Khatami M, Varma RS, Zafarnia N, Yaghoobi H, Sarani M, Kumar VG. Applications of green synthesized Ag, ZnO and Ag/ZnO nanoparticles for making clinical antimicrobial wound-healing bandages. Sustainable Chemistry and Pharmacy. 2018;**10**:9-15

[93] Shao F, Yang A, Yu DM, Wang J, Gong X, Tian HX. Bio-synthesis of *Barleria gibsoni* leaf extract mediated zinc oxide nanoparticles and their formulation gel for wound therapy in nursing care of infants and children. Journal of Photochemistry and Photobiology B: Biology. 2018;**189**: 267-273

[94] Kantipudi S, Sunkara JR, Rallabhandi M, Thonangi CV, Cholla RD, Kollu P, et al. Enhanced wound healing activity of Ag–ZnO composite NPs in Wistar Albino rats. IET Nanobiotechnology. 2017;**12**(4):473-478

[95] Pati R, Mehta RK, Mohanty S, Padhi A, Sengupta M, Vaseeharan B, et al. Topical application of zinc oxide nanoparticles reduces bacterial skin infection in mice and exhibits antibacterial activity by inducing oxidative stress response and cell membrane disintegration in macrophages. Nanomedicine:

Nanotechnology, Biology and Medicine. 2014;**10**(6):1195-1208

[96] Ziv-Polat O, Topaz M, Brosh T, Margel S. Enhancement of incisional wound healing by thrombin conjugated iron oxide nanoparticles. Biomaterials. 2010;**31**(4):741-747

[97] Mir M, Ali MN, Barakullah A, Gulzar A, Arshad M, Fatima S, et al. Synthetic polymeric biomaterials for wound healing: A review. Progress in Biomaterials. 2018;**7**(1):1-21

[98] Perumal G, Pappuru S, Chakraborty D, Nandkumar AM, Chand DK, Doble M. Synthesis and characterization of curcumin loaded PLA—Hyperbranched polyglycerol electrospun blend for wound dressing applications. Materials Science and Engineering: C. 2017;**76**: 1196-1204

[99] Chereddy KK, Coco R, Memvanga PB, Ucakar B, des Rieux A, Vandermeulen G, et al. Combined effect of PLGA and curcumin on wound healing activity. Journal of Controlled Release. 2013;**171**(2):208-215

[100] Liao J, Jia Y, Wang B, Shi K, Qian Z. Injectable hybrid poly (ε-caprolactone)-b-poly (ethylene glycol)-b-poly (ε-caprolactone) porous microspheres/ alginate hydrogel cross-linked by calcium gluconate crystals deposited in the pores of microspheres improved skin wound healing. ACS Biomaterials Science & Engineering. 2018;**4**(3): 1029-1036

[101] Chen FM, Liu X. Advancing biomaterials of human origin for tissue engineering. Progress in Polymer Science. 2016;**53**:86-168

[102] Rath G, Hussain T, Chauhan G, Garg T, Goyal AK. Collagen nanofiber containing silver nanoparticles for improved wound-healing applications. Journal of Drug Targeting. 2016;**24**(6): 520-529

[103] Bilgic HAYATİ, Demiriz M, Ozler M, Ide T, Dogan N, Gumus S, et al. Gelatin based scaffolds and effect of EGF dose on wound healing. Journal of Biomaterials and Tissue Engineering. 2013;**3**(2):205-211

[104] Okamoto Y, Yano R, Miyatake K, Tomohiro I, Shigemasa Y, Minami S. Effects of chitin and chitosan on blood coagulation. Carbohydrate Polymers. 2003;**53**(3):337-342

[105] Xu J, Strandman S, Zhu JX, Barralet J, Cerruti M. Genipin-crosslinked catechol-chitosan mucoadhesive hydrogels for buccal drug delivery. Biomaterials. 2015;**37**:395-404

[106] Lu Z, Gao J, He Q, Wu J, Liang D, Yang H, et al. Enhanced antibacterial and wound healing activities of microporous chitosan-Ag/ZnO composite dressing. Carbohydrate Polymers. 2017;**156**:460-469

[107] Ding L, Shan X, Zhao X, Zha H, Chen X, Wang J, et al. Spongy bilayer dressing composed of chitosan–Ag nanoparticles and chitosan–*Bletilla striata* polysaccharide for wound healing applications. Carbohydrate Polymers. 2017;**157**:1538-1547

[108] Ehterami A, Salehi M, Farzamfar S, Vaez A, Samadian H, Sahrapeyma H, et al. In vitro and in vivo study of PCL/ collagen wound dressing loaded with insulin-chitosan nanoparticles on cutaneous wound healing in rats model. International Journal of Biological Macromolecules. 2018;**117**:601-609

[109] Kim MH, Park H, Nam HC, Park SR, Jung JY, Park WH. Injectable methylcellulose hydrogel containing

silver oxide nanoparticles for burn wound healing. Carbohydrate Polymers. 2018;**181**:579-586

[110] Singla R, Soni S, Kulurkar PM, Kumari A, Mahesh S, Patial V, et al. In situ functionalized nanobiocomposites dressings of bamboo cellulose nanocrystals and silver nanoparticles for accelerated wound healing. Carbohydrate Polymers. 2017a;**155**: 152-162

[111] Singla R, Soni S, Patial V, Kulurkar PM, Kumari A, Mahesh S, et al. In vivo diabetic wound healing potential of nanobiocomposites containing bamboo cellulose nanocrystals impregnated with silver nanoparticles. International Journal of Biological Macromolecules. 2017b;**105**:45-55

[112] Singla R, Soni S, Patial V, Kulurkar PM, Kumari A, Padwad YS, et al. Cytocompatible anti-microbial dressings of *Syzygium cumini* cellulose nanocrystals decorated with silver nanoparticles accelerate acute and diabetic wound healing. Scientific Reports. 2017c; **7**(1):1-13

[113] Sun T, Zhan B, Zhang W, Qin D, Xia G, Zhang H, et al. Carboxymethyl chitosan nanoparticles loaded with bioactive peptide OH-CATH30 benefit nonscar wound healing. International Journal of Nanomedicine. 2018;**13**:5771

[114] Fumakia M, Ho EA. Nanoparticles encapsulated with LL37 and serpin A1 promotes wound healing and synergistically enhances antibacterial activity. Molecular Pharmaceutics. 2016; **13**(7):2318-2331

[115] Yeboah A, Cohen RI, Faulknor R, Schloss R, Yarmush ML, Berthiaume F. The development and characterization of SDF1α-elastin-like-peptide nanoparticles for wound healing. Journal of Controlled Release. 2016;**232**:238-247

[116] Senturk B, Mercan S, Delibasi T, Guler MO, Tekinay AB. Angiogenic peptide nanofibers improve wound healing in STZ-induced diabetic rats. ACS Biomaterials Science & Engineering. 2016;**2**(7):1180-1189

[117] Yergoz F, Hastar N, Cimenci CE, Ozkan AD, Tekinay T, Guler MO, et al. Heparin mimetic peptide nanofiber gel promotes regeneration of full thickness burn injury. Biomaterials. 2017;**134**: 117-127

[118] Deng A, Yang Y, Du S, Yang S. Electrospinning of in situ crosslinked recombinant human collagen peptide/ chitosan nanofibers for wound healing. Biomaterials Science. 2018;**6**(8): 2197-2208

[119] Xi Y, Ge J, Guo Y, Lei B, Ma PX. Biomimetic elastomeric polypeptide-based nanofibrous matrix for overcoming multidrug-resistant bacteria and enhancing full-thickness wound healing/skin regeneration. ACS Nano. 2018;**12**:10772-10784

[120] Santos JCC, Mansur AA, Ciminelli VS, Mansur HS. Nanocomposites of poly (vinyl alcohol)/functionalized-multiwall carbon nanotubes conjugated with glucose oxidase for potential application as scaffolds in skin wound healing. International Journal of Polymeric Materials and Polymeric Biomaterials. 2014;**63**(4):185-196

[121] Mahmoudi N, Eslahi N, Mehdipour A, Mohammadi M, Akbari M, Samadikuchaksaraei A, et al. Temporary skin grafts based on hybrid graphene oxide-natural biopolymer nanofibers as effective wound healing substitutes: Pre-clinical and pathological studies in animal models. Journal of Materials

Science: Materials in Medicine. 2017; **28**(5):73-85

[122] Kawamoto K, Miyaji H, Nishida E, Miyata S, Kato A, Tateyama A, et al. Characterization and evaluation of graphene oxide scaffold for periodontal wound healing of class II furcation defects in dog. International Journal of Nanomedicine. 2018;**13**:2365-2376

[123] Bankoti K, Rameshbabu AP, Datta S, Das B, Mitra A, Dhara S. Onion derived carbon nanodots for live cell imaging and accelerated skin wound healing. Journal of Materials Chemistry B. 2017;**5**(32):6579-6592

[124] Zhou X, Wang H, Zhang J, Li X, Wu Y, Wei Y, et al. Functional poly (ε-caprolactone)/chitosan dressings with nitric oxide-releasing property improve wound healing. Acta Biomaterialia. 2017; **54**:128-137

[125] Lu Z, Dai T, Huang L, Kurup DB, Tegos GP, Jahnke A, et al. Photodynamic therapy with a cationic functionalized fullerene rescues mice from fatal wound infections. Nanomedicine. 2010;**5**(10): 1525-1533

[126] Küchler S, Wolf NB, Heilmann S, Weindl G, Helfmann J, Yahya MM, et al. 3D-wound healing model: Influence of morphine and solid lipid nanoparticles. Journal of Biotechnology. 2010;**148**(1): 24-30

[127] Xu HL, Chen PP, Wang LF, Tong MQ, Ou ZH, Zhao YZ, et al. Skin-permeable liposome improved stability and permeability of bFGF against skin of mice with deep second degree scald to promote hair follicle neogenesis through inhibition of scar formation. Colloids and Surfaces B: Biointerfaces. 2018;**172**:573-585

[128] Gauthier A, Fisch A, Seuwen K, Baumgarten B, Ruffner H, Aebi A, et al. Glucocorticoid-loaded liposomes induce a pro-resolution phenotype in human primary macrophages to support chronic wound healing. Biomaterials. 2018;**178**: 481-495

[129] Gainza G, Bonafonte DC, Moreno B, Aguirre JJ, Gutierrez FB, Villullas S, et al. The topical administration of rhEGF-loaded nanostructured lipid carriers (rhEGF-NLC) improves healing in a porcine full-thickness excisional wound model. Journal of Controlled Release. 2015;**197**:41-47

[130] Gong C, Wu Q, Wang Y, Zhang D, Luo F, Zhao X, et al. A biodegradable hydrogel system containing curcumin encapsulated in micelles for cutaneous wound healing. Biomaterials. 2013;**34** (27):6377-6387

[131] Bonferoni MC, Sandri G, Dellera E, Rossi S, Ferrari F, Mori M, et al. Ionic polymeric micelles based on chitosan and fatty acids and intended for wound healing. Comparison of linoleic and oleic acid. European Journal of Pharmaceutics and Biopharmaceutics. 2014;**87**(1): 101-106

[132] Cardoso AM, de Oliveira EG, Coradini K, Bruinsmann FA, Aguirre T, Lorenzoni R, et al. Chitosan hydrogels containing nanoencapsulated phenytoin for cutaneous use: Skin permeation/ penetration and efficacy in wound healing. Materials Science and Engineering: C. 2019;**96**:205-217

[133] Krausz AE, Adler BL, Cabral V, Navati M, Doerner J, Charafeddine RA, et al. Curcumin-encapsulated nanoparticles as innovative antimicrobial and wound healing agent. Nanomedicine: Nanotechnology, Biology and Medicine. 2015;**11**(1):195-206

[134] Karri VVSR, Kuppusamy G, Talluri SV, Mannemala SS, Kollipara R,

Wadhwani AD, et al. Curcumin loaded chitosan nanoparticles impregnated into collagen-alginate scaffolds for diabetic wound healing. International Journal of Biological Macromolecules. 2016;**93**: 1519-1529

[135] Li L, Xing R, Li J, Li P. Fabrication of guanidinylated chitosan nanoparticles loaded with bioactive factors for facilitating wound healing. International Journal of Polymeric Materials and Polymeric Biomaterials. 2022;**71**(3): 173-179

[136] Liu J, Chen Z, Wang J, Li R, Li T, Chang M, et al. Encapsulation of curcumin nanoparticles with MMP9-responsive and thermos-sensitive hydrogel improves diabetic wound healing. ACS Applied Materials & Interfaces. 2018;**10**(19):16315-16326

[137] Ugazio E, Gastaldi L, Brunella V, Scalarone D, Jadhav SA, Oliaro-Bosso S, et al. Thermoresponsive mesoporous silica nanoparticles as a carrier for skin delivery of quercetin. International Journal of Pharmaceutics. 2016;**511**(1): 446-454

[138] Vedakumari WS, Ayaz N, Karthick AS, Senthil R, Sastry TP. Quercetin impregnated chitosan–fibrin composite scaffolds as potential wound dressing materials—Fabrication, characterization and in vivo analysis. European Journal of Pharmaceutical Sciences. 2017;**97**:106-112

[139] Manconi M, Manca ML, Caddeo C, Cencetti C, di Meo C, Zoratto N, et al. Preparation of gellan-cholesterol nanohydrogels embedding baicalin and evaluation of their wound healing activity. European Journal of Pharmaceutics and Biopharmaceutics. 2018;**127**:244-249

[140] Schaffer MR, Efron PA, Thornton FJ, Klingel K, Gross SS, Barbul A. Nitric oxide, an autocrine regulator of wound fibroblast synthetic function. The Journal of Immunology. 1997;**158**(5): 2375-2381

[141] Englander L, Friedman A. Nitric oxide nanoparticle technology: A novel antimicrobial agent in the context of current treatment of skin and soft tissue infection. The Journal of Clinical and Aesthetic Dermatology. 2010;**3**(6):45

[142] Han G, Martinez LR, Mihu MR, Friedman AJ, Friedman JM, Nosanchuk JD. Nitric oxide releasing nanoparticles are therapeutic for *Staphylococcus aureus* abscesses in a murine model of infection. PloS ONE. 2009;**4**(11):e7804

[143] Zhou Z, Joslin S, Dellinger A, Ehrich M, Brooks B, Ren Q, et al. A novel class of compounds with cutaneous wound healing properties. Journal of Biomedical Nanotechnology. 2010;**6**(5):605-611

[144] Barraud N, Schleheck D, Klebensberger J, Webb JS, Hassett DJ, Rice SA, et al. Nitric oxide signaling in *Pseudomonas aeruginosa* biofilms mediates phosphodiesterase activity, decreased cyclic di-GMP levels, and enhanced dispersal. Journal of Bacteriology. 2009;**191**(23):7333-7342

[145] Pelegrino MT, Weller RB, Chen X, Bernardes JS, Seabra AB. Chitosan nanoparticles for nitric oxide delivery in human skin. MedChemComm. 2017; **8**(4):713-719

[146] Boateng JS, Matthews KH, Stevens HN, Eccleston GM. Wound healing dressings and drug delivery systems: A review. Journal of Pharmaceutical Sciences. 2008;**97**(8):2892-2923

[147] Scales BS, Huffnagle GB. The microbiome in wound repair and tissue

fibrosis. The Journal of Pathology. 2013; **229**(2):323-331

[148] Hurler J, Berg OA, Skar M, Conradi AH, Johnsen PJ, Škalko-Basnet N. Improved burns therapy: Liposomes-in-hydrogel delivery system for mupirocin. Journal of Pharmaceutical Sciences. 2012;**101**(10):3906-3915

[149] Sharma A, Kumar Arya D, Dua M, Chhatwal GS, Johri AK. Nano-technology for targeted drug delivery to combat antibiotic resistance. Expert Opinion on Drug Delivery. 2012;**9**(11): 1325-1332

[150] Cerchiara T, Abruzzo A, Palomino RAÑ, Vitali B, De Rose R, Chidichimo G, et al. Spanish Broom (*Spartium junceum* L.) fibers impregnated with vancomycin-loaded chitosan nanoparticles as new antibacterial wound dressing: Preparation, characterization and antibacterial activity. European Journal of Pharmaceutical Sciences. 2017;**99**: 105-112

[151] Monteiro N, Martins M, Martins A, Fonseca NA, Moreira JN, Reis RL, et al. Antibacterial activity of chitosan nanofiber meshes with liposomes immobilized releasing gentamicin. Acta Biomaterialia. 2015;**18**:196-205

[152] Leung V, Ko F. Biomedical applications of nanofibers. Polymers for Advanced Technologies. 2011;**22**(3): 350-365

[153] Lee K, Silva EA, Mooney DJ. Growth factor delivery-based tissue engineering: General approaches and a review of recent developments. Journal of the Royal Society Interface. 2011;**8** (55):153-170

[154] Vasile BS, Oprea O, Voicu G, Ficai A, Andronescu E, Teodorescu A, et al. Synthesis and characterization of a novel controlled release zinc oxide/ gentamicin–chitosan composite with potential applications in wounds care. International Journal of Pharmaceutics. 2014;**463**(2):161-169

[155] Sabitha M, Rajiv S. Preparation and characterization of ampicillin-incorporated electrospun polyurethane scaffolds for wound healing and infection control. Polymer Engineering & Science. 2015;**55**(3):541-548

[156] Niamlang P, Tongrain T, Ekabutr P, Chuysinuan P, Supaphol P. Preparation, characterization and biocompatibility of poly (vinyl alcohol) films containing tetracycline hydrochloride-loaded quaternized chitosan nanoparticles. Journal of Drug Delivery Science and Technology. 2017;**38**:36-44

[157] Alavarse AC, de Oliveira Silva FW, Colque JT, da Silva VM, Prieto T, Venancio EC, et al. Tetracycline hydrochloride-loaded electrospun nanofibers mats based on PVA and chitosan for wound dressing. Materials Science and Engineering: C. 2017;**77**: 271-281

[158] Tocco I, Zavan B, Bassetto F, Vindigni V. Nanotechnology-based therapies for skin wound regeneration. Journal of Nanomaterials. 2012;**2012**:4

[159] Nosrati H, Aramideh Khouy R, Nosrati A, Khodaei M, Banitalebi-Dehkordi M, Ashrafi-Dehkordi K, et al. Nanocomposite scaffolds for accelerating chronic wound healing by enhancing angiogenesis. Journal of Nanobiotechnology. 2021;**19**(1):1-21

[160] Bigliardi PL, Tobin DJ, Gaveriaux-Ruff C, Bigliardi-Qi M. Opioids and the skin—Where do we stand? Experimental Dermatology. 2009;**18**(5):424-430

[161] Lee CH, Chang SH, Chen WJ, Hung KC, Lin YH, Liu SJ, et al. Augmentation of diabetic wound healing and enhancement of collagen content using nanofibrous glucophage-loaded collagen/PLGA scaffold membranes. Journal of Colloid and Interface Science. 2015;**439**:88-97

[162] Augustine R, Dominic EA, Reju I, Kaimal B, Kalarikkal N, Thomas S. Electrospun poly (ε-caprolactone)-based skin substitutes: In vivo evaluation of wound healing and the mechanism of cell proliferation. Journal of Biomedical Materials Research Part B: Applied Biomaterials. 2015;**103**(7): 1445-1454

[163] Miguel SP, Ribeiro MP, Coutinho P, Correia IJ. Electrospun polycaprolactone/Aloe vera_chitosan nanofibrous asymmetric membranes aimed for wound healing applications. Polymers. 2017;**9**(5):183

[164] Xie Z, Paras CB, Weng H, Punnakitikashem P, Su LC, Vu K, et al. Dual growth factor releasing multi-functional nanofibers for wound healing. Acta Biomaterialia. 2013;**9**(12):9351-9359

[165] Jafari A, Hassanajili S, Karimi MB, Emami A, Ghaffari F, Azarpira N. Effect of organic/inorganic nanoparticles on performance of polyurethane nanocomposites for potential wound dressing applications. Journal of the Mechanical Behavior of Biomedical Materials. 2018;**88**:395-405

[166] Amanzadi B, Mirzaei E, Hassanzadeh G, Mahdaviani P, Boroumand S, Abdollahi M, et al. Chitosan-based layered nanofibers loaded with herbal extract as wound-dressing materials on wound model studies. Biointerface Research in Applied Chemistry. 2019;**9**:3979-3986

[167] Akturk O, Kismet K, Yasti AC, Kuru S, Duymus ME, Kaya F, et al. Collagen/gold nanoparticle nanocomposites: A potential skin wound healing biomaterial. Journal of Biomaterials Applications. 2016;**31**(2):283-301

[168] Wu H, Li F, Wang S, Lu J, Li J, Du Y, et al. Ceria nanocrystals decorated mesoporous silica nanoparticle based ROS-scavenging tissue adhesive for highly efficient regenerative wound healing. Biomaterials. 2018;**151**:66-77

[169] Li Y, Jiang H, Zheng W, Gong N, Chen L, Jiang X, et al. Bacterial cellulose–hyaluronan nanocomposite biomaterials as wound dressings for severe skin injury repair. Journal of Materials Chemistry B. 2015;**3**(17):3498-3507

[170] Sandri G, Aguzzi C, Rossi S, Bonferoni MC, Bruni G, Boselli C, et al. Halloysite and chitosan oligosaccharide nanocomposite for wound healing. Acta Biomaterialia. 2017;**57**:216-224

[171] Kota SK, Meher LK, Jammula S, Kota SK, Krishna SVS, Modi KD. Aberrant angiogenesis: The gateway to diabetic complications. Indian Journal of Endocrinology and Metabolism. 2012; **16**(6):918

[172] Singer AJ, Clark RA. Cutaneous wound healing. New England Journal of Medicine. 1999;**341**(10):738-746

[173] Garcia-Orue I, Pedraz JL, Hernandez RM, Igartua M. Nanotechnology-based delivery systems to release growth factors and other endogenous molecules for chronic wound healing. Journal of Drug Delivery Science and Technology. 2017;**42**:2-17

[174] Pan A, Zhong M, Wu H, Peng Y, Xia H, Tang Q, et al. Topical application of keratinocyte growth factor conjugated gold nanoparticles accelerate wound

healing. Nanomedicine: Nanotechnology, Biology and Medicine. 2018;**14**(5):1619-1628

[175] Goh M, Hwang Y, Tae G. Epidermal growth factor loaded heparin-based hydrogel sheet for skin wound healing. Carbohydrate Polymers. 2016;**147**: 251-260

[176] Mohandas A, Anisha BS, Chennazhi KP, Jayakumar R. Chitosan–hyaluronic acid/VEGF loaded fibrin nanoparticles composite sponges for enhancing angiogenesis in wounds. Colloids and Surfaces B: Biointerfaces. 2015;**127**: 105-113

[177] Luan A, Hu MS, Leavitt T, Brett EA, Wang KC, Longaker MT, et al. Noncoding RNAs in wound healing: A new and vast frontier. Advances in Wound Care. 2018;7(1):19-27

[178] de Kerckhove M, Tanaka K, Umehara T, Okamoto M, Kanematsu S, Hayashi H, et al. Targeting miR-223 in neutrophils enhances the clearance of *Staphylococcus aureus* in infected wounds. EMBO Molecular Medicine. 2018;**10**(10):e9024-e90444

[179] Castleberry SA, Almquist BD, Li W, Reis T, Chow J, Mayner S, et al. Self-assembled wound dressings silence MMP-9 and improve diabetic wound healing in vivo. Advanced Materials. 2016;**28**(9):1809-1817

[180] Whittam AJ, Maan ZN, Duscher D, Wong VW, Barrera JA, Januszyk M, et al. Challenges and opportunities in drug delivery for wound healing. Advances in Wound Care. 2016;**5**(2):79-88

[181] Randeria PS, Seeger MA, Wang XQ, Wilson H, Shipp D, Mirkin CA, et al. siRNA-based spherical nucleic acids reverse impaired wound healing in diabetic mice by ganglioside GM3 synthase knockdown. Proceedings of the National Academy of Sciences. 2015;**112** (18):5573-5578

[182] Wang C, Ma L, Gao C. Design of gene-activated matrix for the repair of skin and cartilage. Polymer Journal. 2014;**46**(8):476-482

[183] Choi JS, Kim HS, Yoo HS. Electrospinning strategies of drug-incorporated nanofibrous mats for wound recovery. Drug Delivery and Translational Research. 2015;**5**(2): 137-145

[184] Kobsa S, Kristofik NJ, Sawyer AJ, Bothwell AL, Kyriakides TR, Saltzman WM. An electrospun scaffold integrating nucleic acid delivery for treatment of full-thickness wounds. Biomaterials. 2013;**34**(15):3891-3901

[185] Ojeh N, Pastar I, Tomic-Canic M, Stojadinovic O. Stem cells in skin regeneration, wound healing, and their clinical applications. International Journal of Molecular Sciences. 2015;**16** (10):25476-25501

[186] Shabbir A, Cox A, Rodriguez-Menocal L, Salgado M, Badiavas EV. Mesenchymal stem cell exosomes induce proliferation and migration of normal and chronic wound fibroblasts, and enhance angiogenesis in vitro. Stem Cells and Development. 2015;**24**(14): 1635-1647

[187] Tartarini D, Mele E. Adult stem cell therapies for wound healing: biomaterials and computational models. Frontiers in Bioengineering and Biotechnology. 2016;**3**:206-212

[188] Li M, Zhao Y, Hao H, Han W, Fu X. Mesenchymal stem cell–based therapy for nonhealing wounds: Today and tomorrow. Wound Repair and Regeneration. 2015;**23**(4):465-482

[189] Ma K, Liao S, He L, Lu J, Ramakrishna S, Chan CK. Effects of nanofiber/stem cell composite on wound healing in acute full-thickness skin wounds. Tissue Engineering Part A. 2011;**17**(9-10):1413-1424

[190] Chueng STD, Yang L, Zhang Y, Lee KB. Multidimensional nanomaterials for the control of stem cell fate. Nano Convergence. 2016;**3**(1):23-38

[191] Tang T, Jiang H, Yu Y, He F, Ji SZ, Liu YY, et al. A new method of wound treatment: Targeted therapy of skin wounds with reactive oxygen species-responsive nanoparticles containing SDF-1α. International Journal of Nanomedicine. 2015;**10**:6571-6585

[192] Yi H, Rehman FU, Zhao C, Liu B, He N. Recent advances in nano scaffolds for bone repair. Bone Research. 2016;**4**: 16050

[193] Guo B, Lei B, Li P, Ma PX. Functionalized scaffolds to enhance tissue regeneration. Regenerative Biomaterials. 2015;**2**(1):47-57

[194] Edwards SL, Werkmeister JA, Ramshaw JA. Carbon nanotubes in scaffolds for tissue engineering. Expert Review of Medical Devices. 2009;**6**(5): 499-505

[195] Shi J, Votruba AR, Farokhzad OC, Langer R. Nanotechnology in drug delivery and tissue engineering: From discovery to applications. Nano Letters. 2010;**10**(9):3223-3230

[196] van Rijt S, Habibovic P. Enhancing regenerative approaches with nanoparticles. Journal of the Royal Society Interface. 2017;**14**(129): 20170093

[197] De Witte TM, Fratila-Apachitei LE, Zadpoor AA, Peppas NA. Bone tissue engineering via growth factor delivery: From scaffolds to complex matrices. Regenerative Biomaterials. 2018;**5**(4): 197-211

[198] Walmsley GG, McArdle A, Tevlin R, Momeni A, Atashroo D, Hu MS, et al. Nanotechnology in bone tissue engineering. Nanomedicine: Nanotechnology, Biology and Medicine. 2015;**11**(5):1253-1263

Chapter 11

Banks of Cryopreserved Skin from Live Donors and Total Skin Allografts in the Surgery of Major Burnt Patients

Marcelo Fonseca Canteros, Aldo Cañete Soto, Dino Ibaceta Orlandini, Jennifer Gómez Aguilera, Paulina Acuña Salazar, Luana Mandriaza Muñoz, Catalina Buchroithner Haase, Manuel Moya Delgado, Giovanni Vivas Rosales, Nicolle Delgado Cárcamo, Florencia Disi Parga, María Belén Larrea Aguilar and María José Pulgar Leyton

Abstract

Scarectomy and prompt coverage are some of the main cornerstones of the actual treatment of major burnt patients. This coverage can be definitive using autologous tissues or temporary with allografts, xenografts, and/or biosynthetic products. Skin allografts (SAs) are the gold standard therapeutic alternative among temporary coverages, since they mimic skin functions. However, cadaveric skin donation and procurement, a common SA source, are infrequent. On the other hand, there is a significant number of patients that, given their health condition, large amounts of skin must be resected for their clinical recovery, including patients submitted to corporal contouring surgeries with esthetic and/or reconstructive motives, usually eliminating the redundant skin as biological waste. This study describes a skin bank model from live donors and cryopreserved total skin cutaneous allografts (CTSCAs), a new type of SA resulting from a particular skin processing.

Keywords: skin allograft, skin bank, burns, cryopreserved total skin cutaneous allografts, Burn Patients

1. Introduction

Since the XX century and due to Janzecovich's contributions, scarectomy and prompt coverage of major burnt patients have become one of the mainstays of the surgical treatment [1–3].

This coverage can be definitive, using autologous tissues, or temporary. The lack of availability of donor areas, infected or doubtful vitality beddings, or graft procurement associated with a morbimortality increase are conditions where temporary coverages are preferred. The latter is done using allografts, xenografts, and/or biosynthetic products, which mimic the skin functions and provide a physiological coverage that permits hydro electrolytic loss control, pain and infection risk reduction, and improvement of the local conditions of the bedding.

Skin allografts (SAs) are the gold standard therapeutic alternative among temporary coverages. Their natural evolution consists of its rejection between days 8 and 10, being retarded in major burnt patients, due to the immune system depression between days 15 and 30 [4–7].

In burnt patients, the use of SA began in 1881, when Girdner treated a patient with severe burns with cadaveric SA [8]. Subsequently, Brown et al. popularized SA as biologic grafts in extensive burns [9–10]. The growing need for SA for managing these patients was responsible for the creation of establishments capable of storing skin during the 50th decade. These centers are usually located inside or near hospitals or burnt centers to satisfy the burnt patient's needs and, on the other hand, promote skin donation with high-quality standards [11–14].

The SA necessity resulted in the emergence of facilities for skin storage during the 1950s. Most of them were located inside or near hospitals or burnt centers, permitting, on the one hand, satisfying the burnt patient's needs and, on the other hand, encouraging skin donation with high-security standards [8, 9].

SAs are usually obtained from cadaveric donors in the context of multiorgan donation. They are obtained with a dermatome as partial skin grafts, preserved with high concentrated glycerol, resulting in cellular death and not viable tissue [15].

The relative shortness of donors encouraged the search and use of other SA sources, as live donors submitted to surgeries resulting in skin redundancy and the need for its resection for reconstructive and/or esthetic motives [16–19].

This study aims to describe the clinical features of SAs, particularly cryopreserved total skin cutaneous allografts (CTSCAs) and a model of skin banks from live donors.

2. Cryopreserved total skin cutaneous allografts (CTSCAs)

CTSCAs emerge from the need and search for coverage for burnt patients and complex wounds associated with a low organ and tissue donation rate. Compared to the classical SAs, CTSCAs have three distinctive features: a) derived from live donors, b) total thickness skin, and c) cryopreserved [20, 21].

2.1 Live donors

It is crucial to emphasize that the skin donation request is done in the context of elective surgery and happiness due to the primary esthetic and functional expected results and not in an environment of familiar sadness of skin procurement in cadaveric donors, where the donor remains with a social altruism sensation secondary to the donation of a tissue that would otherwise be a surgical waste. The extensive inclusion and exclusion criteria for skin donation in cadaveric donors (**Table 1**) in order to guarantee the microbiological safety of the tissues are left aside in live donors, since it is understood that patients submitted to elective body contour surgeries do not have contraindications for the performance of such surgeries and the consequently tissue donation.

Exclusion criteria:
a. For infectious diseases
Patients with history or carriers of HIV/AIDS.
Patients with a history of Hepatitis B or C.
Patients with a history of active Tuberculosis.
Patients diagnosed with Syphilis or positive VDRL.
Patients diagnosed with HTLV I and II.
Patients diagnosed with Chagas disease.
Patients with diagnosis of Rabies, Congenital Rubella and Malaria.
Patients diagnosed with untreated bacterial or fungal endocarditis.
b. For central nervous system diseases
- Degenerative diseases
- Any type or manifestation of Dementia.
- Alzheimer's disease.
- Parkinson's disease.
- Multiple sclerosis.
- Creutzfeldt-Jakob disease.

Infectious diseases
- Bacterial encephalitis.
- Viral, fungal or parasitic meningitis.
- Bacterial meningitis.
- Progressive multifocal leukoencephalopathy.
- Subacute sclerosing panencephalitis.
- Active viral encephalitis or encephalitis of unknown cause.
- Fungal or parasitic encephalitis.

c. For presence of cancer and/or tumors
- History of neoplasia except for cervical uterine cancer in situ.
- Lymphadenopathy for more than one month.
- Lymphomas, lymphosarcomas
- Leukemias.
- Metastasis of primary or secondary malignant tumors (lung, breast, cervical, colon, prostate, squamous cell, melanomas, lymphomas, leukemias, central nervous system, among others).

d. Other pathologies
- Patients who have been treated with growth hormone.
- Patients with Hemophilia.
- Patients carriers of autoimmune diseases or Mesenchymopathies such as Rheumatoid Arthritis, Systemic Lupus Erythematosus.
- Patients who have been treated with prolonged corticosteroid therapy.
- Any suspicious skin alteration.

e. Behavioral:
- Unsafe sexual behavior.
- Drug abuse (including intravenous, intramuscular and subcutaneous).
- Commercial sex workers.
- Inmates.
- Individuals with tattoos, (or) body piercing performed in the last 6 months.
- Individuals from whom no history of sexual behavior can be collected.

f. Specific skin criteria:
- Skin contaminated by toxins.
- Pyoderma.
- Any skin lesion: infectious, traumatic or vascular.
- Psoriasis.
- Epidermolysis bullosa.
- Loxocelism.
- Structurally damaged skin (due to autoimmune or collagen diseases).

HIV, human immunodeficiency virus; HTLV, human T-lymphotropic virus; AIDS, Acquired immunodeficiency syndrome; VDRL, Venereral Disease Research Laboratory.

Table 1.
Exclusion criteria for skin donation.

Besides, there are multiple myths around the organ and tissue donation process; thus, the skin procurement in live donors permits the breakdown of two important myths: a) cadaveric body disfigurement secondary to the skin extraction, a factor that affects the low skin donation rates in many countries, which becomes a "refinement" obtained after a body contour surgery, and b) poor patients donate their tissues and organs to wealthy patients, since people with higher incomes have more access to body contour surgeries and burns are more common in the poor population [22, 23].

2.2 Total thickness skin

Skin resection in body contour surgeries allows the procurement of a cutaneous-subcutaneous flap, which is defatted with scissors, obtaining total skin cutaneous allografts (TCSAs) (**Figures 1** and **2**) compared to classical SA, which are procured with a dermatome, obtaining only partial skin allografts. The amount of TCSA obtained is variable. In an adult abdominoplasty, 3–4% of the total body surface is resected, and once the skin is processed, the valuable surface is of approximately 250–300 cm^2. The skin surface obtained is more extensive in patients submitted to body contour surgeries post-bariatric surgery. However, histologically, the skin presents chronic inflammation areas, sebaceous gland infections, lower collagen fiber organization, elastin and fibroblast concentration, and metalloproteinase levels similar to oncologic or burnt patients [24, 25].

Even if the skin surface obtained compared to a cadaveric skin procurement is smaller, its potential is associated with the number of patients submitted to these

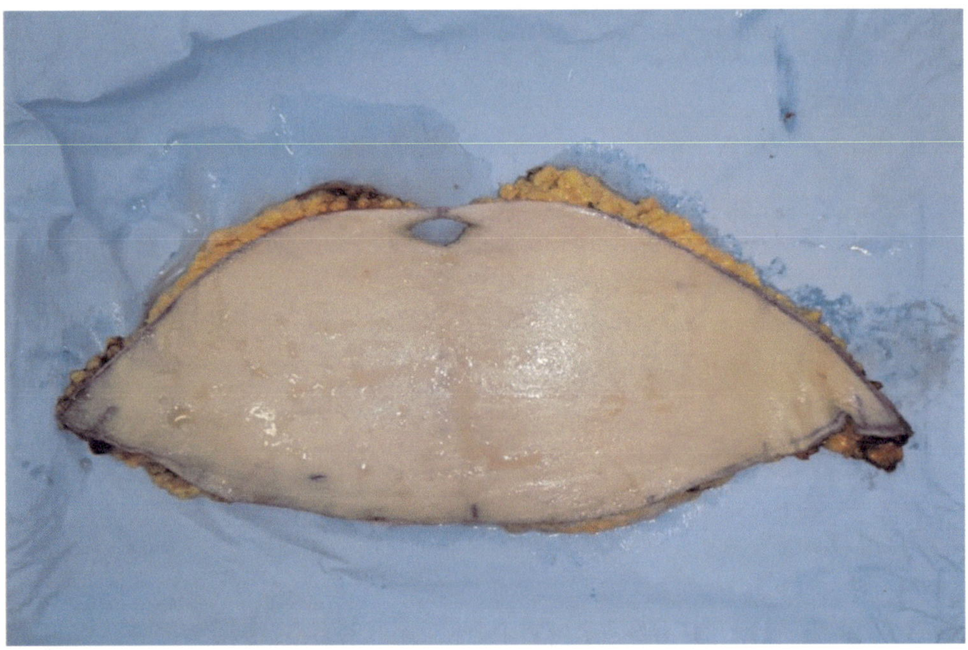

Figure 1.
Abdominal cutaneous-subcutaneous flap.

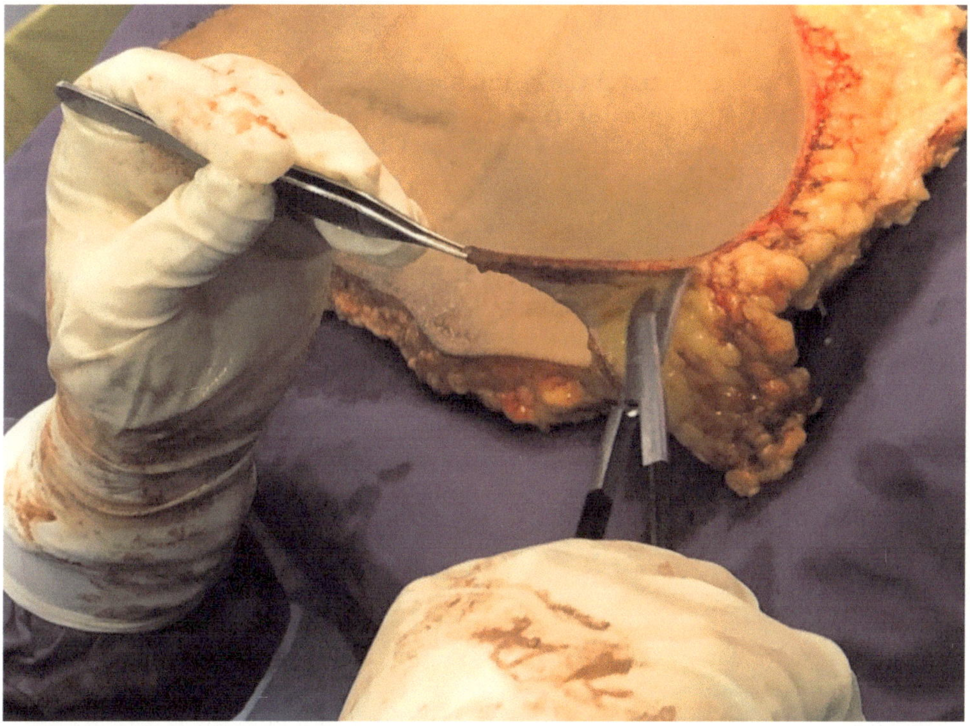

Figure 2.
Procurement of total skin with scissors from redundant adipose skin flap.

types of surgeries and the possibility of obtaining all the skin layers, making it an attractive option [26, 27].

2.3 Cryopreservation

There are multiple forms to preserve tissues: high-concentration glycerol and cryopreservation are the most used techniques in skin banks [28, 29]. The main difference among both techniques is that in the first case, the tissue is nonviable but maintains its structural and mechanical properties, generating a biological dressing. In contrast, the second preserves some cellular viability, and the tissue can be integrated into a wound bedding.

Preservation with high-concentration glycerol is the predominant method in most skin banks since its lower cost and easier storage and distribution. Cryopreservation freezes the TCSA in the presence of a cryoprotectant (glycerol 10%), which prevents the crystallization effects, maintaining the viability of keratinocytes, fibroblasts, endothelial, and Langerhans cells over the time following the freezing. The viability of the obtained tissues is crucial for the clinical results [30–34].

Dimethyl sulfoxide (DMS) is another cryoprotectant frequently used in cryopreservation procedures; however, there are contradictory publications regarding the best alternative for cryopreservation compared to glycerol 10% [35–36].

Precisely, both partial and total skin allografts can be cryopreserved, but the viability is one of the features of CTSCA.

3. Technical aspects of skin banks

Human skin storage started at the beginning of the XX century, following the description of skin transplant after its refrigeration, but modern skin banks began in 1949, after the creation of the Tissue Bank of the United States Marine. However, Tissue Banks arrived in developing countries three decades later than the developed world [37–43].

According to the American Association of Tissue Banks, a Tissue Bank is defined as "an entity that provides or is dedicated to one or more services related with tissues from live or dead persons, with a transplant objective. These services include obtaining authorization and/or informed consent, evaluating donor eligibility, recuperation, harvest, acquisition, processing, storage, labeling, distribution, and dispensing tissues" [41].

Skin donation, a source of SA and CTSCA, is mainly influenced by cultural and religious factors but regulated by specific laws depending on each country and can be divided into seven big stages: 1) donor selection, 2) procurement, 3) processing, 4) storage, 5) radiation, 6) distribution, and 7) clinical use [42–45].

3.1 Donor selection

The appropriate donor selection allows the generation of safe tissues, primarily reducing the risk of disease transmission during the CTSCA transplant [46].

When deciding the body contour surgery, mainly abdominoplasty, patients are invited to be donors of redundant skin flaps, which would otherwise be a surgical waste. A health survey, verification of exclusion criteria absence, and routine laboratory tests related to organ and tissue donation (hepatitis B surface antigen, hepatitis C antibodies, HIV antibodies, VDRL, HTLV I and II, Chagas, and cytomegalovirus) (**Table 2**) are done. As previously mentioned, most exclusion criteria for organ and tissue donation are usually inexistent in the live donor submitted to elective surgery.

3.2 Procurement

The skin procurement takes place in the surgical ward, with the same surgical team and time of the body contour surgery, respecting all the asepsis and antisepsis

1. Hepatitis B surface antigen.
2. Antibodies against Hepatitis C.
3. Antibodies against HIV.
4. VDRL
5. HTLV I and II.
6. Chagas.
7. Citomegalovirus

HIV, human immunodeficiency virus; HTLV, human T-lymphotropic virus; VDRL, Venereral Disease Research Laboratory.

Table 2.
Laboratory tests.

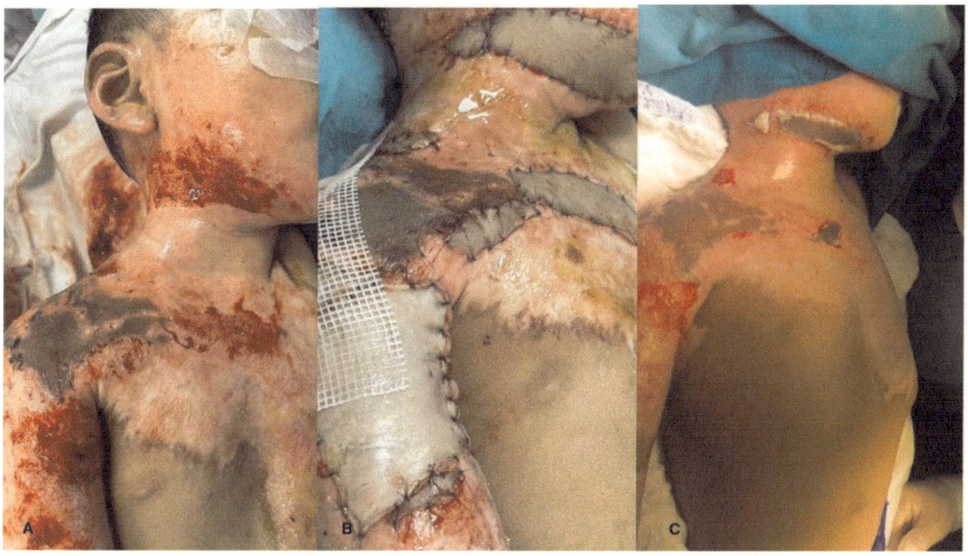

Figure 3.
A. Patient with intermediate and deep burns. B. Burnt patient following a CTSCA use, immediate postoperative. C. Burnt patient, 14 days postoperative with CTSCA coverage.

measures. In the particular case of abdominoplasty (the most frequent CTSCA source), the redundant skin is demarcated in a transverse-infra umbilical-ellipse form, followed by dissection and resection of the skin flap. The abdominoplasty is developed independently, and the skin procurement is done in a separate surgical table.

The subcutaneous component of the cutaneous-subcutaneous flap is resected using scissors, exposing the deeper dermis (**Figures 3** and **4**). Three tissue samples are taken for current (aerobic), anaerobic, and fungal cultures. Procured skin is placed in a sterile recipient with 500 cc of physiological serum, Cloxacillin 1 g, and Gentamicin 80 mg, hermetically closed, promoting the complete skin submersion. The same receipt is saved in a double sterile bag and stored at 2 and 8°C until processing. All the information needed to guarantee the traceability and biosecurity of the tissues is consigned.

3.3 Processing

The skin processing is subdivided into three stages: 1) cutting, b) cleaning, and c) packing/labeling, all of them take place in a clean room, with rigorous aseptic technique and a biosecurity cabinet.

3.3.1 Cutting

Once the skin flap is measured (length, width, and thickness), cuts using a scalpel and scissors are done according to the requested or standardized measures (**Figure 2**). Standard measures are 10 x 10 cm, 10 x 5 cm, and 5 x 5 cm. According to the redundant skin, other dimensions cuts are done, and the smallest size accepted is 2 x 2 cm.

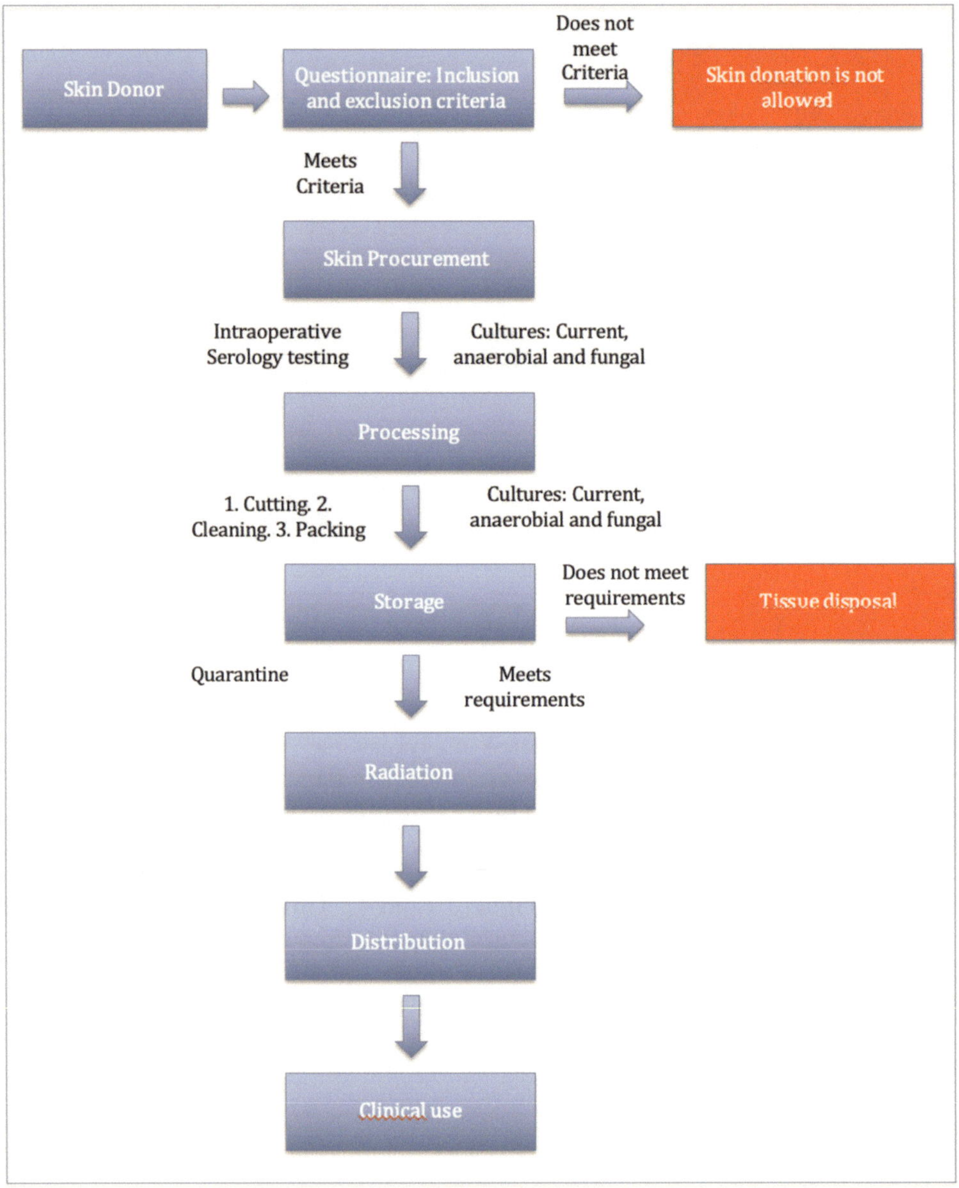

Figure 4.
CTSCA processing flow chart.

3.3.2 Cleaning

The cleaning takes place by depositing the skin in sterile jars with 10% glycerol, followed by a manual agitation for 5 minutes. The process is repeated five times in different jars. During this procedure, jars change from a tainted red color to transparent. Concomitant, new samples are taken for culture. Finally, the last jar with skin sheets in a cryopreserving solution (glycerol 10%) is carefully transferred to refrigeration (between 2 and 8°) for at least 1 hour.

3.3.3 Final packing and labeling

This phase includes measuring, packing, and labeling each piece of the skin set. It is done once the tissue has been immersed in the cryopreserved solution (glycerol 10%) for at least 1 hour.

Samples for culture (current, anaerobic, and fungal) are taken at the beginning and end of the packing. The packing used to pack the skin is completely transparent, allowing the tissue visualization with its features and conditions. The obtained tissue is then labeled according to internal codes, with the information needed for their traceability. It is important to emphasize that in contrast to organ transplant, where a donor usually benefits one receptor, tissue transplants from one donor may benefit many receptors.

3.4 Storage

The processed skin is kept in quarantine in an ultra freezer at −80°C until the skin cultures, and donor serology results are obtained. Following the entrance of the samples, the clinical laboratory usually informs the results of the aerobic cultures in 72 hours and the fungal cultures in 15 to 18 days. If any culture develops any microorganism (positive result), the table of microorganisms allowed in the skin for radiation (**Table 3**) is consulted to determine if the skin set will complete the final phase of radiation or will be discarded.

3.5 Radiation

The objective is the sterilization of the CTSCA and bacterial contamination risk reduction, using gamma radiation (25 to 30 kGy). Dry ice must be used to keep the cold chain during the skin transportation from the skin bank to the radiation center.

Twenty-five kilograms of gamma radiation to an ultra-frozen skin with low glycerol concentration sterilize the tissue with no histological, cytotoxic, or physical alteration, in contrast to normal cryopreserved skin [47, 48]. Only tissues with a negative serology from the patient and negative cultures or accepted microorganisms for radiation will complete the final radiation process.

3.6 Distribution

Facing the CTSCA requirements, the skin sets must be transferred in dry ice, in a pellet-like presentation, keeping the temperature between −76 and − 80°C from skin banks to the different hospitals for their clinical use.

Microorganisms allowed in skin for radiation	Microorganisms not allowed in skin for radiation
Staphylococcus aureus, beta hemolytic streptococcus, enterococcus, yeast	Aerobic and anaerobic Gram-negative bacilli, Gram-negative cocaceae, clostidium, anthacis bacilli

Table 3.
List of microorganisms allowed in skin for radiation.

3.7 Clinical use

In the preoperative phase, the size of the defect to be covered must be calculated to request the appropriate amount and size of skin sheets. All the information that guarantees tissue traceability and biovigilance from the donor and the final receptors must be consigned.

It is essential to emphasize the elasticity of the CTSCA, which may also expand doing small incisions on its epidermal layer, so the cover surface of the CTSCA is more extensive than its size.

In the preoperative, the size of the defect to be covered must be calculated to request the appropriate amount and size of skin sheets. It is essential to emphasize the elasticity of the CTSCA, which may also expand doing small incisions on its epidermal layer, so the cover surface of the CTSCA is more extensive than its size.

Prior to clinical use, the CTSCAs are washed three times with warm physiological saline (without exceeding 40°C) to remove the cryoprotectants (glycerol 10%).

The receptor bedding is prepared with scarectomy of the necrotic, devitalized, and disorganized granulation tissue; subsequently, the CTSCA is fixed in our case with stitches and/or medical clasps associated with negative pressure therapy [49].

All the skin processing, from donation to clinical use, is resumed in the flow diagram of **Figure 4**.

4. Clinical indications

Scarectomy and prompt coverage have increased the survival of major burnt patients. However, on many occasions, the available skin for autografts is limited, and the lack of donor areas impedes grafting the totality of the excised areas. In the latter conditions, the SA has become the reference cutaneous substitute, which can be used alone or combined with autografts. Other SA clinical indications among burnt patients are bedding with doubtful vitality or infection, or when the autograft procurement significantly increases the morbimortality of the patient.

The current role of the SA in treating burns varies among the burnt units or centers, where most of them lack the access or experience of using this product [50].

4.1 Sole skin allografts use

4.1.1 Lack of donor areas

When donor areas are minimal or lacking, a scarectomy and coverage with SA are done directly on the residual bedding, which is replaced after the healing of intermediate burns, and the donor areas allow the harvesting of new autografts.

It is vital to emphasize that in burnt inpatients, the hospitalization time and economic costs are lower in the group of patients who first receive an SA followed by an autograft than in the group that only receives autografts. The latter could probably be since the autograft obtention generates new bloody areas and that the autograft in a non-completely defined vitality could imply its loss [51].

4.1.2 Engraftment test

When the bedding to cover has a doubtful vitality, the use of SA is preferred, since it permits an engraftment evaluation before using autografts. As autologous skin grafts, CTSCAs suffer revascularization, providing the wound bedding with crucial growth factors and cytokines, promoting cellular chemotaxis and proliferation.

The increased wound bedding vascularization stimulates angiogenesis and favors the bedding preparation for an autologous skin graft.

Another indication for using allografts in burns surgery could be in the context of infected burns when the risk of losing the autograft is considered significant [52, 53].

4.1.3 Unstable patient

Scarectomy of extensive body surfaces, mainly associated with the autografts harvesting in the same surgical time, produces significant bleeding. Using SA, scarectomy may be done alone and the graft harvesting during a second time, reducing the bleeding and hemodynamic instability.

4.2 Use of SA associated with autografts

Alexander et al. described the “In sandwich compound graft.” Following the scarectomy of the burnt patient, the bedding was covered with expanded autografts (meshed 1/6 or higher), which were then covered by a SA expanded in smaller meshes (1/1, 5, or 1/3). The latter worked as tutors and avoided the autograft dissection. This technique allows the coverage of extensive body surfaces with high success rates. Besides, Cuono et al. demonstrated that the engraftment of keratinocyte culture grafts improved significantly using dermic bedding provided by allografts [54, 55].

5. Clinical evolution

CTSCAs have initial engraftment, similar to an autologous skin graft, subsequently evolving to rejection. The rejection is clinically manifested as a gradual color change and formation of a necrotic scar in a 21-day average interval, when removed, exposing a vital tissue adhered to the receptor (**Figures 1–3**). The latter is histologically evidenced in the CTSCA as necrotis foci with mainly neutrophils and the receptor bedding exposing an interface rich in fibroblasts and neoformation vessels.

CTSCA acts as a scaffold and biological inductor, which becomes colonized by cells from the receptor, creating a neodermis. This model has been verified in xenograft models, where CTSCAs promote angiogenesis and collagen type 1 production without causing a significant fibrotic response.

Secondary to an immunologic phenomenon, the cellular elements of the skin allografts are rejected; however, the dermal components can persist and incorporate into the healing dermis of the receptor. The biologic mechanisms underlying this integration are not fully understood [56, 57].

6. Conclusions

Live donor skin donation is an alternative and readily available source of SA, particularly in countries with a low rate of cutaneous donation. Besides, total skin SA can be obtained, maintaining their vitality after cryopreservation, resulting in CTSCA.

Even if the total surface skin obtained is lower than in cadaveric procurement, this may be compensated by the high number of patients submitted to body contour surgeries. The clinical indications of CTSCA in burnt patients are multiple, including patients with lack of donor areas, infected or with doubtful vitality beddings, or when the graft harvesting process increases the morbimortality of the patient.

Conflict of interest

The authors declare no conflicts of interest.

Author details

Marcelo Fonseca Canteros[1*], Aldo Cañete Soto[1,2,3], Dino Ibaceta Orlandini[1], Jennifer Gómez Aguilera[2,3], Paulina Acuña Salazar[4], Luana Mandriaza Muñoz[5], Catalina Buchroithner Haase[6], Manuel Moya Delgado[1], Giovanni Vivas Rosales[1], Nicolle Delgado Cárcamo[1], Florencia Disi Parga[7], María Belén Larrea Aguilar[8] and María José Pulgar Leyton[8]

1 Department of Plastic Surgery and Burns, Hospital Dr. Ernesto Torres Galdames, Iquique, Chile

2 Unit of Organs and Tissue Procurement, Hospital Dr. Ernesto Torres Galdames, Iquique, Chile

3 Regional Bank of Tissues, Iquique, Chile

4 Department of the Coordination of Organs and Tissue Procurement and Transplant, Ministerio de Salud, Chile

5 National Bank of Tissues, Santiago, Chile

6 Department of Dermatology, Hospital Dr. Ernesto Torres Galdames, Iquique, Chile

7 Department of Pathology, Hospital Dr. Ernesto Torres Galdames, Iquique, Chile

8 Centro de Cirugía Plástica Terranova, Iquique, Chile

*Address all correspondence to: mfon777@hotmail.com

References

[1] Janzecovich Z. A new concept in early excision and immediate grafting of burns. The Journal of Trauma. 1970; **10**:110

[2] Miller TA, Switzer WE, Foley FD, Moncrief JA. Early homografting of second degree burns. Plastic and Reconstructive Surgery. 1967;**40**: 117-125

[3] Burd A, Chiu T. Allogenic skin in the treatment of burns. Clinics in Dermatology. 2005;**23**(4):376-387

[4] Lazzeri D, Pantaloni M, Agostini T. Homografts and the rejection phenomenon: From burn care to organ transplantation. Plastic and Reconstructive Surgery. 2010;**126**(5): 1802-1803

[5] Roa R, Piñeros JL. Coberturas transitorias en quemaduras. Cirugía Plástica Ibero-Latinoamericana. 2020; **46**:17-22

[6] Dantzer E. Indicaciones de los sustitutos cutáneos y de los aloinjertos. EMC-Cirugía Plástica Reparadora y Estética. 2015;**23**(1):1-14

[7] Gaucher S, Jarraya M. Aloinjertos cutáneos en la cirugía del gran quemado. EMC-Cirugía Plástica Reparadora y Estética. 2009;**17**(1):1-10

[8] Girdner JH. Skin grafting with grafts from a dead subject. Medical Record NY. 1881;**20**:119-120

[9] Brown JB, McDowell F. Massive repairs of burns with thick split-skin grafts: Emergency "dressings" with homografts. Annals of Surgery. 1942;**115**: 658-674

[10] Brown JB, Fryer MP. Postmortem homografts to reduce mortality in extensive burns: Early biological closure and saving of patients for permanent healing; use in mass casualties and in national disaster. Journal of the American Medical Association. 1954;**156**: 1163-1166

[11] Bondoc CC, Burke JF. Clinical experience with viable frozen human skin and a frozen skin bank. Annals of Surgery. 1971;**174**:371-382

[12] Kagan R, Winter R, Robb E. The Skin Bank. Total Burn Care. 4th ed. Edinburgh: Saunders Elsevier; 2012. pp. 199-208

[13] Martínez-Flores F, Sandoval-Zamora H, Machuca-Rodriguez C, Barrera-López A, García-Cavazos R, Madinaveitia-Villanueva J. Banco de piel y tejidos: un modelo operativo para la recuperación y preservación de aloinjertos de piel y tejidos. Cirugía y Cirujanos. 2016;**84**(1):85-92

[14] Wang C, Zhang F, Lineaweaver W. Clinical applications of allograft skin in burn care. Annals of Plastic Surgery. 2020;**84**(3S):S158-S160

[15] Khoo TL, Halim AS, Saad AM, Dorai AA. The application of glycerol-preserved skin allograft in the treatment of burn injuries: An analysis based on indications. Burns. 2010;**36**(6):897-904

[16] González F, Vera F, Alcayaga R, González F. Análisis crítico de la baja tasa de donación de órganos en Chile. Review Medicine Chile. 2020;**148**: 242-251

[17] Zúñiga-Fajuri A, Merino M, Urtubia M. *Una* mirada al origen,

funcionamiento y desafíos del nuevo sistema de donación y trasplantes chileno. Review Medicine Chile. 2018; **146**:780-785

[18] Zidan S, Eleowa S. Banking and use of glycerol preserved full-thickness skin allograft harvested from body contouring procedures. Burns. 2014; **40**(4):641-647

[19] Friedland J, Maffi T. MOC-PS (SM) CME article: Abdominoplasty. Plastic and Reconstructive Surgery. 2008; **121**(4):1-11

[20] Fonseca M, Cañete A, Ibaceta D, Gomez J, Santander M, Acuña P, et al. Procuramiento y uso de aloinjertos cutáneos de piel total criopreservados obtenidos de pacientes sometidas a abdominoplastía. Reviews Cirugia. 2022; **74**(1):61-72. DOI: 10.35687/s2452-4549% Y00%i1227

[21] Fonseca M, Cañete A, Ibaceta D, Buchroithner C, Disi F, Olivares J. Procurement and use of cryopreserved total skin allograft in complex wounds. In: Gore M, editor. Skin grafts - Role in Successful Wound Closure. London: IntechOpen; 2021 [cited 11 May 2022]. Available from: https://www.intechopen.com/chapters/77727. DOI: 10.5772/intechopen.99125

[22] Smolle C, Cambiaso-Daniel J, Forbes A, Wurzer P, Hundeshagen G, Branski L, et al. Recent trends in burn epidemiology worldwide: A systematic review. Burns. 2017;**43**(2):249-257

[23] Albornoz C, Villegas J, Peña V, Whittle S. Epidemiología del paciente gran quemado adulto en Chile: experiencia del Servicio de Quemados del Hospital de la Asistencia Pública de Santiago. Review Medicine Chile. 2013; **141**(2):181-186

[24] Morales-Olivera JM, Plasencia Beltrán JC, Vázquez Mendoza X, Ricón Rubio LL. Cambios histológicos dérmicos tras pérdida masiva de peso y su repercusión en la herida quirúrgica en abdominoplastia. Cirugía Plástica Ibero-Latinoamericana. 2019;**45**(3):275-283

[25] Light D, Arvanitis G, Abramson D, Glasberg S. Effect of weight loss after bariatric surgery on skin and the extracellular matrix. Plastic and Reconstructive Surgery. 2010;**125**(1): 343-351

[26] American Society of Plastic Surgeons Public Surgery Statistics. 2020. https://www.plasticsurgery.org/documents/News/Statistics/2020/plastic-surgery-statistics-full-report-2020.pdf

[27] Heidekrueger PI, Juran S, Patel A, et al. Plastic surgery statistics in the US: Evidence and implications. Aesthestic Plastic Surgery. 2016;**40**:293-300

[28] Van Baare J, Cameron PU, Vardaxis N, et al.. Comparison of glycerol preservation with cryopreservation methods on HIV-1 inactivation. The Journal of Burn Care & Rehabilitation. 1998;**19**:494-500

[29] Blondet R, Gibert-Thevenin MA, Pierre C, et al. Skin preservation by programmed freezing. British Journal of Plastic Surgery. 1982;**35**:530-536

[30] Pegg DE. Viability assays for preserved cells, tissues, and organs. Cryobiology. 1989;**26**:212-231

[31] Castagnoli C, Alotto D, Cambieri I, Casimiri R, Aluffi M, Stella M, et al. Evaluation of donor skin viability: Fresh and cryopreserved skin using tetrazolioum salt assay. Burns. 2003;**29**: 759-767

[32] Cleland H, Wasiak J, Dobson H, Paul M, Pratt G, Paul E, et al. Clinical application and viability of cryopreserved cadaveric skin allografts in severe burn: A retrospective analysis. Burns. 2014;**40**(1):61-66

[33] Blome-Eberwein S, Jester A, Kuentscher M, Raff T, Germann G, Pelzer M. Clinical practice of glycerol preserved allograft skin coverage. Burns. 2002;**28**:10-12

[34] Ge L, Huang Z, Wei H. Skin graft preservation. In: Spear M, editor. Skin Grafts-Indications, Applications and Current Research. London, UK: IntechOpen; 2011. DOI: 10.5772/23084

[35] Gaucher S, Elie C, Vérola O, Jarraya M. Viability of cryopreserved human skin allografts: Effects of transport media and cryoprotectant. Cell and Tissue Banking. 2012;**13**(1):147-155

[36] Ock S, Rho G. Effect of dimethyl sulfoxide (DMSO) on cryopreservation of porcine mesenchymal stem cells (pMSCs). Cell Transplantation. 2011; **20**(8):1231-1239

[37] Wentscher J. A further contribution about the survivability of human epidermal cells. Dtsch Z Chir. 1903;**70**: 21-44

[38] Strong D, The US. Navy tissue Bank: 50 years on the cutting edge. Cell and Tissue Banking. 2000;**1**(1):9-16

[39] Meshram H, Chauhan S, Kute V. Development of tissue banks in developing nations: A journey from past to future. Burn Care and Prevention. 2021;**1**:10-15

[40] Cai L, Long C, Karki B, Nakarmi K, Iqbal A, Casertano M, et al. Creation of Nepal's first skin bank: Challenges and outcomes. Plastic and Reconstructive Surgery Global Open. 2017;**5**(11)

[41] American Association of Tissue Banks. [Accessed: January 09, 2022]. https://www.aatb.org/

[42] Guerrero L. Vigencia de los bancos de tejidos laminares. Cirugía Plástica Ibero-Latinoamericana. 2020;**46**:23-30

[43] Pianigiani E, Ierardi F, Di Simplicio FC, Andreassi A. Skin bank organization. Clinics in Dermatology. 2005;**23**(4):353-356

[44] Tognetti L, Pianigiani E, Ierardi F, Mariotti G, Perotti R, Di Lonardo A, et al. Current insights into skin banking: Storage, preservation and clinical importance of skin allografts. Journal of Biorepository Science for Applied Medicine. 2017;**5**:41-56

[45] Ministerio de Salud. Gobierno de Chile. Norma general técnica para el procuramiento, preservación e implante de tejidos. 2018

[46] Clark JA. HIV transmission and skin grafts. Lancet. 1987;**329**(8539):983

[47] Rooney P, Eagle M, Hogg P, Lomas R, Kearney J. Sterilisation of skin allograft with gamma irradiation. Burns. 2008;**34**(5):664-673

[48] Johnston C, Callum J, Mohr J, Duong A, Garibaldi A, Simunovic N, et al. Disinfection of human skin allografts in tissue banking: A systematic review report. Cell and Tissue Banking. 2016;**17**(4):585-592

[49] Gupta S. Optimal use of negative pressure wound therapy for skin grafts. International Wound Journal. 2012;**9**: 40-47

[50] Vera M, Alegría L, Domínguez J, Rebolledo R, Dib M. Donación y trasplante de órganos: análisis y propuestas para avanzar hacia una cultura de donación. Temas de la Agenda Pública. 2019;**14**(117):1-20 Centro de Políticas Públicas UC

[51] Chua A, Song C, Chai A, Chan L, Tan KC. The impact of skin banking and the use of its cadaveric skin allografts for severe burn victims in Singapore. Burns. 2004;**30**(7):696-700

[52] Kitala D, Kawecki M, Klama-Baryła A, Łabuś W, Kraut M, Glik J, et al. Allogeneic vs. autologous skin grafts in the therapy of patients with burn injuries: A restrospective, open-label clinical study with pair matching. Adv. Clinical and Experimental Medicine. 2016;**25**(5):923-929

[53] Rogers A, Allorto N, Adams S, Adams K, Hudson D, Rode H. Isn't it time for a cadaver skin bank in South Africa? Annals of Burns and Fire Disasters. 2013;**26**(3):142

[54] Alexander JW, Mac Millan BG, Law E, Kittur DS. Treatment of severe burns with widely mesh skinautograft and Meshed skin allograft overlay. The Journal of Trauma. 1981;**21**:433-438

[55] Cuono CB, Langdon R, Birchall N, Barttelbort S, McGuire J. Composite autologous-allogenic skin replacement: Development and clinical application. Plastic and Reconstructive Surgery. 1987; **80**:626-635

[56] Henn D, Chen K, Maan Z, Greco A, Moortgat Illouz S, Bonham C, et al. Cryopreserved human skin allografts promote angiogenesis and dermal regeneration in a murine model. International Wound Journal. 2020; **17**(4):925-936

[57] Ge L, Huang Z, Wei H. Skin graft preservation, Skin Grafts - Indications, Applications and Current Research; 2011 Marcia Spear (Ed.), InTech, London, UK, ISBN: 978-953-307-509-9, Available from: http://www.intechopen.com/books/skin-grafts-indications-applications-and-current-research/skin-graft-preservation

Chapter 12

Integrated Optical Coherence Tomography and Deep Learning for Evaluating of the Injectable Hydrogel on Skin Wound Healing

Qingliang Zhao and Lin Chen

Abstract

Recently hydrogels and the treatment of skin wounds based on hydrogel dressings have become one of the research hotspots in the field of skin trauma. In this chapter, we focus on the materials and methods of hydrogel preparation, and discuss the properties that hydrogels should possess for the treatment of wounds. Moreover, we discuss the potential of non-invasive optical imaging techniques in the assessment of cutaneous wound healing. The research results of the application of non-invasive optical techniques such as diffuse reflectance spectroscopy (DRS) and optical coherence tomography (OCT) in scar identification, skin bruising, and skin and vascular structure identification are reviewed. Furthermore, we further discuss the superiority and potential of current artificial intelligence (AI) technology in dermatological diagnosis, and analyze the application status of hydrogel in skin wound treatment. Finally, we believe that the combination of AI and optical imaging technology in the development and efficacy monitoring of hydrogels will be a promising research direction in the future.

Keywords: hydrogel, OCT, *in vivo* imaging, artificial intelligence, wound healing

1. Introduction

As the largest organ system in the human body, the skin plays a vital role in maintaining the body's physiological stability, protecting the skin from external stimuli, preventing infection, and maintaining fluid balance. Therefore, skin wound healing is an important step in the survival to complete wound closure [1]. Although human skin can heal itself after injury, this is limited to superficial wounds. In cases such as deep burns or diabetes, the wound's self-healing ability is limited, and supportive methods are needed to accelerate and protect the wound healing process. Current conventional approaches to wound treatment including the application of different types of dressings, electrical stimulation therapy, skin grafting, and negative pressure wound therapy (NPWT) have proven beneficial, but they also have certain limitations [2].

Since O. Wichterle et al., reported the first case of hydrophilic gel in 1960, the results of the application of hydrogel in wound healing have become increasingly abundant [3–9]. More and more research results show that hydrogels have the ability to deliver drugs, cytokines, and growth factors as carriers, which will greatly accelerate wound healing. In addition, compared with traditional dressings, the non-adhesive nature of the hydrogel avoids secondary damage, and its 3D network structure is conducive to absorbing wound exudate while maintaining an ideal moist environment [10–13]. In view of this, hydrogels have gradually become ideal wound dressings in recent years and show good prospects in the treatment of burns and other skin injuries [14, 15]. In this chapter, we describe advanced hydrogels for wound healing and enhanced skin repair.

1.1 Development of injectable hydrogel

To date, a plethora of biomaterials as wound dressings for different clinical treatment protocols have been developed, which may be composed of synthetic or natural materials, or may be a hybrid of the two. Naturally occurring polymers, such as sodium alginate (SA), chitosan (CS), gelatin, and hyaluronic acid (HA), are biocompatible and biodegradable, which allow adhesion and coordination of cellular responses [16]. Unfortunately, natural hydrogels suffer from some limitations, such as not having strong mechanical properties and significant batch-to-batch variability [17]. In contrast, synthetic polymers such as polyvinyl alcohol (PVA), polyacrylamide (PAM), and polyethylene glycol (PEG) have become increasingly popular due to their strong mechanical properties, customizable structures and low immunogenicity [18]. However, the application of synthetic polymers in the field of biomedicine should pay attention to the rejection of the body. Therefore, more complex hydrogels were synthesized. Currently, the material design of hydrogels usually combines natural biopolymers and synthetic polymers to overcome the limitations brought by a single polymer [18]. Hydrogels are formed by cross-linking polymer chains dispersed in an aqueous medium, and the cross-linking methods mainly include physical entanglement, ionic interactions, and chemical cross-linking (**Figure 1**) [19]. Physical cross-linking is usually non-permanent, not as stable as chemical cross-linking, and has cross-linking reversibility, but it is sufficient for polymer chains to aggregate to form gel substances that are insoluble in aqueous media. Due to the covalent bonds between different polymer chains, chemically cross-linked gels have excellent mechanical strength because they are mainly connected by covalent bonds, but their preparation requires the addition of chemical initiators or cross-linking agents. It has been reported that the cross-linking agent has certain toxicity, so the cross-linking agent used to prepare the hydrogel should be extracted from the hydrogel before use, which increases the complexity of the use of chemically cross-linked gel [20]. Electron beam (EB) radiation cross-linking technology can overcome the above defects, which belongs to the grafting in chemical cross-linking and is more stable than the physical cross-linking network structure. Furthermore, when using radiation crosslinking, neither initiators nor crosslinking agents are required, making it safer, softer, and more stretchable than traditional chemical crosslinking [21]. Work in the late 1990s showed that hydrogel precursors can be injected via standard syringes without the need for pre-molding and the use of highly invasive surgical procedures to deliver the material to the target site. Injectable hydrogels have received increasing attention in recent years due to their excellent self-healing ability and minimal invasiveness [22]. Injectable hydrogel technology can better reproduce the complex extracellular

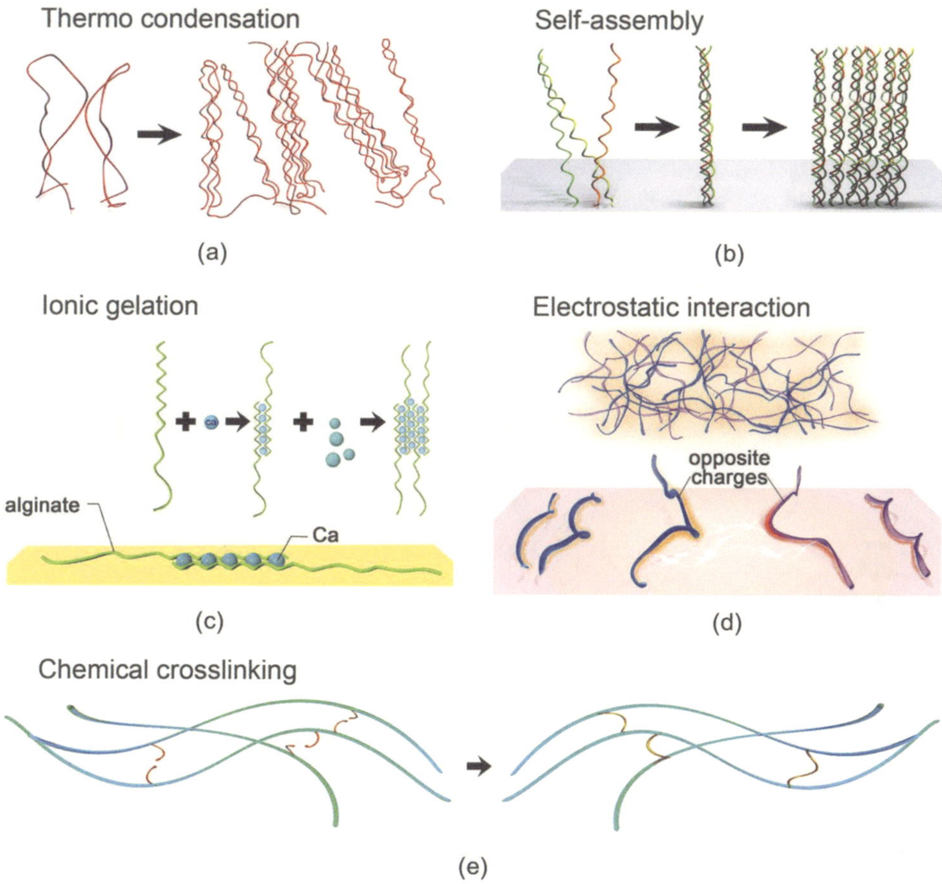

Figure 1.
Cross-linking of hydrogels. (a to d) physical cross-linking. (a) Thermally induced entanglement of polymer chains. (b) Molecular self-assembly. (c) Ionic gelation. (d) Electrostatic interaction. (e) Chemical cross-linking. Reprinted with permission from reference [19].

environment and maintain cell viability, thereby enabling adequate delivery of cells and therapeutic small molecules, which enables the development and optimization of novel therapeutic injectable Hydrogels [23, 24].

Gelatin is inexpensive and readily available and has good cell adhesion [25]. Alginates are commonly used in the treatment of deep second-degree burns due to their excellent biological properties, exudate absorption potential, and ability to maintain a moist wound environment [26–28]. In addition, carboxymethyl cellulose (CMC) contains a large number of carboxymethyl groups, which facilitates polymerization with other material [29, 30]. Their combined strengths make up for the deficiencies of one or both of these natural polymers for applications.

The EB radiation cross-linking mechanism in **Figure 2** is proposed for cross-linking of injectable 3D-PH. The radiation energy of EB is mainly absorbed by water in aqueous solution, and the radiation decomposition of water mainly produces reactive species such as hydroxyl radicals (OH) (**Figure 2a**) [32]. Amino acid residues in gelatin molecules are easily self-oxidized to form aldehyde groups, and aldehyde groups can cross-link with amino acids on gelatin molecules to form Schiff bases (**Figure 2b**), which is the first cross-linked network. Injectable 3D-PH

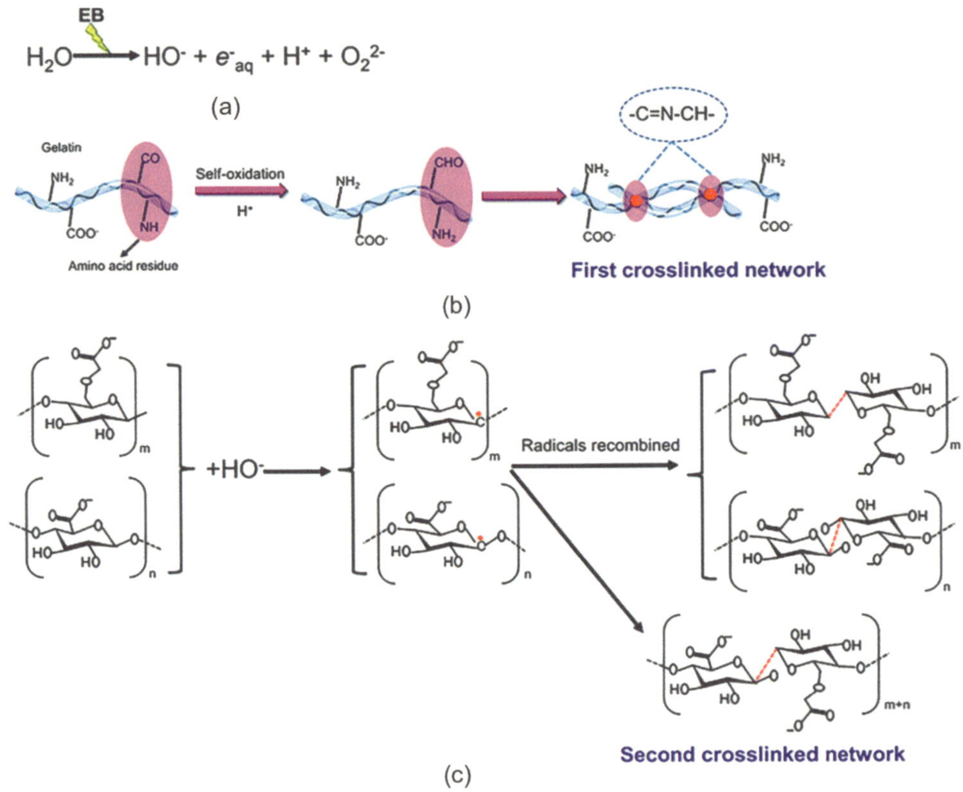

Figure 2.
Mechanism of EB radiation crosslinking of injectable 3D-PH. (a) Ionizing radiation reaction equation of water in polymer aqueous solution. (b) Gelatin self-crosslinking to form the fifirst network of injectable 3D-PH. (c) the crosslinking mechanism of alginate and CMC under EB irradiation. Reprinted with permission from reference [31].

Furthermore, OH- is considered to be a very reactive species, which can remove H from alginate and CMC carbon chains, inducing the formation of alginate-derived radicals, CMC-derived radicals, and HO. Subsequently, the radicals recombine to form new covalent bonds between the carbon chains (**Figure 2c**), which is a second cross-linked network. Hydrogen bonds formed between the injectable 3D-PH stabilize the chemical structure of the hydrogel. The new bonds formed during electron beam irradiation made the molecular chains of the hydrogel connect more tightly. The double-crosslinked network structure triggered by EB and Schiff base can significantly strengthen the hydrogel. These results demonstrate that EB irradiation cross-linking injectable 3D-PH can form a stable double-cross-linked network structure [31].

In view of this, our team designed an injectable 3D-PH via EB radiation crosslinking gelatin-alginate-carboxymethyl cellulose solution, which developed by green materials and facile applicable method (**Figure 3a**). In another study, Zhang et al. synthesized dopamine-modified gelatin@Ag nanoparticles (Gel-DA@Ag NPs) by chemical grafting for wound healing as shown in **Figure 3b** [33]. For the first time, they found that the biomineralization ability of gelatin can be enhanced with dopamine-modified gelatin (Gel-DA). This biomineralization-enhancing strategy provides a new strategy for developing organic and inorganic hybrid multifunctional

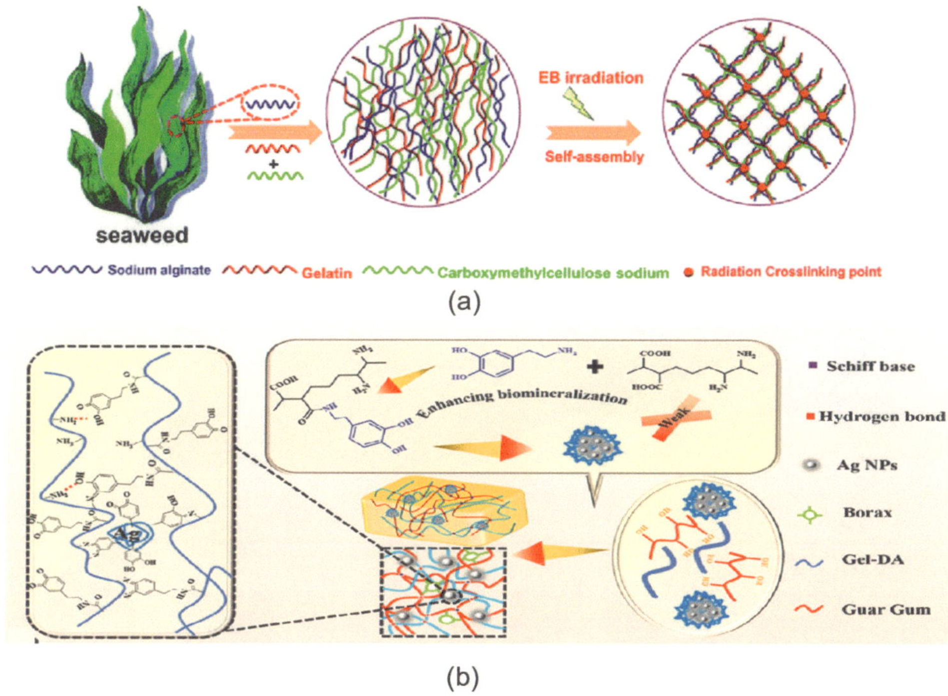

Figure 3.
Schematic diagram of the preparation of hydrogels. (a) 3D-PH. (b) Gel-DA/GG@Ag hydrogels. Reprinted with permission from reference [31, 33].

hydrogels. Among the two different materials, gelatin plays different roles, the former mainly induces platelet activation for wound hemostasis and the latter mainly acts as a biomineralizer combined with metal nanoparticles, resulting in different functional localization.

1.2 Design points of hydrogels for wound treatment

Given the characteristics of the wound surface, the goals of wound management seem obvious, including providing temporary wound coverage, preventing infection, and relieving scarring [34]. Because bacterial infection can hinder the regeneration of epithelial cells and the synthesis of collagen, the prevention of wound infection is an important function of wound dressings [35]. To achieve this function, some broad-spectrum antimicrobial agents are often added to hydrogels, such as silver ions/nanoparticles (AgNPs) [36]. Zhang et al. compared the antibacterial properties of Gel-DA/GG@Ag hydrogels by spread plate method using two hydrogels with only guar gum (GG) and without silver ions (Gel-DA hydrogel) as the control group. As shown in **Figure 4b**, in the three treatments, the number of bacterial colonies in the GG and Gel-DA hydrogel did not change significantly, but in the GG@Ag hydrogel treatment group, the number of colonies of *Escherichia coli* and *Staphylococcus aureus* was significantly reduced, reflecting the antibacterial effect of AgNPs." Guo et al. synthesized a hydrogel TS-Gel-Ag-col with antibacterial and anti-inflammatory functions for wound treatment, which was prepared by muco-mimetic poloxamer 407 (F-107), polyvinylpyrrolidone, and dencichine/chitosan dialdehyde synergistic cross-linked aggregated collagen nanofibers decorated with silver nanoparticles [37]. The

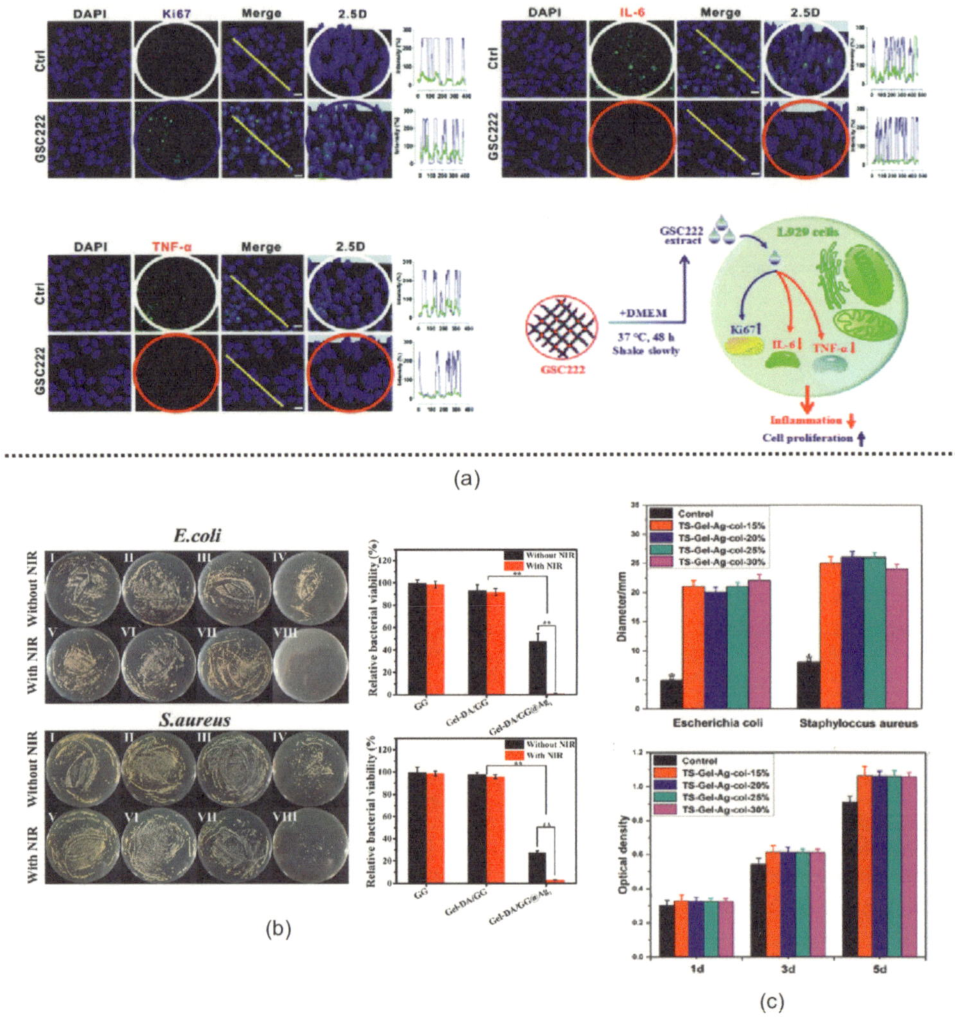

Figure 4.

Antibacterial and anti-inflammatory properties of hydrogels. (A) 3D-PH stimulate cell proliferation and suppresses inflammation in L929 cells. (B) Photographs of E. coli and S. aureus colonies after treatments and the relative survival rates with I) PBS, II) GG, III) gel-DA/GG, IV) gel-DA/GG@Ag1, V) PBS + NIR, VI) GG + NIR, VII) gel-DA/GG + NIR, and VIII) gel-DA/GG@Ag1 + NIR. Power density: 2 W cm^{-2}, 10 min. (C) Antimicrobial effect of TS-gel-Ag-col with different F-107 contents against E. coli and S. aureus and effect of F-107 contents on the proliferation of fibroblasts on TS-gel-Ag-col at different time intervals (1 d, 3 d, and 5 d). Reprinted with permission from reference [31, 33, 37].

addition of F-107 will make the hydrogel have a heat-reverse gelation and enhance biocompatibility, which can overcome the loss of the original native hierarchical aggregated structure present in living tissue fabricated by post-functionalization of collagen molecules [38, 39]. By comparing the inhibition zone diameters of *E. coli* and *S. aureus* affected by different types of gels, the authors found that the amount of F-107 had no significant effect on the bacteriostatic properties of TS-Gel-Ag-col. In addition, although TS-Gel-Ag-col without silver nanoparticles (AgNPs) also exhibited certain antibacterial properties due to the presence of dialdehyde chitosan, the antibacterial effect of AgNPs was more significant (**Figure 4c**). It can be seen that TS-Gel-Ag-col also enhanced the antibacterial effect of the hydrogel through AgNPs.

The high concentration of silver in this silver-containing hydrogel can provide a faster rate of bacterial inhibition, but at the same time cause cytotoxicity, and low concentrations have no significant cytotoxicity to cells, but the rate of inhibition is slow [40]. Therefore, when designing wound dressings, the silver content in the hydrogel needs to be carefully considered to achieve the optimal balance between low cytotoxicity and high antibacterial activity. However, given the oxidative damage and potential toxicity of silver nanoparticles in tissues, researchers prefer to directly synthesize hydrogels from materials with antibacterial properties rather than adding antibacterial agents [41–43].

The occurrence of inflammation is the basis of wound healing, but excessive expression of inflammatory mediators will cause some cells and tissues to atrophy and form chronic inflammation, thereby impairing the healing of skin wounds [44]. Therefore, the anti-inflammatory functional design of hydrogels is equally important. To investigate whether 3D-PH can block inflammatory signaling activation and promote cell proliferation, we used confocal laser scanning microscopy to quantify the expression of cell proliferation-related protein Ki-67 and inflammatory factors (IL- 6, TNF-α, etc.).The results showed that injectable 3D-PH successfully blocked inflammatory signaling activation and stimulated dermal fibroblast proliferation and migration in vitro (**Figure 4a**). Specifically, the level of Ki-67 was increased, while the expression of inflammatory factors was decreased. All of these are beneficial to accelerate the healing process of deep second-degree burn wounds in vivo [31].

Scars often appear after an injury, and scarring of various types can have long-term psychological and physical effects on patients, especially those located in frequently exposed areas [45]. Therefore, scar management is also an important part of wound management, and the ideal result is a dressing that minimizes scarring while allowing the wound to heal quickly. Injectable 3D-PH has the ability to accelerate necrotic tissue removal and wound healing [31]. As shown in **Figure 5a**, the injectable 3D-PH, coloplast wound dressing and blank control were injected into the wounds of second-degree scald. The results showed that after 20 days of treatment, the wounds treated with 3D-PH injection were almost invisible, and the healing rate was significantly higher than the other two groups (**Figure 5b**). Two other hydrogels, Gel-DA@AgNPs and TS-Gel-Ag-col, also have great potential to repair skin tissue (**Figure 5c** and **d**). The researchers used a mouse full-thickness Staphylococcus aureus-infected wound model to demonstrate the properties of Gel-DA@Ag in promoting wound healing. It can be seen that among the groups, the gel DA/GG@Ag1 + NIR group had the best wound regeneration effect, showing an advantage on the fourth day of treatment, and significant epidermal regeneration could be observed, proving that Gel-DA/GG @Ag has the effect of intrinsically accelerating wound healing [33]. **Figure 5d** shows three types of traumatic bleeding models were synthetically utilized to evaluate the hemostatic performance of TS-Gel-Ag-col *in vivo* [37]. The results clearly showed that TS-Gel-Ag-col presented significantly faster hemostasis as compared to the commercial Helitene collagen hemostatic material. And due to the injectable nature of these two hydrogels, when a sol–gel transition occurs, the wound can be easily covered comprehensively and fit well to the injury site. In addition, the 3D porous structure of the hydrogel is important for wound healing, because the denseness of the porous material can prevent the escape of red blood cells and platelets. At the same time, the presence of hydrophilic residues in the 3D grid of the hydrogel enables the hydrogel to further absorb wound exudate and provide a hypoxic and humid healing environment, shortening the healing time of the epidermis [46, 47].

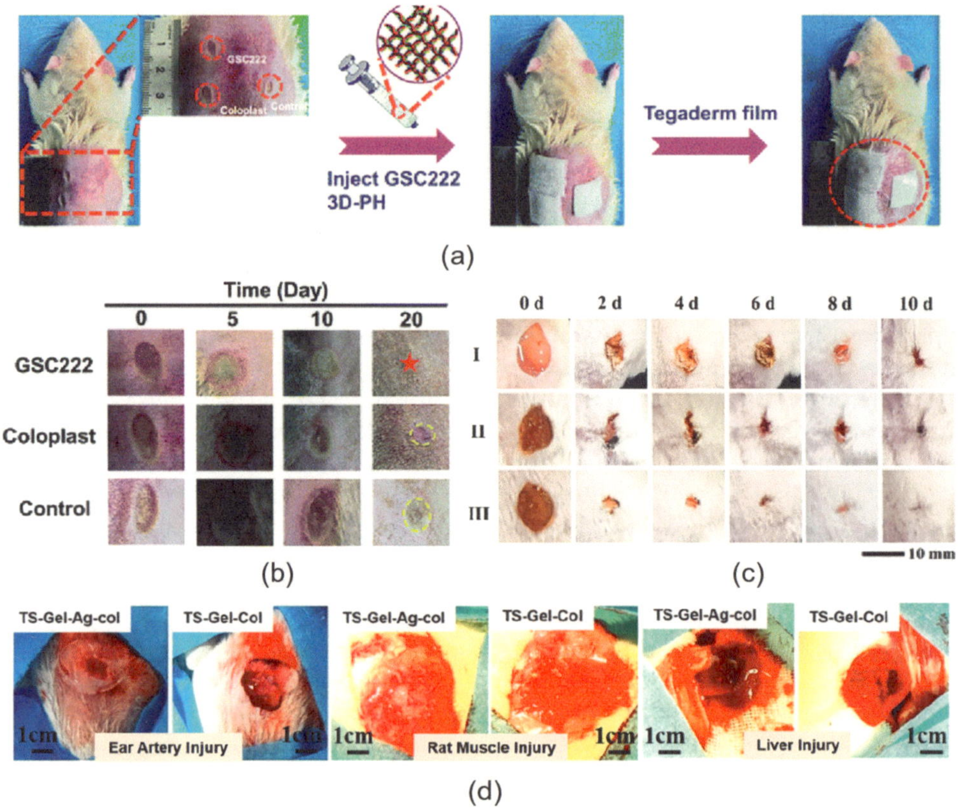

Figure 5.
Healing of animal wounds treated with hydrogels. (a) schematic diagram of the surgical procedure. (b) Coloplast wound dressing, 3D-PH, and control group recovery of scalded wounds in rats on days 0, 5, 10, and 20. (c) Photographs of S. aureus-infected wounds with different treatments. I) Control, II) gel-DA/GG@Ag1, and III) gel-DA/GG@Ag1 + NIR. (d) Photographs of rat muscle trauma, liver and rabbit ear artery injury after TS-gel-Ag-col and TS-gel-col treatment. Reprinted with permission from reference [31, 33, 37].

Most importantly, the 3D porous network structure of the hydrogel resembles the natural extracellular matrix, which will facilitate the adhesion of cells, tissue factors and growth factors for delivery [24].

2. Optical technology applying on the skin *in vivo*

Histology remains the most accurate method for wound healing assessment, including biopsy and chamber-embedding, re-epithelization, epithelial thickness index, granulation tissue thickness, remodeling, and scarring can be obtained by histological analysis. Moreover, visual inspection also can evaluate woundswhich is based on observations such as wound size, color, odor, and level of pain [48–51]. The limitations of the histological analysis method are mainly invasive and destructive, the method generates new wounds during the examination, which delays the time of wound healing and is not suitable for patients at high risk of wound infection, thus reducing the accuracy of wound assessment. Therefore, non-invasive monitoring techniques are a safer way to assess and monitor wound healing, which can help clinicians and researchers more objectively determine and assess whether healing is improving or deteriorating [50–52]. DRS is a non-invasive technique, and the general configuration of a DRS system includes a light source, a photodetector, and a fiber optic probe for light transmission. The DRS can measure the characteristic diffuse reflectance spectrum of tissue in the visible to near-infrared wavelength range. The tissue structure was restored by diffuse reflectance using photon transmission model and least squares curve fitting algorithm. In addition, DRS can also obtain information such as chromophore concentration, absorption and scattering properties of tissues such as breast and skin [53–55]. OCT provides a non-invasive method for obtaining optical cross-sections of the superficial cortex [56, 57], which uses the light scattering characteristics of tissue to construct high-resolution subsurface images. OCT is based on the same echolocation principle as an ultrasound but uses light waves instead of acoustic waves. **Figure 6** shows schematic diagram of the DRS and OCT system.

2.1 Evaluation of skin scars and structure by DRS

Hsu, Chao-Kai et al. assessed the severity of scarring by measuring the diffuse reflectance of the skin. **Figure 7a** shows the representative clinical pictures of keloid (KS, black solid circle) and normal scars (NS, red solid circle) of one of such patients. The uninjured skin located 3 cm away from the keloid (CKS, black dashed circle) and normal scars (CNS, red dashed circle) were used as control groups. It can be seen that in the range of 500–600 nm, the absorption rate of keloids is higher than that of normal scars and uninjured skin, and the magnitude of the reduced scattering spectrum of keloids is the lowest (**Figure 6b** and **c**) [53]. The results of this study demonstrate that the DRS system can not only quantify collagen concentration, water content,

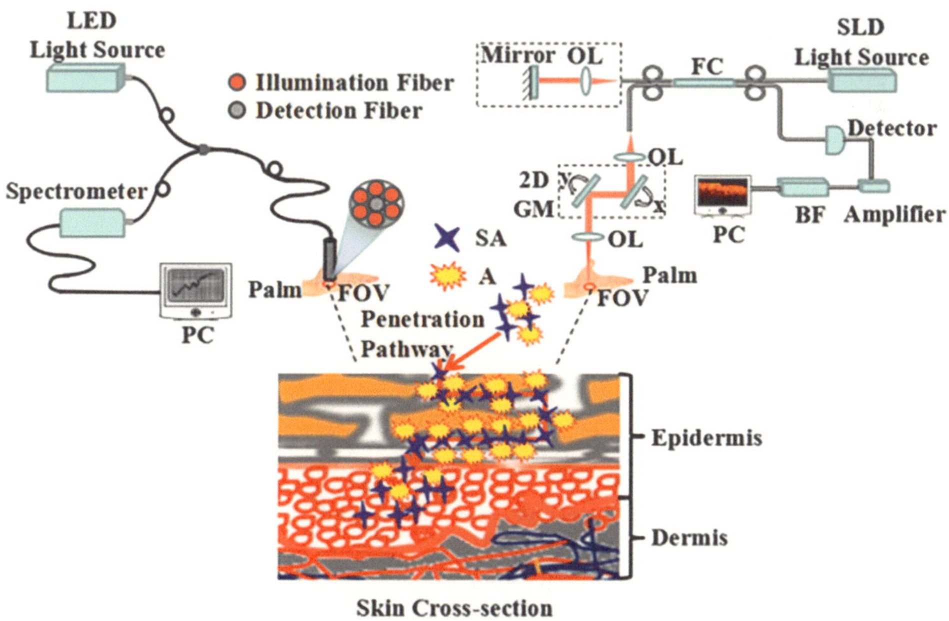

Figure 6.
Schematic diagram of the DRS and OCT system. SLD: Super-luminescent diodes, FC: Fiber coupler, GM: Galvo mirrors, OL: Objective lens, PC: Personal computer, BF: Bandpass filter, FOV: Field of view, SA: Salicylic acid, a: Azone. Reprinted with permission from reference [58].

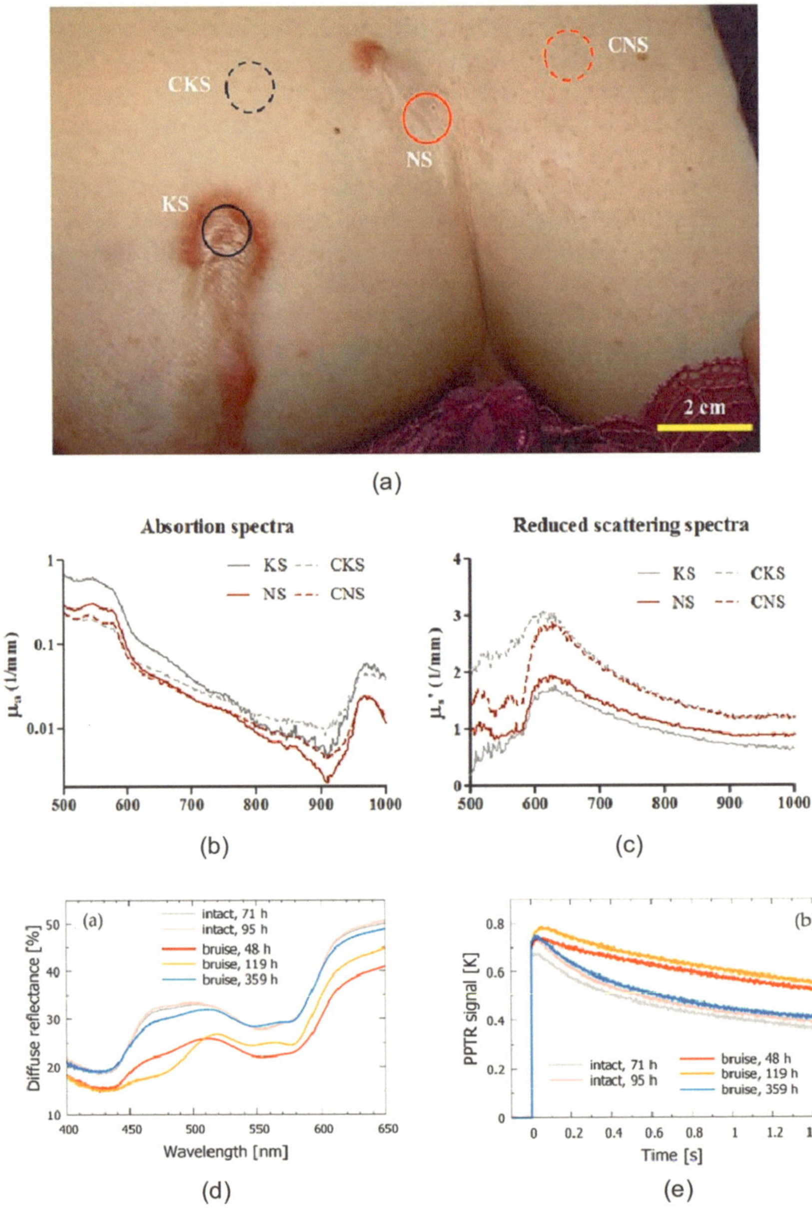

Figure 7.
(a) The clinical picture of a keloid patient containing keloid scar (KS), normal scar (NS)the uninjured skin (CKS), and normal scars (CNS). (b) Typical absorption and (c) reduced scattering spectra in KS, NS, CNS and CKS, (d) DRS spectrum and (f) PPTR signal as obtained from the intact skin site near the bruise in subject a (solid orange curves) and the best-fitting model predictions (dashed lines). Reprinted with permission from reference [53, 59].

and oxygen saturation, but also determine the alignment of collagen bundles in keloid scars. In another study, Bin Chen et al. developed a DRS-based inverse method to extract structural parameters of skin tissue. The model was experimentally validated by constructing a skin model and performing spectral measurements, which demonstrated the agreement between the measured and calculated spectral data [60]. Marin, Ana et al. combined diffuse reflectance spectroscopy and pulsed photothermal radiometry (PPTR) in the visible spectral range to examine the dynamic process of traumatic bruising recovery, while using a numerical model of light and heat transport in a four-layer model of human skin from data for both techniques. **Figure 6d** and **f** shows both DRS spectra and PPTR signals obtained from the bruised site display large differences with respect to the nearby intact site.We can see a significant reduction in diffuse reflectance can be seen throughout the presented spectral range, mainly due to the higher blood content in the dermis [59]. These tasks show that DRS should also be able to quantitatively evaluate the wound healing during the treatment of wounding gel, including the scar condition after wound healing, whether the wound ulcers occurs.

2.2 Investigating the wound healing by OCT and OMAG

In recent years, how to extract the blood flow information in tissue capillaries and image the microcirculation blood flow of tissue capillaries has become a hotspot in the field of OCT research. Compared with OCT, OCT microangiography (OMAG) is a novel technique that can provide microcirculatory imaging enabled by processing OCT data [61].

For this reason, OCT technology has been extended to develop OMAG. OMAG uses the structural imaging of OCT to extract tissue blood flow information through algorithms, so as to achieve non-invasive, non-contact, and no need for contrast agents to image blood flow in tissue capillaries [62, 63]. Wang et al. [64] used an imaging system that combined dual wavelength laser speckle imaging (DW-LSI) with DOMAG to image the ears of mouse, which monitored hemodynamic changes during acute wound healing. After the wound was created using the biopsy punch, the blood flow in the first-order branches of the affected arteries and veins in the laser speckle image was markedly reduced as can be seen from the orange circles in **Figure 8B**. In addition, detailed changes in axial blood flow velocity can be found in the DOMAG image (**Figure 8C**). 10 min after perforation, compared with the baseline image at the white circle in **Figure 8C** (b), the two venous branches of the involved vessel and its downstream disappeared. At the same time, the left collateral vein was significantly increased to compensate for blood flow (white arrows in **Figure 8C** (b). Finally, changes in blood flow were quantified by integrating the flow velocity in the projection plane to obtain arterial flow maps.

Furthermore, blood vessel images can be obtained by incorporating OMAG technique into PS-OCT instrument [65]. Both Jung-Taek Oh and Kwan S Park used PS-OCT for quantitative assessment and monitoring of wound healing. Epidermis (E) and dermis layers (D), blood vessel (V), and cartilage (C) in the tissue of the pinna is observable in the reflectivity images. And blood vessels can be separately visualized in the blood vessel images by OMAG technique (**Figure 8D**) [65, 66]. The phase retardation image represents cumulative phase retardation due to the birefringence inside the tissue because the difference in phase shift between two characteristic polarization states of backscattered light from the tissue is altered by the tissue birefringence. Therefore, PS-OCT can characterize the amount of collagen by measuring the polarization parameters of the sample, such as phase retardation and degree of polarization (DOP), which will help us to observe the growth direction and recovery of the wound [67].

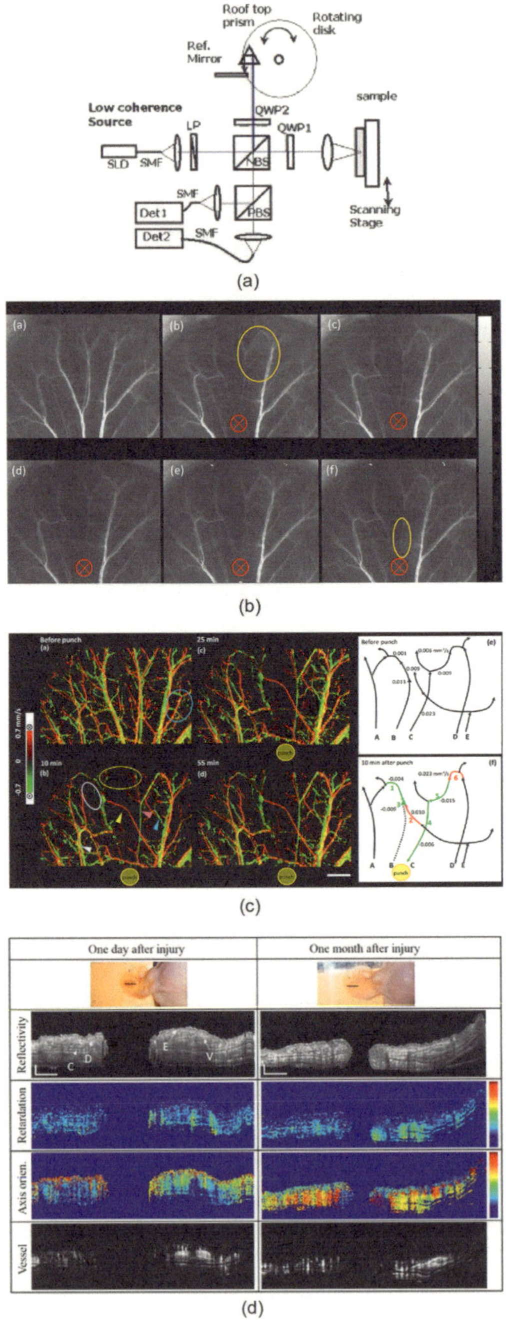

Figure 8.
(a) Schematic of the bulk-type PS-OCT system. (b) Images acquired from the laser speckle imaging system showing the large-scale blood flow changes of the mouse ear following a punch biopsy. (a) Baseline image of the mouse ear before punch; (b)-(f) are images taken at 10 s, 5 min, 10 min, 25 min, and 55 min after punch, respectively. Scale bar: 1 mm. (c) Changes in blood flow velocity and direction of the mouse ear following a punch biopsy. (a) Baseline DOMAG image of the mouse ear; (b), (c) and (d) are DOMAG images taken at before punch, 10 min, 25 min and 55 min after the punch, respectively. (e) and (f) are skeletonized arterial network at baseline and at 10 min after he punch, respectively. 1–6 denote the blood vessel segments that have shown significant blood flow changes, A-E denote the five main arterial branches. Scale bar: 1 mm. (D) Multifunctional PS-OCT imaging of the punch biopsy wound model of a mouse. Reprinted with permission from reference [64–66].

3. AI for extracting and quantitating the feature information of skin

Artificial intelligence (AI) came out in 1956. This technology is widely used in various fields, and realizes intelligent diagnosis and treatment in the medical field through the screening, diagnosis, and management of diseases. Machine learning (ML), which is a subset of artificial intelligence, is represented by mathematical algorithms that improve learning through experience. There are two main types of machine learning algorithms (**Figure 9**): (i) unsupervised (ability to spot patterns), (ii) supervised (classification and prediction algorithms based on previous examples) [68–70]. ML has gradually become a common method for solving difficult problems in artificial intelligence because computer algorithms can be automatically improved through previous experience [71]. There are dozens of algorithms in ML, including deep learning, decision trees, clustering, and Bayesian. For example, the use of decision trees to monitor the depth of anesthesia is a type of ML [72]. Artificial neural networks (ANNs) are mathematical models of information processing based on structures similar to the brain's synaptic connections. ANNs have performances such as self-learning, associative storage, and fast finding optimal solutions, which are far superior to ML algorithms, and are especially suitable for dealing with cluttered and unstructured data (such as images, audio, and text) [73]. As researchers delved into the structure of ANNs, Deep neural networks (DNN) with more and more complex network hierarchies were produced [74]. It also means that DNNs are more capable of modeling or abstract representations of things, as well as simulating more complex models.

3.1 Supervised learning for dermatology

Skin cancer is a common cancer type [75]. Melanoma and non-melanoma are the two main types of skin cancer, with melanoma being the most dangerous type of skin cancer with a high mortality rate [76]. Traditional methods for early detection of skin cancer include skin self-examination and skin clinical examination [77]. However, skin self-examination is a random method and its accuracy depends on how well people know about skin cancer. In addition, the use of professional medical tools such as dermoscopy and microspectroscopy for clinical examinations is not only expensive but also requires professionals to operate [78]. Therefore, using AI to identify patients and upload shared images for diagnosis has become a more convenient method.

The most commonly used machine learning algorithm in dermatology is supervised learning. It is mainly related to retrieval-based AI, where we need to input already labeled data in advance [79]. The goal is to analyze this training data and produce an inferred feature that can be used to map out new instances. For example, when identifying benign and malignant skin lesions, we need to label the skin lesions images as benign and malignant in advance. In this approach, automatic classification of new and unlabeled images can be achieved once training on these images is complete. Esteva et al. explored the accuracy of this skin cancer classification algorithm by comparing deep-learning diagnoses with labeled results from 21 dermatologists. They used approximately 1.28 million images (1000 object categories) from the 2014 ImageNet Large-Scale Visual Recognition Challenge as pre-training objects to form validation and testing datasets. **Figure 10** shows the working system. The area under the curve (AUC) of the CNN algorithm exceeds 91%, indicating that the sensitivity and specificity in the classification of epidermal and melanocytic lesions is superior to

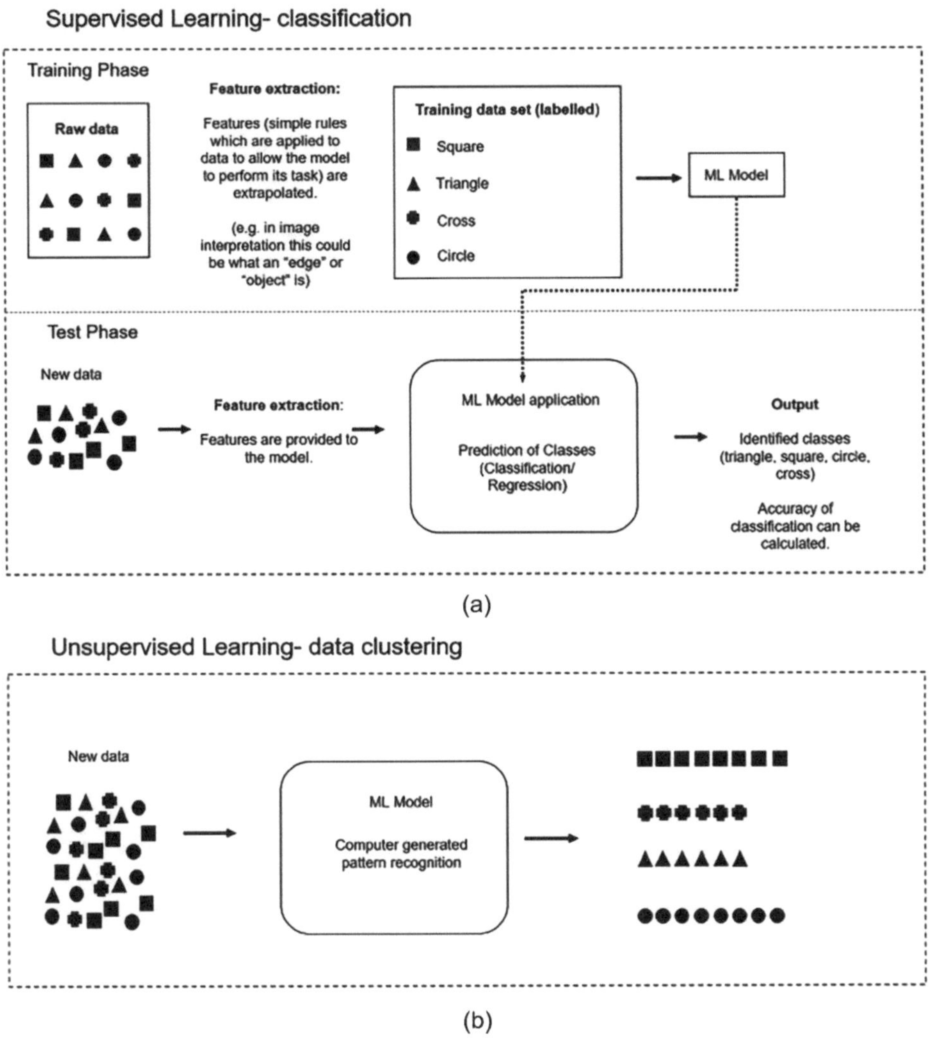

Figure 9.
Machine learning algorithms (a) supervised learning (b) unsupervised learning. Reprinted with permission from reference [68].

that of dermatologists. The results of this study show that, well-trained deep learning enables highly accurate diagnostic classification [80]. At present, ML has been gradually applied in combination with optical technology, which is mainly manifested in the use of AI-assisted analysis of OCTA data to achieve advanced diagnosis and correction of dispersion problems in OCT images to improve axial resolutio [81, 82]. These findings will help advance the application of AI in wound healing monitoring.

3.2 Unsupervised learning for dermatology

Unsupervised learning means that the algorithm is only given input data without corresponding output values. This type of algorithm is more of an exploration and does not have the correct output value [83]. Therefore, unsupervised methods are often suitable for situations where the statistics vary widely. For example, in a study

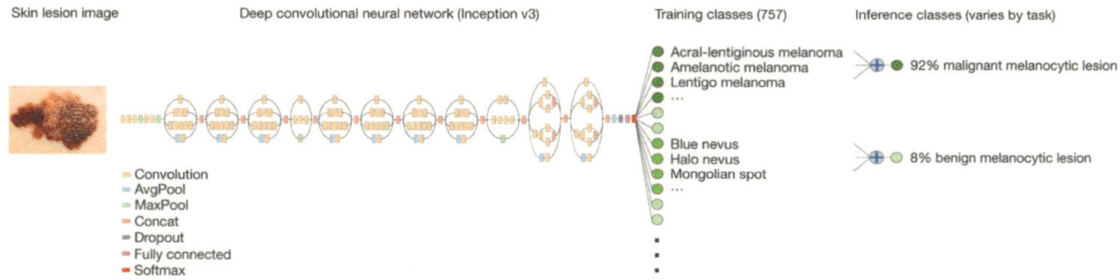

Figure 10.
Deep CNN layout. Reprinted with permission from reference [80].

by Kharazmi et al. [84] detecting basal cell carcinoma (BCC), unsupervised learning was used to classify vascular features in BCC dermoscopy for automatic cancer detection. The results show that the framework outperforms the state-of-the-art norm supervised learning results by 7% in Area Under Curve (AUC), with a sensitivity of 98.1% for BBC detection. This approach eliminates the need for supervised learning to use large and dense datasets at multiple scales to find appropriate images to build blocks of visual content [85]. So the advantage over supervised learning is that the algorithm is free to act in order to learn more about the data and present interesting findings. It is popular in clustering applications or the behavior of discovering groups in data and associations or predicting the behavior of rules that describe data.

3.3 Deep learning for classification of OCT images

OCT is also often used to detect BBC at the dermis-epidermal junction due to its ability to sub-epidermally visualize the skin structure and any underlying lesions [86]. Li et al. [87] used an image-based approach to identify the skin surface and normalized the skin image by surface flattening, then used pre-trained AlexNet, VGG-16, VGG-19 and GoogLeNet for deep feature extraction, and finally used SVM for BCC Classification. The experimental results show that the system based on the VGG-16 image descriptor is the best with a sensitivity of 0.935.

In the current research, image-based deep learning is mainly used in medical image noise reduction and reconstruction processing. Disease diagnosis mainly focuses on tumor detection, brain nervous system disease classification, and cardiovascular disease detection. There are few related studies in the field of skin [88–93]. For example, Kermany D et al. applied deep learning to a dataset of optical coherence tomography images to form a diagnostic tool for screening patients with common treatable blind retinal diseases. The trial results showed that the diagnostic tool was as accurate as hospital specialists in classifying age-related macular degeneration and diabetic macular edema [94]. Abdolmanafi et al. also used intra-coronary tomography images provided by intravascular optical coherence tomography (IV-OCT) as a deep learning library, and extracted the features of convolutional neural network features and fully convolutional network. The accuracy of the diagnostic models can be as high as 90% [95].

4. Challenges and perspectives

In conclusion, most current studies consider hydrogels to be ideal candidates for synthetic wound dressings because of their 3D structure and high water content similar to skin, which ensures a moist environment for wounds [96, 97]. A wide variety of polymers have been used alone or in blends to create hydrogels designed for biomedical applications, with a focus on wound healing and less scarring [98–101]. In addition, most of the current research shows that non-invasive optical technology DRS and OCT may be useful for research related to abnormal wound healing. Although artificial intelligence has only realized the diagnosis of skin diseases [49, 52–55, 102], it will be gradually applied to the management of wound healing in the future.

Although the application of multifunctional composite hydrogels has obvious advantages, most of them are in the basic research stage of animal experiments, and there is still a lack of large-scale clinical studies to prove their efficacy and safety. In order to prevent and reduce the occurrence of adverse reactions, the indications and correct operation methods of each material hydrogel should be strictly mastered, and a comprehensive analysis of individuals should be carried out to remove adverse factors. We still have a long way to go in clinical application of wounds [103].

Dayong Yang et al. prepared persistent luminescent nanoparticles (PLNPs) containing a hydrogel (PL-gel) for targeted, sustained, and autofluorescence-free tumor metastasis imaging [104]. Professor Yu Lin's team develop a tri-modal bioimaging technique, they longitudinally and non-invasively track the degradation behavior of materials by designing and synthesizing thermosensitive hydrogels containing macromolecular fluorescent probes and magnetic resonance imaging (MRI) contrast agents, utilizing the collaborative application of optical techniques such as ultrasound, fluorescence, and MRI [105]. At present, the combination of hydrogel and optical technology mainly focuses on the tracking function. There are relatively few studies on the monitoring function of hydrogel in vivo efficacy, and there is still a lot of room for improvement.

The past few years have witnessed many changes in the fields of ML and Computer Science. Following this long progress, one may see many exciting developments in the next few years, but there are challenges before it can become more robust and be widely adopted in the clinic. AI is constrained by a lack of high quality, high volume, longitudinal, outcomes data [106]. Even the same image modality on the same disease site, the parameters of the imaging setting and protocols might be different in different clinical settings [91, 107]. But we believe that AI can play an important role in medical imaging and disease diagnosis when we master how to organize and preprocess data generated from different institutions and can encourage more sharing of image data.

Although there are relatively few studies on the use of deep learning in skin OCT and DRS imaging, current research on disease diagnosis systems combining AI and OCT leads us to believe that optical technology can be fully integrated with AI for wound healing monitoring [108]. This not only helps us to better detect the recovery of wounds treated with hydrogel dressings, but also more accurately evaluate the effectiveness of hydrogel treatment. In addition, AI based on optical images also helps to determine the type and depth of wounds, and can better design corresponding hydrogel wound dressings. Finally, we also believe that more and more new and safe wound dressings will be developed and applied with the aid of AI and optical imaging technology.

Acknowledgments and funding

This work was supported by the Natural science Foundation of Guangdong Province (2021A1515011654), Fundamental Research Funds for the Central

Universities of China (20720210117), Joint Funds for the Innovation of Science and Technology of Fujian province (2019Y9128), Xiamen Key Laboratory of Endocrine-Related Cancer Precision Medicine (XKLEC2021KF03, XKLEC2020KF04). Key Laboratory of OptoElectronic Science and Technology for Medicine of Ministry of Education, Fujian Provincial Key Laboratory of Photonics Technology (JYG2105). XMU Undergraduate Innovation and Entrepreneurship Training Programs (202210384051S202210384404, 2021X1119, 2021Y1119, S202110384391), and Shenzhen Bay Laboratory (SZBL2019062801005).

Conflict of interest

The authors declare that they have no known competing financial interests or personal relationships that could have appeared to influence the work reported in this paper.

Author details

Qingliang Zhao* and Lin Chen
Department of Laboratory Medicine, Shenzhen Research Institute of Xiamen University, Xiamen University, State Key Laboratory of Molecular Vaccinology and Molecular Diagnostics, Center for Molecular Imaging and Translational Medicine, School of Public Health, Xiamen, China

*Address all correspondence to: zhaoql@xmu.edu.cn

References

[1] Sorg H, Tilkorn DJ, Hager S, Hauser J, Mirastschijski U. Skin wound healing: An update on the current knowledge and concepts. European Surgical Research. 2017;**58**(1-2):81-94. DOI: 10.1159/000454919

[2] Hassanshahi A, Hassanshahi M, Khabbazi S, Hosseini-Khah Z, Peymanfar Y, Ghalamkari S, et al. Adipose-derived stem cells for wound healing. Journal of Cellular Physiology. 2019;**234**(6):7903-7914. DOI: 10.1002/jcp.27922

[3] Wichterle O, Lím D. Hydrophilic gels for biological use. Nature. 1960;**185**:117-118. DOI: 10.1038/185117a0

[4] Boucard N, Viton C, Agay D, Mari E, Roger T, Chancerelle Y, et al. The use of physical hydrogels of chitosan for skin regeneration following third-degree burns. Biomaterials. 2007;**28**(24):3478-3488. DOI: 10.1016/j.biomaterials.2007.04.021

[5] Kirker KR, Luo Y, Nielson JH, Shelby J, Prestwich GD. Glycosaminoglycan hydrogel films as bio-interactive dressings for wound healing. Biomaterials. 2002;**23**(17):3661-3671. DOI: 10.1016/s0142-9612(02)00100-x

[6] Balakrishnan B, Mohanty M, Umashankar PR, Jayakrishnan A. Evaluation of an in situ forming hydrogel wound dressing based on oxidized alginate and gelatin. Biomaterials. 2005;**26**(32):6335-6342. DOI: 10.1016/j.biomaterials.2005.04.012

[7] Griffin DR, Weaver WM, Scumpia PO, Di Carlo D, Segura T. Accelerated wound healing by injectable microporous gel scaffolds assembled from annealed building blocks. Nature Materials. 2015;**14**(7):737-744. DOI: 10.1038/nmat4294

[8] Cheng B, Yan Y, Qi J, Deng L, Shao ZW, Zhang KQ, Li B, Sun Z, Li X. Cooperative assembly of a peptide Gelator and silk fibroin afford an injectable hydrogel for tissue engineering. ACS Applied Materials & Interfaces 2018;**10**(15):12474-12484. DOI: 10.1021/acsami.8b01725

[9] Qu J, Zhao X, Liang Y, Zhang T, Ma PX, Guo B. Antibacterial adhesive injectable hydrogels with rapid self-healing, extensibility and compressibility as wound dressing for joints skin wound healing. Biomaterials. 2018;**183**:185-199. DOI: 10.1016/j.biomaterials.2018.08.044

[10] Kiyozumi T, Kanatani Y, Ishihara M, Saitoh D, Shimizu J, Yura H, et al. Medium (DMEM/F12)-containing chitosan hydrogel as adhesive and dressing in autologous skin grafts and accelerator in the healing process. Journal of Biomedical Materials Research. Part B, Applied Biomaterials. 2006;**79**(1):129-136. DOI: 10.1002/jbm.b.30522

[11] Jones AM, Vaughan DE. Hydrogel dressings in the management of a variety of wound types: A review. Journal of Orthopaedic Nursing. 2005;**9**(4):234-238. DOI: 10.1159/000085725

[12] Gennari O, Rega R, Mugnano M. A skin-over-liquid platform with compliant microbumps actuated by pyro-EHD pressure. NPG Asia Materials. 2019;**11**(1):1-8. DOI: 10.1038/s41427-018-0100-z

[13] Caló E, Khutoryanskiy VV. Biomedical applications of hydrogels: A review of patents and commercial

products - ScienceDirect. European Polymer Journal. 2015;**65**:252-267. DOI: 10.1016/j.eurpolymj.2014.11.024

[14] Li Z, Zhou F, Li Z, Lin S, Chen L, Liu L, et al. Hydrogel cross-linked with dynamic covalent bonding and Micellization for promoting burn wound healing. ACS Applied Materials & Interfaces. 2018;**10**(30):25194-25202. DOI: 10.1021/acsami.8b08165

[15] Sun G, Zhang X, Shen YI, Sebastian R, Dickinson LE, Fox-Talbot K, et al. Dextran hydrogel scaffolds enhance angiogenic responses and promote complete skin regeneration during burn wound healing. Proceedings of the National Academy of Sciences of the United States of America. 2011;**108**(52):20976-20981. DOI: 10.1073/pnas.1115973108

[16] Boateng J, Catanzano O. Advanced therapeutic dressings for effective wound healing--a review. Journal of Pharmaceutical Sciences. 2015;**104**(11):3653-3680. DOI: 10.1002/jps.24610

[17] Catoira MC, Fusaro L, Di Francesco D, Ramella M, Boccafoschi F. Overview of natural hydrogels for regenerative medicine applications. Journal of Materials Science. Materials in Medicine. 2019;**30**(10):115. DOI: 10.1007/s10856-019-6318-7

[18] Dimatteo R, Darling NJ, Segura T. In situ forming injectable hydrogels for drug delivery and wound repair. Advanced Drug Delivery Reviews. 2018;**127**:167-184. DOI: 10.1016/j.addr.2018.03.007

[19] Zhang YS, Khademhosseini A. Advances in engineering hydrogels. Science. 2017;**356**(6337):eaaf3627. DOI: 10.1126/science.aaf3627

[20] Patenaude M, Smeets NM, Hoare T. Designing injectable, covalently cross-linked hydrogels for biomedical applications. Macromolecular Rapid Communications. 2014;**35**(6):598-617. DOI: 10.1002/marc. 201300818

[21] Lu L, Yuan S, Wang J, Shen Y, Deng S, Xie L, et al. The formation mechanism of hydrogels. Current Stem Cell Research & Therapy. 2018;**13**(7):490-496. DOI: 10.2174/1574888X12666170612102706

[22] Mo C, Xiang L, Chen Y. Advances in injectable and self-healing polysaccharide hydrogel based on the Schiff Base reaction. Macromolecular Rapid Communications. 2021;**42**(10):e2100025. DOI: 10.1002/marc.202100025

[23] Elisseeff J, Anseth K, Sims D, McIntosh W, Randolph M, Langer R. Transdermal photopolymerization for minimally invasive implantation. Proceedings of the National Academy of Sciences of the United States of America. 1999;**96**(6):3104-3107. DOI: 10.1073/pnas.96.6.3104

[24] Tu Y, Chen N, Li C, Liu H, Zhu R, Chen S, et al. Advances in injectable self-healing biomedical hydrogels. Acta Biomaterialia. 2019;**90**:1-20. DOI: 10.1016/j.actbio.2019.03.057

[25] Liu SQ, Ee PL, Ke CY, Hedrick JL, Yang YY. Biodegradable poly(ethylene glycol)-peptide hydrogels with well-defined structure and properties for cell delivery. Biomaterials. 2009;**30**(8):1453-1461. DOI: 10.1016/j.biomaterials. 2008. 11. 023

[26] Stubbe B, Mignon A, Declercq H, Van Vlierberghe S, Dubruel P. Development of gelatin-alginate hydrogels for burn wound treatment. Macromolecular Bioscience. 2019;**19**(8):e1900123. DOI: 10.1002/mabi.201900123

[27] Rowley JA, Madlambayan G, Mooney DJ. Alginate hydrogels as

synthetic extracellular matrix materials. Biomaterials. 1999;**20**(1):45-53. DOI: 10.1016/s0142-9612(98)00107-0

[28] Wiegand C, Heinze T, Hipler UC. Comparative in vitro study on cytotoxicity, antimicrobial activity, and binding capacity for pathophysiological factors in chronic wounds of alginate and silver-containing alginate. Wound Repair and Regeneration. 2009;**17**(4):511-521. DOI: 10.1111/j.1524-475X.2009.00503.x

[29] Zheng WJ, Gao J, Wei Z, Zhou JX, et al. Facile fabrication of self healing carboxymethyl cellulose hydrogels. European Polymer Journal. 2015;**72**(72):514-522. DOI: 10.1016/j.eurpolymj.2015.06.013

[30] Capanema NSV, Mansur AAP, de Jesus AC, Carvalho SM, de Oliveira LC, Mansur HS. Superabsorbent crosslinked carboxymethyl cellulose-PEG hydrogels for potential wound dressing applications. International Journal of Biological Macromolecules. 2018;**106**:1218-1234. DOI: 10.1016/j.ijbiomac.2017.08.124

[31] Xu X, Che L, Xu L, Huang D, Wu J, Du Z, et al. Green preparation of anti-inflammation an injectable 3D porous hydrogel for speeding up deep second-degree scald wound healing. RSC Advances. 2020;**10**(59):36101-36110. DOI: 10.1039/d0ra04990e

[32] Zhang X, Xu L, Huang X, Wei S, Zhai M. Structural study and preliminary biological evaluation on the collagen hydrogel crosslinked by γ-irradiation. Journal of Biomedical Materials Research. Part A. 2012;**100**(11):2960-2969. DOI: 10.1002/jbm.a.34243 Epub 2012 Jun 14

[33] Zhang H, Sun X, Wang J, Zhang Y, Wang L. Multifunctional injectable hydrogel dressings for effectively accelerating wound healing: Enhancing biomineralization strategy. Advanced Functional Materials. 2021:**31**(23):2100093. DOI: 10.1002/adfm.202100093

[34] Stone Ii R, Natesan S, Kowalczewski CJ, Mangum LH, Clay NE, Clohessy RM, et al. Advancements in regenerative strategies through the continuum of burn care. Frontiers in Pharmacology. 2018;**9**:672. DOI: 10.3389/fphar.2018.00672

[35] Homaeigohar S, Boccaccini AR. Antibacterial biohybrid nanofibers for wound dressings. Acta Biomaterialia. 2020;**107**:25-49. DOI: 10.1016/j.actbio.2020.02.022

[36] Chen H, Cheng R, Zhao X, Zhang Y, Tam A, Yan Y, et al. An injectable selfhealing coordinative hydrogel with antibacterial and angiogenic properties for diabetic skin wound repair. NPG Asia Materials. 2019;**11**(1):3. DOI: 10.1038/s41427-018-0103-9

[37] Liu X, Hou M, Luo X, Zheng M, Wang X, Zhang H, et al. Thermoresponsive hemostatic hydrogel with a biomimetic nanostructure constructed from aggregated collagen nanofibers. Biomacromolecules. 2021;**22**(2):319-329. DOI: 10.1021/acs.biomac.0c01167

[38] Ting YH, Chen HJ, Cheng WJ, Horng JC. Zinc(II)-histidine induced collagen peptide assemblies: Morphology modulation and hydrolytic catalysis evaluation. Biomacromolecules. 2018;**19**(7):2629-2637. DOI: 10.1021/acs.biomac.8b00247

[39] Zhu S, Yuan Q, Yin T, You J, Gu Z, Xiong S, et al. Self-assembly of collagen-based biomaterials: Preparation, characterizations and biomedical applications. Journal of Materials Chemistry B. 2018;**6**(18):2650-2676. DOI: 10.1039/c7tb02999c

[40] Yao Y, Zhang A, Yuan C, Chen X, Liu Y. Recent trends on burn wound care: Hydrogel dressings and scaffolds. Biomaterials Science. 2021;**9**(13):4523-4540. DOI: 10.1039/d1bm00411e

[41] Boonkaew B, Barber PM, Rengpipat S, Supaphol P, Kempf M, He J, et al. Development and characterization of a novel, antimicrobial, sterile hydrogel dressing for burn wounds: Single-step production with gamma irradiation creates silver nanoparticles and radical polymerization. Journal of Pharmaceutical Sciences. 2014;**103**(10):3244-3253. DOI: 10.1002/jps.24095

[42] Kim MH, Park H, Nam HC, Park SR, Jung JY, Park WH. Injectable methylcellulose hydrogel containing silver oxide nanoparticles for burn wound healing. Carbohydrate Polymers. 2018;**181**:579-586. DOI: 10.1016/j.carbpol.2017.11.109

[43] Hashmi MU, Khan F, Khalid N, et al. Hydrogels incorporated with silver nanocolloids prepared from antioxidant rich Aerva javanica as disruptive agents against burn wound infections. Colloids & Surfaces A Physicochemical & Engineering Aspects. 2017;**529**(20):475- 486. DOI:10.1016/j.colsurfa.2017.06.036

[44] Lohmann N, Schirmer L, Atallah P, Wandel E, Ferrer RA, Werner C, et al. Glycosaminoglycan-based hydrogels capture inflammatory chemokines and rescue defective wound healing in mice. Science Translational Medicine. 2017;**9**(386):eaai9044. DOI: 10.1126/scitranslmed.aai9044

[45] Schulz A, Fuchs PC, Rothermundt I, Hoffmann A, Rosenberg L, Shoham Y, et al. Enzymatic debridement of deeply burned faces: Healing and early scarring based on tissue preservation compared to traditional surgical debridement. Burns. 2017;**43**(6):1233-1243. DOI: 10.1016/j.burns.2017.02.016

[46] Behrens AM, Sikorski MJ, Li T, Wu ZJ, Griffith BP, Kofinas P. Blood-aggregating hydrogel particles for use as a hemostatic agent. Acta Biomaterialia. 2014;**10**(2):701-708. DOI: 10.1016/j.actbio.2013.10.029

[47] Hong Y, Zhou F, Hua Y, Zhang X, Ni C, Pan D, et al. A strongly adhesive hemostatic hydrogel for the repair of arterial and heart bleeds. Nature Communications. 2019;**10**(1):2060. DOI: 10.1038/s41467-019-10004-7

[48] Weingarten MS, Neidrauer M, Mateo A, Mao X, McDaniel JE, Jenkins L, et al. Prediction of wound healing in human diabetic foot ulcers by diffuse near-infrared spectroscopy: A pilot study. Wound Repair and Regeneration. 2010;**18**(2):180-185. DOI: 10.1111/j.1524-475x.2010.00583.x

[49] Cutting KF, White R. Defined and refined: Criteria for identifying wound infection revisited. British Journal of Community Nursing. 2004;**9**(3):S6-S15. DOI: 10.12968/bjcn.2004.9.Sup1.12495

[50] Zhou A. A survey of optical imaging techniques for assessing wound. The International Journal of Intelligent Control and Systems. 2012;**17**:79-85

[51] Neidrauer M, Papazoglou E. Optical non-invasive characterization of chronic. Bioengineering Research of Chronic Wounds. 2009;**1**:381-404

[52] Kaiser M, Yafi A, Cinat M, Choi B, Durkin AJ. Noninvasive assessment of burn wound severity using optical technology: A review of current and future modalities. Burns. 2011;**37**(3):377-386. DOI: 10.1016/j.burns.2010.11.012

[53] Hsu CK, Tzeng SY, Yang CC, Lee JY, Huang LL, Chen WR, et al. Non-invasive evaluation of therapeutic response in keloid scar using diffuse reflectance spectroscopy. Biomedical Optics Express. 2015;**6**(2):390-404. DOI: 10.1364/BOE.6.000390

[54] Cappon DJ, Farrell TJ, Fang Q, Hayward JE. Fiber-optic probe design and optical property recovery algorithm for optical biopsy of brain tissue. Journal of Biomedical Optics. 2013;**18**(10):107004. DOI: 10.1117/1.JBO.18.10.107004

[55] Cerussi A, Shah N, Hsiang D, Durkin A, Butler J, Tromberg BJ. In vivo absorption, scattering, and physiologic properties of 58 malignant breast tumors determined by broadband diffuse optical spectroscopy. Journal of Biomedical Optics. 2006;**11**(4):044005. DOI: 10.1117/1.2337546

[56] Onozato ML, Andrews PM, Li Q, Jiang J, Cable A, Chen Y. Optical coherence tomography of human kidney. The Journal of Urology. 2010;**183**(5):2009-2004. DOI: 10.1016/j.juro.2009.12.091

[57] Wierwille J, Andrews PM, Onozato ML, Jiang J, Cable A, Chen Y. In vivo, label-free, three-dimensional quantitative imaging of kidney microcirculation using Doppler optical coherence tomography. Laboratory Investigation. 2011;**91**(11):1596-1604. DOI: 10.1038/labinvest.2011.112

[58] Zhao Q, Dai C, Fan S, Lv J, Nie L. Synergistic efficacy of salicylic acid with a penetration enhancer on human skin monitored by OCT and diffuse reflectance spectroscopy. Scientific Reports. 2016;**6**:34954. DOI: 10.1038/srep34954

[59] Marin A, Verdel N, Milanič M, Majaron B. Noninvasive monitoring of dynamical processes in bruised human skin using diffuse reflectance spectroscopy and pulsed Photothermal radiometry. Sensors (Basel). 2021;**21**(1):302. DOI: 10.3390/s21010302

[60] Chen B, Zhang Y, Gao S, Li D. Extraction of the structural properties of skin tissue via diffuse reflectance spectroscopy: An inverse methodology. Sensors (Basel). 2021;**21**(11):3745. DOI: 10.3390/s21113745

[61] Fujimoto J, Swanson E. The development, commercialization, and impact of optical coherence tomography. Investigative Ophthalmology & Visual Science. 2016;**57**(9):OCT1-OCT13. DOI: 10.1167/iovs.16-19963

[62] Wang RK, Jacques SL, Ma Z, Hurst S, Hanson SR, Gruber A. Three dimensional optical angiography. Optics Express. 2007;**15**(7):4083-4097. DOI: 10.1364/oe.15.004083

[63] An L, Qin J, Wang RK. Ultrahigh sensitive optical microangiography for in vivo imaging of microcirculations within human skin tissue beds. Optics Express. 2010;**18**(8):8220-8228. DOI: 10.1364/OE.18.008220

[64] Wang H, Shi L, Qin J, Yousefi S, Li Y, Wang RK. Multimodal optical imaging can reveal changes in microcirculation and tissue oxygenation during skin wound healing. Lasers in Surgery and Medicine. 2014;**46**(6):470-478. DOI: 10.1002/lsm.22254

[65] Park KS, Choi WJ, Song S, Xu J, Wang RK. Multifunctional in vivo imaging for monitoring wound healing using swept-source polarization-sensitive optical coherence tomography. Lasers in Surgery and Medicine. 2018;**50**(3):213-221. DOI: 10.1002/lsm.22767

[66] Oh JT, Lee SW, Kim YS, Suhr KB, Kim BM.Quantification of the wound

healing using polarization-sensitive optical coherence tomography. Journal of Biomedical Optics. 2006;**11**(4):041124. DOI: 10.1117/1.2338826

[67] Adams DC, Szabari MV, Lagares D, McCrossan AF, Hariri LP, Tager AM, et al. Assessing the progression of systemic sclerosis by monitoring the tissue optic axis using PS-OCT. Scientific Reports. 2020;**10**(1):2561. DOI: 10.1038/s41598-020-59330-7

[68] Tack C. Artificial intelligence and machine learning | applications in musculoskeletal physiotherapy. Musculoskeletal Science & Practice. 2019;**39**:164-169. DOI: 10.1016/j.msksp.2018.11.012

[69] Hamet P, Tremblay J. Artificial intelligence in medicine. Metabolism. 2017;**69S**:S36-S40. DOI: 10.1016/j.metabol.2017.01.011

[70] Singh Pathania Y, Budania A. Artificial intelligence in dermatology: "unsupervised" versus "supervised" machine learning. International Journal of Dermatology. 2021;**60**(1):e28-e29. DOI: 10.1111/ijd.15288

[71] Shafique M, Theocharides T, Bouganis CS, Hanif MA, Rehman S. An overview of next-generation architectures for machine learning: Roadmap, opportunities and challenges in the IoT Era. In: 2018 Design, Automation & Test in Europe Conference & Exhibition (DATE). 2018;**1558**(1101):827-832. DOI: 10.23919/DATE.2018.8342120

[72] Khan FH, Ashraf U, Altaf M, Saadeh W. A patient-specific machine learning based EEG processor for accurate estimation of depth of anesthesia. In: 2018 IEEE Biomedical Circuits and Systems Conference (BioCAS). IEEE; 2018

[73] He K, Zhang X, Ren S, Sun J. Delving deep into rectifiers: Surpassing human-level performance on ImageNet classification. Computer Vision and Pattern Recognition. In: Proceedings of the IEEE International Conference on Computer Vision. Santiago, Chile; 2015. pp. 7-13

[74] LeCun Y, Bengio Y, Hinton G. Deep learning. Nature. 2015;**521**(7553):436-444. DOI: 10.1038/nature14539

[75] Marsland S. Machine Learning: An Algorithmic Perspective. 1st. ed. Chapman and Hall/CRC: Massey University Manawatu; 2009. DOI: 10.1016/S0967-2109(97)89838-9

[76] Ray A, Gupta A, Amutha AL. Skin lesion classification with deep convolutional neural network: Process development and validation. JMIR Dermatology. 2020;**3**(1):e18438. DOI: 10.2196/18438

[77] Carvalho TMD, Noels E, Wakkee M, Udrea A, Nijsten T. Development of smartphone apps for skin cancer risk assessment: Progress and promise. JMIR Dermatology. 2019;**2**(1):e13376. DOI: 10.2196/13376

[78] Loescher LJ, Janda M, Soyer HP, Shea K, Curiel-Lewandrowski C. Advances in skin cancer early detection and diagnosis. Seminars in Oncology Nursing. 2013;**29**(3):170-181. DOI: 10.1016/j.soncn.2013.06.003

[79] Lieber CA, Majumder SK, Ellis DL, Billheimer DD, Mahadevan-Jansen A. In vivo nonmelanoma skin cancer diagnosis using Raman microspectroscopy. Lasers in Surgery and Medicine. 2008;**40**(7):461-467. DOI: 10.1002/lsm.20653

[80] Esteva A, Kuprel B, Novoa RA, Ko J, Swetter SM, Blau HM, et al.

Dermatologist-level classification of skin cancer with deep neural networks. Nature. 2017;**542**(7639):115-118. DOI: 10.1038/nature21056

[81] Hormel TT, Hwang TS, Bailey ST, Wilson DJ, Huang D, Jia Y. Artificial intelligence in OCT angiography. Progress in Retinal and Eye Research. 2021;**85**:100965. DOI: 10.1016/j.preteyeres.2021.100965

[82] Dan Y, Wenxin G, Tonglei C, Zhulin W, Bin X. Artificial neural network (ANN) for dispersion compensation of spectral domain – Optical coherence tomography (SD-OCT). Instrumentation Science & Technology. 2022. DOI: 10.1080/10739149.2022.2048008

[83] Haenssle HA, Fink C, Schneiderbauer R, Toberer F, Buhl T, Blum A, et al. Man against machine: Diagnostic performance of a deep learning convolutional neural network for dermoscopic melanoma recognition in comparison to 58 dermatologists. Annals of Oncology. 2018;**29**(8):1836-1842. DOI: 10.1093/annonc/mdy166

[84] Arevalo J, Cruz-Roa A, Arias V, Romero E, González FA. An unsupervised feature learning framework for basal cell carcinoma image analysis. Artificial Intelligence in Medicine. 2015;**64**(2):131-145. DOI: 10.1016/j.artmed.2015.04.004

[85] Kharazmi P, Kalia S, Lui H, Wang ZJ, Lee TK. A feature fusion system for basal cell carcinoma detection through data-driven feature learning and patient profile. Skin Research and Technology. 2018;**24**(2):256-264. DOI: 10.1111/srt.12422

[86] Boone M, Suppa M, Miyamoto M, Marneffe A, Jemec G, Del Marmol V. In vivo assessment of optical properties of basal cell carcinoma and differentiation of BCC subtypes by high-definition optical coherence tomography. Biomedical Optics Express. 2016;**7**(6):2269-2284. DOI: 10.1364/BOE.7.002269

[87] Li A, Cheng J, Yow AP, Srivastava R, Wong DW, Hong Liang T, et al. Automated basal cell carcinoma detection in high-definition optical coherence tomography. In: 2016 38th Annual International Conference of the IEEE Engineering in Medicine and Biology Society (EMBC). 2016. pp. 2885-2888. DOI: 10.1109/EMBC.2016.7591332

[88] Yang Y, Sun J, Li HB. ADMMCS net: A deep learning approach for image compressive sensing. IEEE Transactions on Pattern Analysis and Machine Intelligence. 2020;**42**(3):521-538

[89] Adler J, Öktem O. Learned primal-dual reconstruction. IEEE Transactions on Medical Imaging. 2018;**37**(6):1322-1332

[90] Chen H, Zhang Y, Kalra MK, et al. Low-dose CT with a residual encoderdecoder convolutional neural network. IEEE Transactions on Medical Imaging. 2017;**36**(12):2524-2535

[91] Huang S, Yang J, Fong S, Zhao Q. Artificial intelligence in cancer diagnosis and prognosis: Opportunities and challenges. Cancer Letters. 2020;**471**:61-71. DOI: 10.1016/j.canlet.2019.12.007

[92] Cao C, Liu F, Tan H, Song D, Shu W, Li W, et al. Deep learning and its applications in biomedicine. Genomics, Proteomics & Bioinformatics. 2018;**16**(1):17-32. DOI: 10.1016/j.gpb.2017.07.003

[93] Wang LH, Qin YB. State of the art and future perspectives of the applications of deep learning in the

medical image analysis. Big Data Research. 2020;**6**(6):83-104

[94] Kermany DS, Goldbaum M, Cai W, Valentim CCS, Liang H, Baxter SL, et al. Identifying medical diagnoses and treatable diseases by image-based deep learning. Cell. 2018;**172**(5):1122-1131.e9. DOI: 10.1016/j.cell.2018.02.010

[95] Abdolmanafi A, Cheriet F, Duong L, Ibrahim R, Dahdah N. An automatic diagnostic system of coronary artery lesions in Kawasaki disease using intravascular optical coherence tomography imaging. Journal of Biophotonics. 2020;**13**(1):e201900112. DOI: 10.1002/jbio.201900112

[96] Li J, Yu F, Chen G, Liu J, Li XL, Cheng B, et al. Moist-retaining, self-recoverable, bioadhesive, and transparent in situ forming hydrogels to accelerate wound healing. ACS Applied Materials & Interfaces. 2020;**12**(2):2023-2038. DOI: 10.1021/acsami.9b17180

[97] Korting HC, Schöllmann C, White RJ. Management of minor acute cutaneous wounds: Importance of wound healing in a moist environment. Journal of the European Academy of Dermatology and Venereology. 2011;**25**(2):130-137. DOI: 10.1111/j.1468-3083.2010.03775.x

[98] Feng P, Qiu H, Luo Y, Hu J, Cao Y, Pang Q, et al. Development of Poloxamer hydrogels containing antibacterial guanidine-based polymers for healing of full-thickness skin wound. ACS Biomaterials Science & Engineering. 2021;**7**(9):4557-4568. DOI: 10.1021/acsbiomaterials.1c00600

[99] Shanmugapriya K, Kim H, Kang HW. EGFR-conjugated hydrogel accelerates wound healing on ulcer-induced burn wounds by targeting collagen and inflammatory cells using photoimmunomodulatory inhibition. Materials Science & Engineering. C, Materials for Biological Applications. 2021;**118**:111541. DOI: 10.1016/j.msec.2020.111541

[100] Chen K, Sivaraj D, Davitt MF, Leeolou MC, Henn D, Steele SR, et al. Pullulan-collagen hydrogel wound dressing promotes dermal remodelling and wound healing compared to commercially available collagen dressings. Wound Repair and Regeneration. 2022;**30**(3):397-408. DOI: 10.1111/wrr.13012

[101] Yang L, Lan Y, Guo H, Cheng L, Fan J, Cai X, et al. Ophthalmic drug-loaded N, O-carboxymethyl chitosan hydrogels: Synthesis, in vitro and in vivo evaluation. Acta Pharmacologica Sinica. 2010;**31**(12):1625-1634. DOI: 10.1038/aps.2010.125

[102] Lazarus GS, Cooper DM, Knighton DR, Margolis DJ, Pecoraro RE, Rodeheaver G, et al. Definitions and guidelines for assessment of wounds and evaluation of healing. Archives of Dermatology. 1994;**130**(4):489-493

[103] Zarrintaj P, Khodadadi Yazdi M, Youssefi Azarfam M, Zare M, Ramsey JD, Seidi F, et al. Injectable cell-laden hydrogels for tissue engineering: Recent advances and future opportunities. Tissue Engineering. Part A. 2021;**27**(11-12):821-843. DOI: 10.1089/ten.TEA.2020.0341

[104] Zhao H, Liu C, Gu Z, Dong L, Li F, Yao C, et al. Persistent luminescent nanoparticles containing hydrogels for targeted, sustained, and autofluorescence-free tumor metastasis imaging. Nano Letters. 2020;**20**(1):252-260. DOI: 10.1021/acs.nanolett.9b03755

[105] Chen X, Zhang J, Wu K, Wu X, Ding J. Visualizing the In Vivo Evolution

of an Injectable and Thermosensitive Hydrogel Using Tri-Modal Bioimaging. Small Methods. 2020;**4**(9):2000310. DOI: 10.1002/smtd.202000310

[106] Schwalbe N, Wahl B. Artificial intelligence and the future of global health. Lancet. 2020;**395**(10236):1579-1586. DOI: 10.1016/S0140-6736(20)30226-9

[107] Feng H, Gu ZY, Li Q, Liu QH, Yang XY, Zhang JJ. Identification of significant genes with poor prognosis in ovarian cancer via bioinformatical analysis. Journal of Ovarian Research. 2019;**12**(1):35. DOI: 10.1186/s13048-019-0508-2

[108] Yow AP, Srivastava R, Cheng J, Li A, Liu J, Schmetterer L, et al. Techniques and applications in skin OCT analysis. Advances in Experimental Medicine and Biology. 2020;**1213**:149-163. DOI: 10.1007/978-3-030-33128-3_10

Chapter 13

Minimally Invasive Microneedle: A Novel Approach for Drug Delivery System and Infected Wound Care Management

Bidhan Pramanick and Aishwarya G. Patil

Abstract

Chronic wound healing has become an area of fundamental research. Wound healing for a diabetic patient is one of the significant challenges in the biomedical field. Diabetes is a globally challenging disease that has affected around 400 million people. Many therapeutic factors are introduced to treat chronic wounds, with minimal success due to difficulty in delivery of the drug to the wound location. Microneedle patches are considered an efficient medical treatment procedure to address wound healing problems. The wound healing is accelerated, and the bacterial infection is inhibited by the devices based on microneedle with the loaded active drugs (including hemostatic drugs, bacterial drugs, and anti-inflammatory drugs). The wound healing process is generally divided into three steps: inflammation, proliferation, and tissue remodeling. This chapter will discuss the significant challenges and the advantages of microneedle applications in chronic wound healing.

Keywords: wounds, wound healing, microneedle, drug delivery, disease diagnostic

1. Introduction

A wound can be defined as a disruption of the functioning and anatomical structure of the tissues. This disruption ranges from more severe damage to the subcutaneous tissue with tendons, vessels, nerves, parenchymal organs, muscles, and bones being affected or a small break in the epithelial tissue [1].

Wound healing is a process of recovery, and it has three phases: inflammation, proliferation, and maturation. However, if the process is not thoroughly studied, this is not enough to understand wound healing. Wound healing involves complicated continuous interactions between cells and mediators. Recently, there has been an increase in the understanding of cellular interactions and inflammatory mediators, as new mediators are discovered every year [1, 2].

The complicated and organized cascade of biochemical and cellular events is triggered by an injury resulting in a wound. The nonclosure of the wound or delay in healing is the result of prolongation or failure in any one of the phases of wound

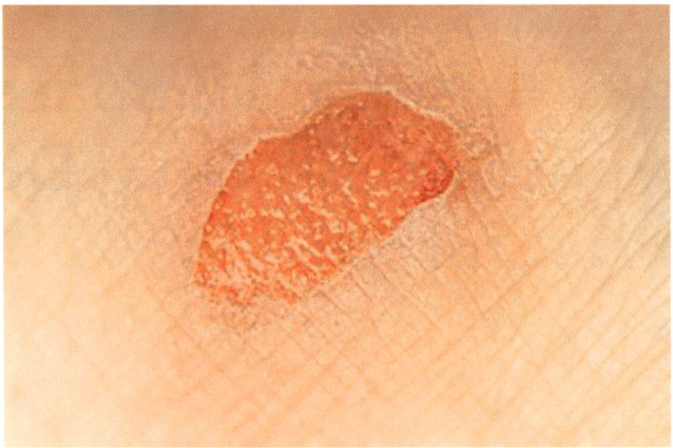

Figure 1.
The macroscopic appearance of an open wound [3].

healing. This delay is one of the significant clinical issues affecting health care expenditure. A better understanding of the pathophysiologic process can better grasp the fundamentals of wound healing physiology [3]. The macroscopic appearance of an open wound is shown in **Figure 1**.

The damaged tissue is restored after the tissue lesion occurs, followed by the tissue repair and regeneration process involving a series of cellular and molecular events. The amalgamation of different dynamic processes involving blood cells, parenchymal cells, and soluble mediators gives rise to different wound healing phases. The tissue edema is developed due to soluble mediators. The area of the tissue injury is reduced by contracting the myofibroblasts and fibroplasia in the proliferative stage. Re-epithelialization and angiogenesis are still observed at this stage. The mesenchymal components are generated by the endothelial cells, which are adequately orchestrated by the signaling proteins. This process is called as Hedgehog pathway [4].

This chapter focuses on the applications of microneedles for wound care management. However, it is also imperative to understand the types of wounds, different stages of the healing process, and available treatments before discussing microneedle-based treatments. Details on wounds and their treatments are presented in the next sections, followed by microneedle application for wound healing [5].

2. Classifications of wounds

Wounds are classified based on many criteria. An essential factor in managing the injury and the wound repair is the time elapsed since the injury. Thus, depending upon the time frame of healing, wounds are clinically categorized as acute or chronic [6].

2.1 Acute wounds

The self-repairing wounds that proceed with an orderly healing process, with an anatomical and functional restoration as the end result, are called acute wounds. A total of 5–10 days or a maximum of 30 days is the duration of time needed for acute wounds to heal. The surgical procedure or traumatic loss of tissue gives rise to acute

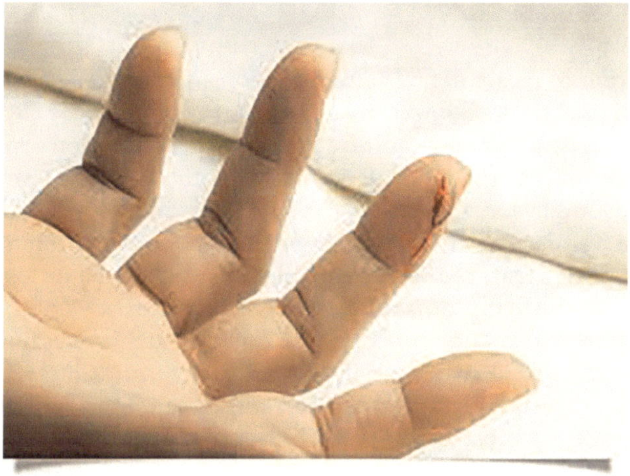

Figure 2.
A photograph of an acute wound or self-repairing wound [6].

wounds. Traumatic wounds usually involve bone fractures or only soft tissue [6]. An image of the acute wound can be a small cut on the finger, as shown in **Figure 2**.

2.2 Chronic wounds

The wounds that are not repaired in a timely or orderly manner and fail to follow the typical healing stages are called chronic wounds. Many factors cause the disturbance in the healing process of the four stages of the wound, such as tissue hypoxia, necrosis, exudate, infection, and excessive levels of inflammatory cytokines. A nonhealing state is perpetuated due to the cascading of tissue responses to the continuous state of inflammation in the wound. Chronic wounds relapse frequently, and the functional and anatomical outcomes are inferior. Pressure, burns, vasculitis, naturopathic, arterial, and venous insufficiency are causes of chronic wounds [6]. An example of a chronic wound is shown in **Figure 3**.

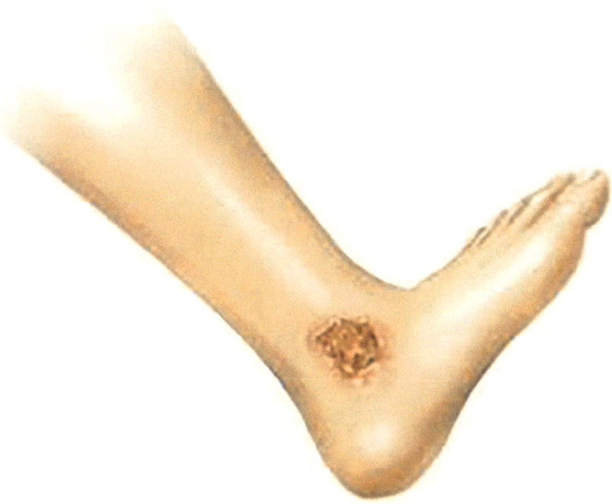

Figure 3.
An example of a chronic wound [6].

2.3 Complicated wounds

The combination of tissue defects and infections is classified as a complicated wound. It is a unique entity. Complicated wounds are affected by different types of infections. A wide tissue resection and traumatic or postinfectious etiology are a few of the causes of complicated wounds. Irrespective of the size, management, cause, and location, every wound is contaminated. The infection that develops depends on the number and type of microorganisms, virulence, the patient's inherent resistance, and the local blood supply. Heat, redness, pain, edema, and limited or loss of function of the affected part are the symptoms or the typical characteristics of infection. The wound classification is also done based on the criteria, such as degree of contamination, morphological characteristics, etiology, and communication with solid or hollow organs [6]. Wounds are also classified as open and closed. In the case of open wounds, the underlying tissue is exposed, and the skin layer is damaged. In the case of a closed wound, the skin is not severed, but the underlying tissue is damaged [7]. The image shown in **Figure 4** depicts a complicated, open, and contaminated wound.

3. Wound healing process

The wound healing process mainly consists of four stages: Hemostasis, inflammatory, proliferative, and remodeling [8]. The graphical representation of this sequence is shown in **Figure 5**.

- **Hemostasis:** In this phase, blood clotting causes the wound to close. The moment blood outflows the body (due cut or some other reason), this phase starts and restricts the blood flow by constricting the blood vessels. When the blood vessel's epithelial wall ruptures, the aggregation and adherence of platelets to the subendothelium surface take place within seconds. Within sixty seconds after the above event, the adherence of the first fibrin strand takes place. The blood gets converted from liquid to gel by releasing prothrombin and procoagulants when the fibrin mesh begins. The wound area contains the trapped blood cells and platelets due to the formation of thrombus or clot. Thrombus is vital in wound healing, but if it gets detached from the vessel wall and travels through the

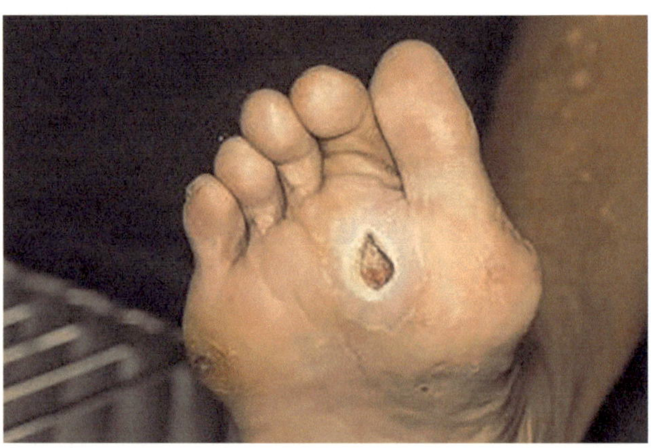

Figure 4.
A photograph of a complicated wound [7].

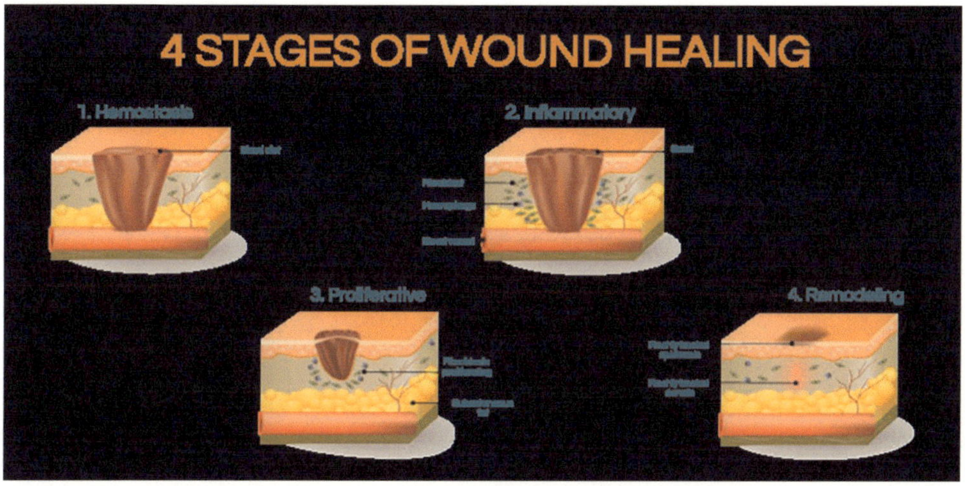

Figure 5.
A diagrammatic representation of wound healing phases: Hemostasis phase, inflammatory phase, proliferative phase, and remodeling [8].

circulatory system, it might cause strokes or pulmonary embolism [9]. The process of hemostasis is shown in **Figure 6**.

- **Inflammation:** It begins immediately after the injury, which causes localized swelling due to leakage of a transudate. Infection and bleeding are prevented by inflammation. The bacteria, damaged cells, and pathogens are removed from the wound area in this phase. The common symptoms observed in this phase are heat, pain, redness, and swelling, which are caused due to growth factors, nutrients, enzymes, and white blood cells. This phase is a problem if it is excessive or prolonged, even if it is a part of the natural process of wound healing [10]. **Figure 7** depicts the inflammatory phase.

- **Proliferation**: The new tissue made up of extracellular matrix and collagen is rebuilt in the wound. With the new tissues being developed, the wound starts contracting. To ensure the granulation tissue is healthy so that it receives enough nutrients and oxygen, the construction of new blood vessels must take place. The contraction of the wound takes place by the myofibroblasts, which grip the wound at its edges, similar to the smooth muscle cells. If the granulation tissue is healthy, it does not bleed easily. The granulation tissue is red or pink in the healthy stages of healing of the wound, and also the texture is uneven. Poor perfusion, ischemia, and infection are caused due to dark granulation tissue. Epithelial cells finally reappear in the injury. Keeping the wound hydrated and moist enhances the process of epithelialization. In order to maintain optimum humidity and improve epithelialization, semiocclusive and occlusive dressings are applied within 48 hours of the injury [11] **Figure 8** shows the graphical representation of all the stages of wound healing.

- **Maturation or remodeling**: The complete closure of the wound takes place. Remodeling of collagen from type 3 to type 1 occurs. Apoptosis is also called programmed cell death, in which the cells that are no longer needed but were

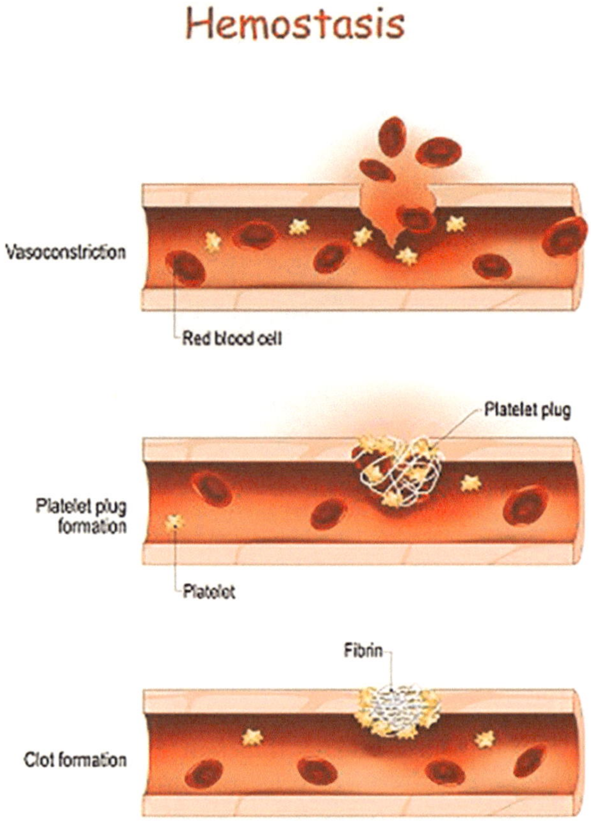

Figure 6.
An image indicating different stages of hemostasis: vessel constriction, primary hemostasis, and fibrin clot conversion [9].

used for repairing the wound are removed [12]. Disorganization of the collagen, which was laid down during the proliferative phase, takes place; the wound becomes thicker. The tensile strength of the healing tissue is increased by remodeling the collagen into a more organized structure along the lines of stress. Matrix metalloproteinases are secreted by fibroblasts. Type III collagen is remodeled into type I collagen by enzymes. After around 21 days of the injury has taken place, the remodeling begins and may continue for a year or more. The wound areas, which are healed, are weaker than the uninjured skin, even with cross-linking. They have only 80% of the tensile strength of healthy skin [13]. **Figure 9** is the diagrammatic representation of the remodeling phase.

4. Chronic wound

Chronic wounds do not follow the timely fashion of wound healing. Burns are included in chronic wounds as they take a long duration to heal than acute wounds. A large variety of surgically induced wounds and traumatic wounds are considered as chronic wounds by surgeons, as they heal unexpectedly slow. These chronic wounds

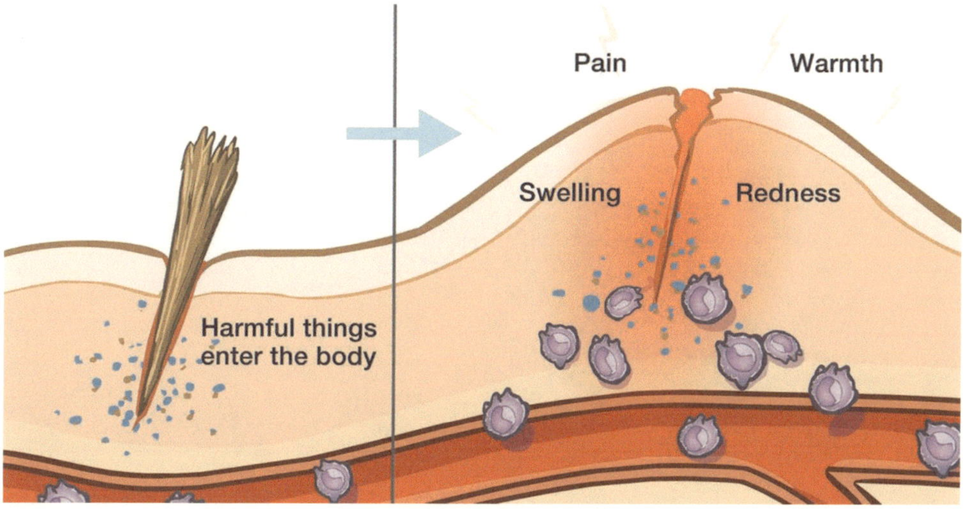

Figure 7.
A picture of the inflammatory phase indicating the inflammation and the action of fibrin and phagocyte [10].

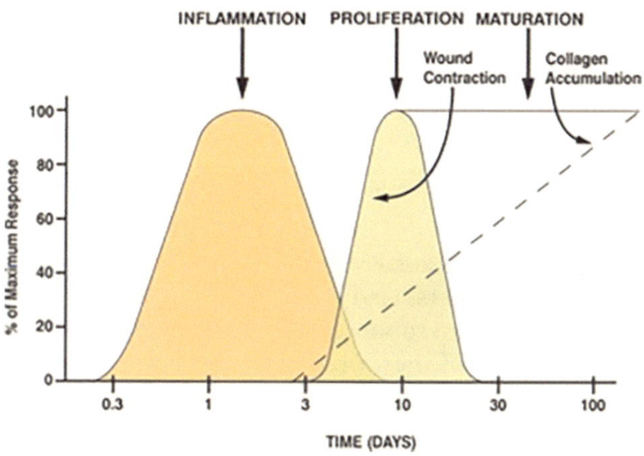

Figure 8.
Graphical representation of four stages of wound healing and their mutual relation is depicted in the figure above [11].

are also considered as vascularly compromised or infected. Chronic wounds also include the entire category of skin ulcers [14].

Despite good wound management, chronic wounds remain intractable, and they fail to follow the orderly phases of healing. Chronic wounds are detained in a self-perpetuating inflammatory stage. There are a high number of factors that delay wound healing, such as vascular insufficiency, chronic disease, malnutrition, diabetes, and aging. It is also affected by local factors, such as infection, edema, and pressure [15]. The wound gets locked in a prolonged and heightened inflammatory state due to the subsequent tissue damage, which is characterized by reactive oxygen species (ROS) and destructive enzymes perpetuating the cycle associated with neutrophil infiltration. If the primary noxious factor is eliminated, many chronic wounds can be effectively healed [16].

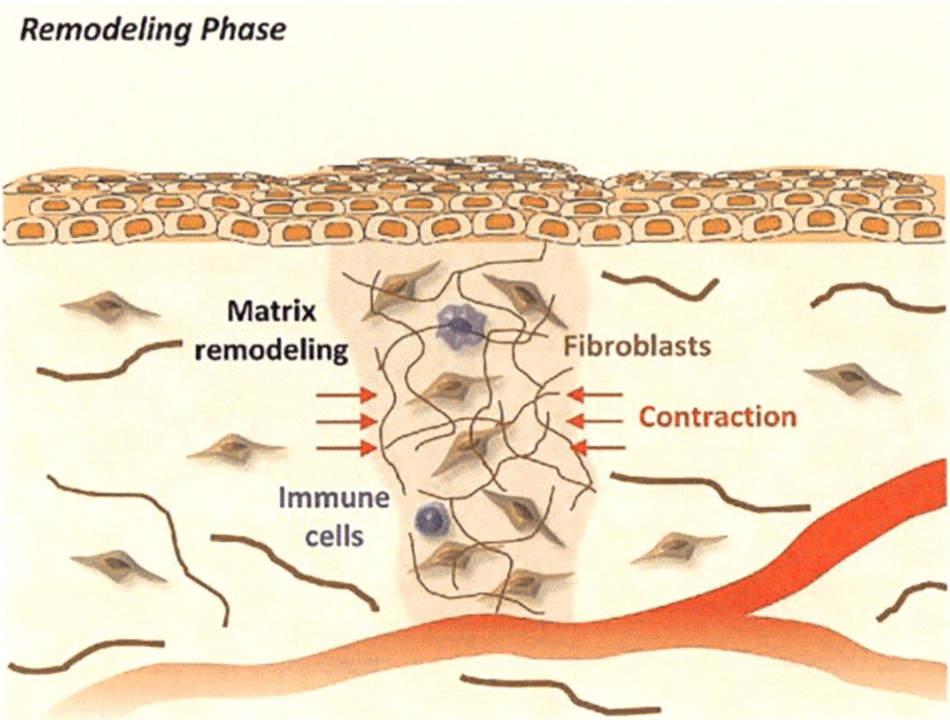

Figure 9.
A diagrammatic representation of the remodeling phase and the process involved in maturation or remodeling [13].

Patients with chronic wounds suffer the loss of function, financial costs, pain, and infections due to nonhealing ulcers, leading to sepsis or amputations. Diabetes, obesity, and the aging population are some of the high-profile issues that give rise to chronic wounds. In most parts of the world, these health issues are on the rise, and with this, the occurrence of diabetic, venous, and nonhealing pressure ulcers also increases. Unfortunately, the appropriate care and education about chronic wounds are lacking. The causes of chronic wounds overshadow their significance, and also, their costs are poorly documented. However, the quality of life of around 40 million people is impacted adversely and persists as a silent epidemic [17].

There are three main categories of chronic wounds: diabetic ulcers, pressure ulcers, and venous ulcers. There exists a fourth small group secondary to arterial ischemia [14].

4.1 Venous ulcers

Venous stasis ulcers affect around 1–2% of the adult population, primarily women and the elderly. They occur mainly in the lower limb and account for more than half. Venous hypertension and congestion are mainly responsible for venous ulcers caused due to venous thrombosis or valvular incompetence [18]. The blood vessel permeability is increased due to back pressure, which leads to leakage of red blood cells and macromolecules into the perivascular space. These then act as chemoattractants for leukocyte infiltration. Inflammatory processes associated with reperfusion exacerbate the injury, and leg elevation restores the effective loss of circulation. Venous ulcers

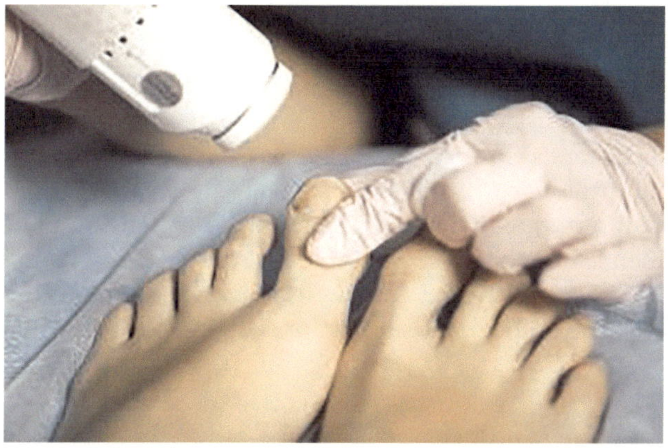

Figure 10.
Various stages of venous ulcers: from skin redness, inflammation of the subcutaneous tissue in the area of the lower leg progresses to formation of wound on the surface [19].

commonly occur in the medial malleolus. They tend to be shallower and more prominent and are irregular with ill-defined margins [19]. **Figure 10** depicts the various stages involved in the formation of venous ulcers.

4.2 Arterial ulcers

Arterial ulcers are rare when compared to venous ones. The consequence of arterial insufficiency, which is caused by atherosclerosis or rarely thromboembolic or radiation damage, gives rise to arterial ulcers. When the arterial lumen narrows down, it reduces perfusion, which leads to ischemia and hypoxia [18]. Peripheral vascular disease is defined as the blockage of arteries other than those supplying blood to the heart and brain. An increase in age, hypertension, diabetes, smoking, and hypercholesterolemia are the significant risk factors for these ulcers. The management of risk factors and reconstructive surgery or angioplasty to restore the peripheral flow is a part of wound therapy. These ulcers usually occur distally over bony prominences and are present with a round and the sharply demarcated border [20]. **Figure 11** is an image representing an arterial ulcer.

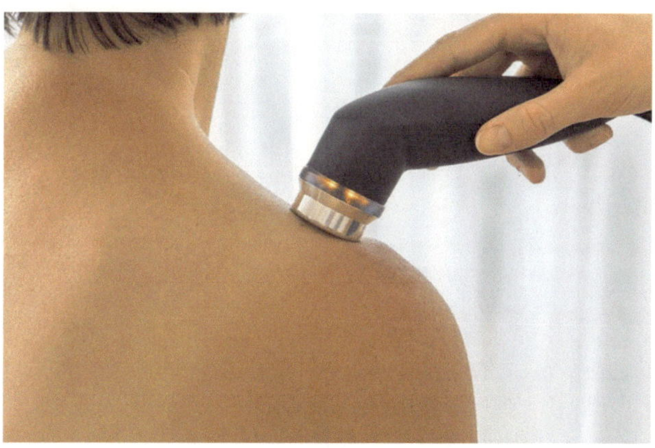

Figure 11.
An image representing an arterial ulcer [5].

4.3 Pressure ulcers

These kinds of ulcers are common in patients who have compromised sensory perception and mobility, are either paralyzed or unconscious, and cannot respond to the periodic need for repositioning. When the capillary pressure is exceeded by tissue compression due to prolonged, unrelieved pressure or shear leads to ischemia necrosis. This is the result of tissue hypoxia and ischemia-reperfusion injury. Usually, skin over bony prominences, such as the sacrum, hips, and malleoli, is vulnerable to pressure ulcers. This may be caused after as little as two hours of immobility [18]. **Figure 12** shows the four different stages of pressure ulcers.

4.4 Diabetic ulcers

Around 382 million people worldwide suffer from diabetes mellitus, which is one of the leading causes of death. Diabetic foot ulcers are a common serious complication of diabetes and are very common. Diabetes associated with peripheral neuropathy increases the risk of ulceration due to repeated mechanical stress, which creates a weakened, insensate foot, heightened by disrupted perfusion. Wound healing is directly disrupted by metabolic derangements caused due to hyperglycemia in diabetic patients [18]. There is a higher risk of re-ulceration, amputation, and death in patients suffering from diabetic foot ulcers. This has drawn greater attention to diabetic wound healing and limb salvage in the recent past [21]. **Figure 13** shows patients suffering from diabetic ulcers.

5. Treatments for faster wound healing

Techniques like cushions, magnetic fields, pressure-relieving beds, ultrasound, and electric fields are also used along with conventional medications. The healing and prevention of pressure wounds are addressed by the aforementioned methods [22].

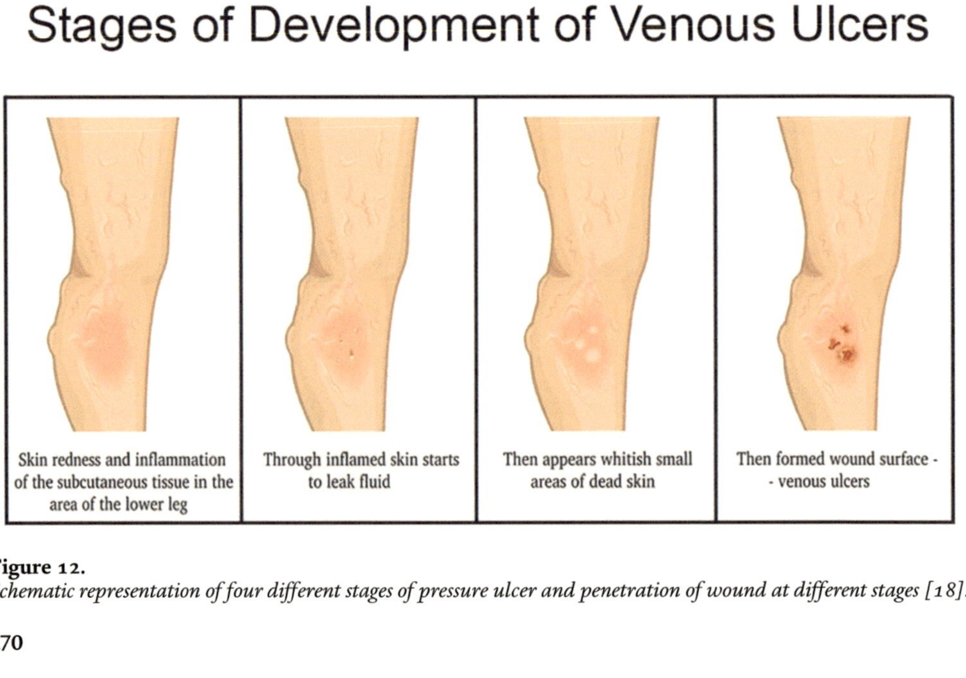

Figure 12.
Schematic representation of four different stages of pressure ulcer and penetration of wound at different stages [18].

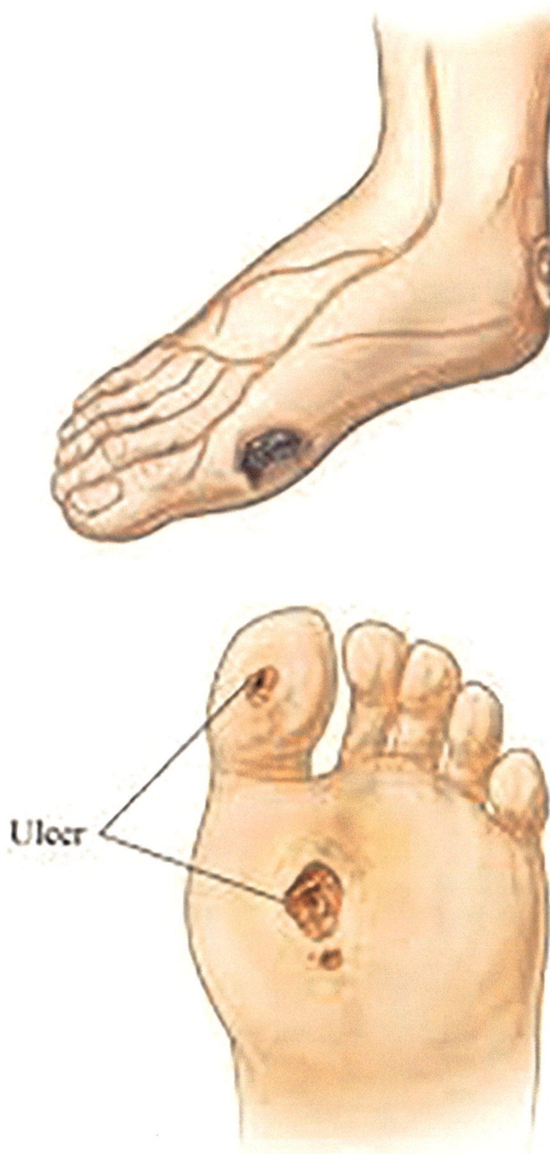

Figure 13.
A photograph of diabetic ulcers caused due to repeated mechanical stress, which creates a weakened, insensate foot, heightened by disrupted perfusion [21].

5.1 Wound healing using laser therapy

LASER (light amplification by stimulated emission of radiation) therapy is one of the potential methods. The efficiency of LASER therapy is affected by different parameters. There has been a variety of studies to develop this technique for various medical applications [23]. **Figure 14** shows the wound healing procedure using laser therapy.

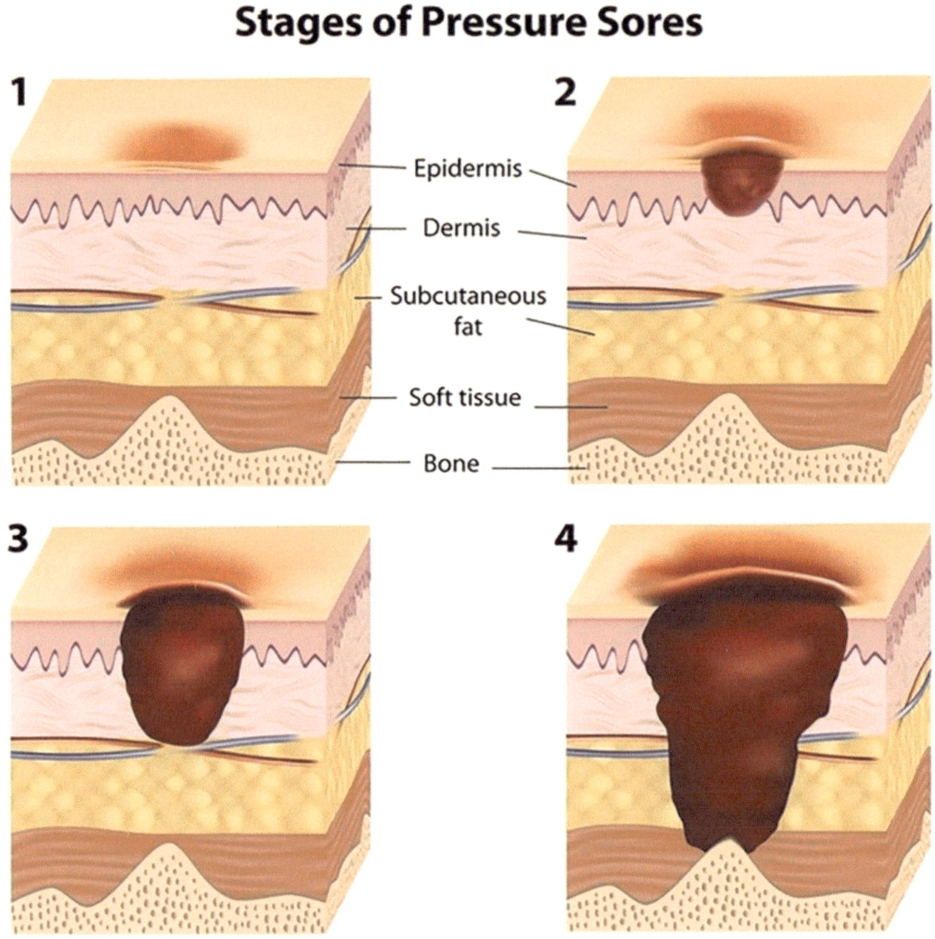

Figure 14.
A picture of a device used in laser therapy for wound healing application [23].

Recently, lasers have enhanced the nonsurgical method of the wound healing procedure. A therapy of low-power light is a great approach to treat lesions of wounds using light devices like LASER (light amplification by stimulated emission of adiation). A laser is used to repair the biological injury. However, it is not entirely understood the role of laser in reducing pain and repairing tissue. The parameters like optical properties of the tissue, wavelength, and dosage of light affect the interaction of biological tissues and light. Laser has features like various active media types, including solid, liquid, and gaseous materials and also resonant optical cavity [24]. A wide range of therapeutic effects is produced with an account of different irradiation conditions, such as frequency, duration of treatment, and exposure time, and also other laser parameters, such as energy, pulse frequency, pulse duration, power, and wavelength. The wounded cells are affected with suboptimal growth with laser therapy without affecting normal cells [10].

When the dosage of laser therapy was more than 5 J/cm^2, it revealed more considerable biological effects. It is also shown that at lower doses, no biological effects were observed, and at very high doses, the cell function is inhibited. Hence an optimum dosage of laser gives better results in wound healing [18].

5.2 Ultrasound therapy for wound healing

Ultrasound (US) waves have always proven promising therapeutic outcomes for various wounds. The main advantages of US in healing the wound are as follows: highly steering, focusable and high penetration into the wound bed. The physiological mechanisms of US in wound healing are based on its antimicrobial effects. There is no definite dose response observed in the clinical trials of this technique, despite evidence of therapeutic efficiency for chronic wounds in particular. To better understand the dose response and mechanism of action of US methods, more clinical trials and *in vitro* trials are required. **Figure 15** shows the device used for ultrasound therapy [25].

The low US frequencies in the range of 20–120 kHz are used in wound healing applications. The process of producing heat in the tissue by delivering nonionizing radiation in the form of mechanical sound waves is called the therapeutic US, which is a physical method. When the frequencies 1.0 MHz and 3.0 MHz are used to exert the therapeutic US, it attains a depth of 5 cm and even more beneath the body surface. It is also the often used deep-heating modality.

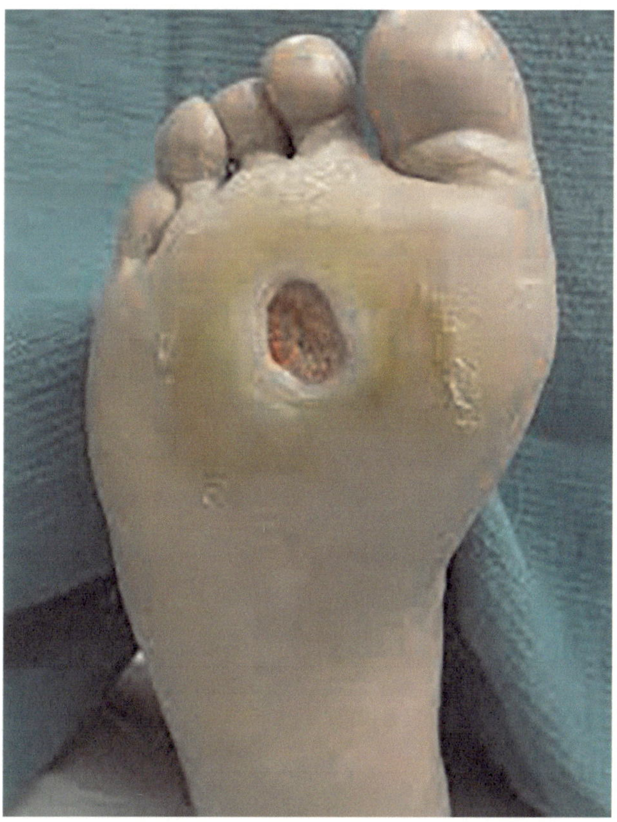

Figure 15.
A photograph of a device used for ultrasound therapy [25].

Very high frequencies of US may cause cell death, whereas low frequencies of US have beneficial effects on the wound [26]. The wound healing procedures, such as gene treatment, fracture repair, sonoporation, sonophoresis, and physiotherapy, use low power of US. By altering the wave intensity and wavelength, the US dosage could be changed. US therapy can either be pulsed or continuous. More heating effects are exerted by continuous US therapy. The pulsed US has on and off cycles; this variation changes the dosage of US therapy [27].

6. Wound healing treatment using microneedle

A different level of success has been achieved using various technologies to treat chronic wounds. Additional treatments like the application of fillers such as collagen sponges, usage of negative wound pressure, hyperbaric oxygen therapy, application of select growth factors, advanced wound dressings, systemic or local antibiotic therapy, and, more recently, the use of cell-based tissue-engineered products have been applied depending on the type and severity of the wound that is being treated [28]. In this section, we have mainly focused on the details of the microneedle, followed by the wound treatment using microneedles.

This technique is based on the use of tiny needles, so small that they are measured in micrometers (millionths of a meter/μm). These microneedles are designed to deliver medicines. In terms of how they work, microneedles are similar to that transdermal patch, for example, the ones used for nicotine delivery that helps people give up smoking compared to the traditional hypodermic needles [17].

The epidermis plays an essential role in acting like a protective layer and keeping things out and protecting all the penetrants. It forms the 10–50 μm layer. When we talk about drug delivery, we mainly aim to get the medicine across this layer. It is this issue from where the concept of the microneedle was developed [29].

Microneedles were made worldwide using the materials like silicon, glass, and metal by the researchers during late 1990s. Microneedles are capable of creating an easier passage to reach the bloodstream in the lower dermal layers. This is a pain-free and easy way of delivering a wide range of medicines across the skin. **Figure 16** is an image of an array of microneedles. **Figure 17** shows the penetration of a conventional needle and a microneedle [30]. The dimensions of the microneedle are as shown in **Figure 18**.

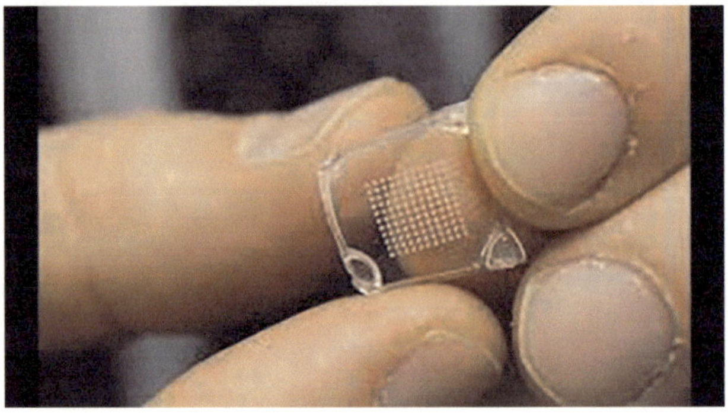

Figure 16.
A photograph of a microneedle array [30].

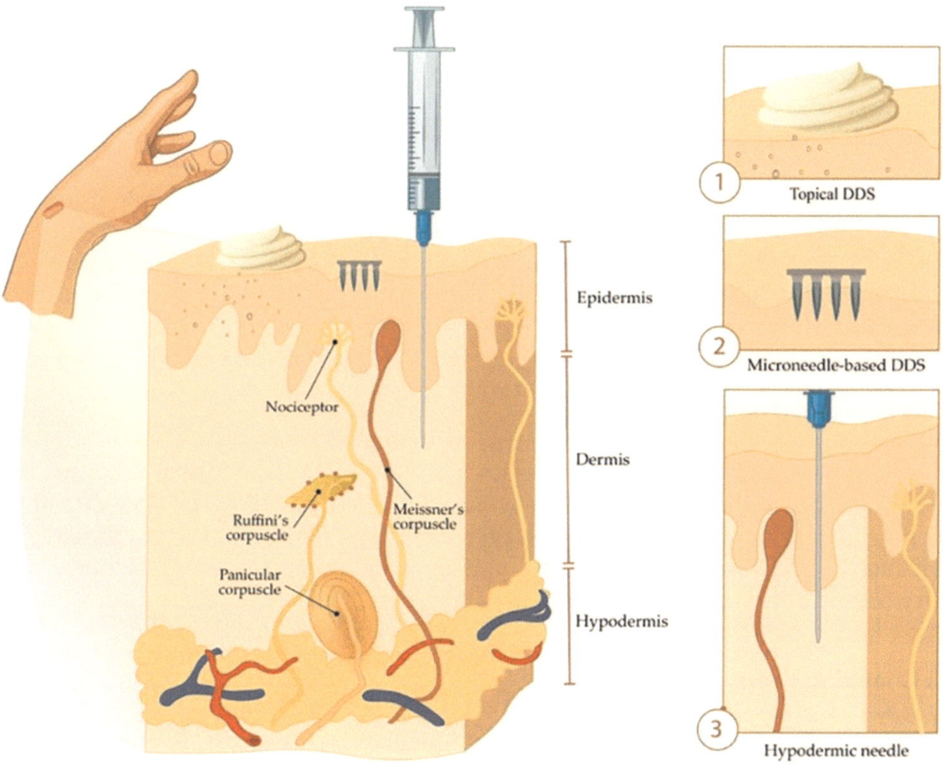

Figure 17.
Diagrammatic representation of three DDS delivering drugs through various layers of skin: Topical DDS, microneedles-based DDS, and hypodermic needle [31].

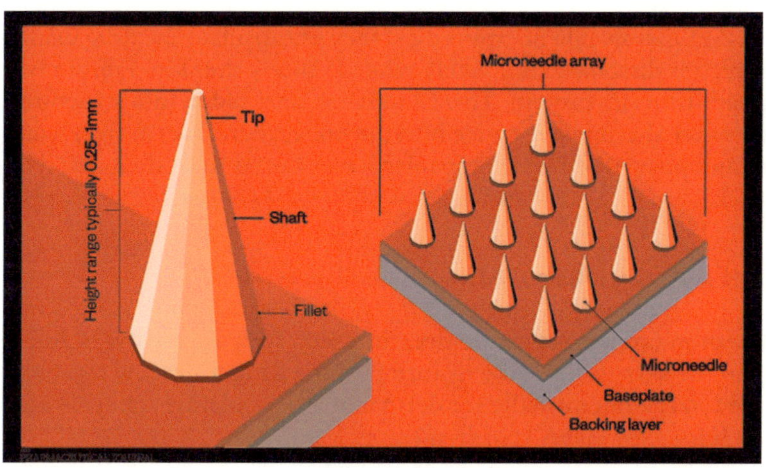

Figure 18.
A schematic representation of a microneedle and various sections of a microneedle array [31].

7. Types of microneedles

7.1 Solid microneedle

Solid microneedles are arranged as an array in a two-part system; microscopic wells are created on the skin using this microneedle just deep enough to penetrate the outermost layer of the skin, and then a transdermal patch is used to apply the drug. Collagen induction therapy is a method in dermatology, which uses solid microneedles. This method involves the repeated puncturing of the skin with microneedles, wherein the expression and deposition of elastin and collagen proteins are induced [32].

7.2 Hollow microneedle

These are similar to solid microneedles with respect to the material. They act like a reservoir containing the drug to be delivered to the site directly. The flow rate of the microneedle influences the drug delivery; therefore, a flawed design or excessive swelling may cause clogging of the array. Hollow microneedles have a higher probability of collapsing under pressure, thus failing to deliver drugs [32].

7.3 Coated microneedle

Coated microneedles are designed using metals or polymers, similar to that of solid microneedles. Here the drug is directly applied to the microneedle, unlike in other cases where patches or applicators are used. To ensure the proper delivery of the drug, thickening agents or surfactants are used to cover coated microneedles. The chemicals that are used on coated microneedles are known as irritants. There is sometimes the risk of local inflammation in the area where the array was used. In such cases, the array can be removed immediately without harming the patient [32].

7.4 Dissolvable microneedle

In the case of dissolvable microneedles, they encapsulate the drug using a nontoxic polymer, which is dissolved completely when it enters the skin. Fibroin is a polymer that is derived from silk protein. This fibroin can be molded into structures of microneedles and also dissolves once into the body; therefore, in the recent past, researchers and pharmaceutical companies have started to study its mechanisms and potential [32].

7.5 Hydrogel-forming microneedles

This type of microneedles has no drug in itself. They follow the technique of swelling in the skin to allow the diffusion of the drug inside the reservoir layer attached to the microneedle for dermal microcirculation for systemic absorption [32].

The various types of microneedles explained above are shown in **Figure 19**.

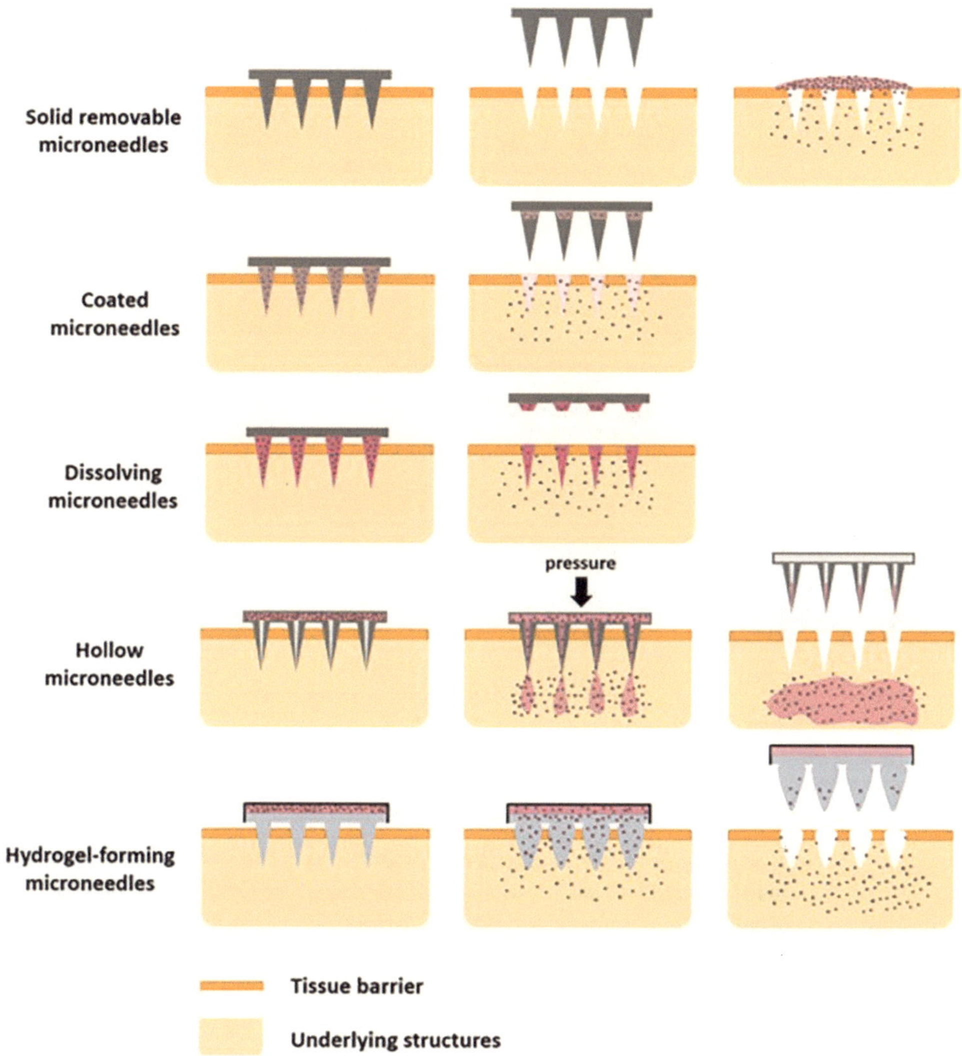

Figure 19.
A schematic representation of five different types of microneedles: solid removable, coated, dissolving, hollow, and hydrogel-forming microneedles [32].

8. Applications of microneedles

The applications of microneedles in different domains are shown below in the chart in **Figure 20** [33].

9. Recent work in chronic wound healing using microneedles

In the case of chronic wounds, the delivery of topically administered therapeutics is disrupted due to the discharge of exudate, the presence of eschar, and a harsh

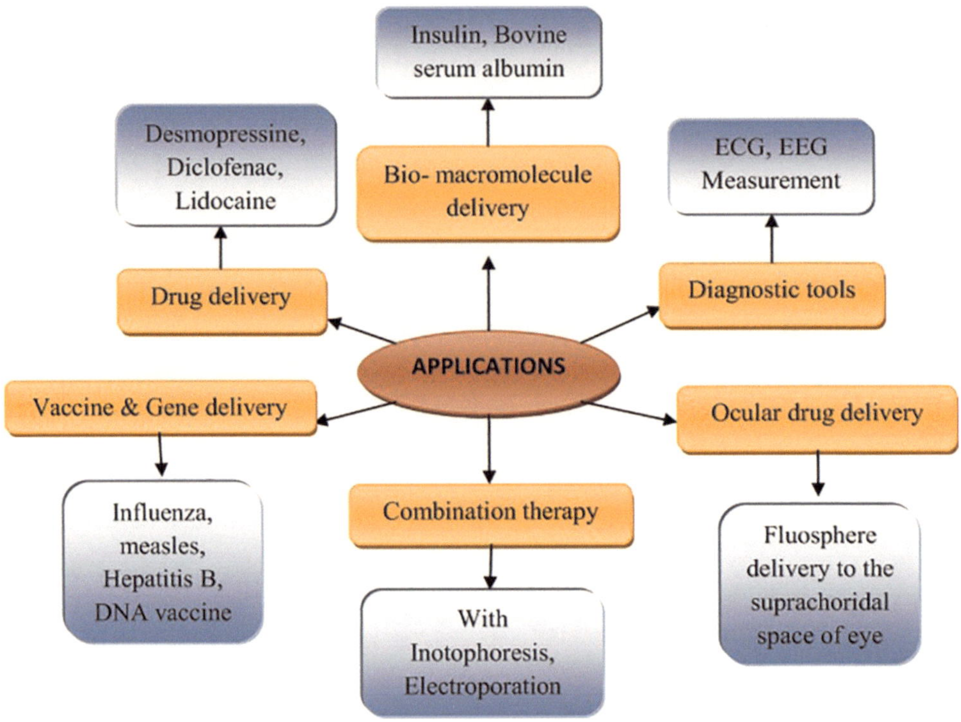

Figure 20.
A flow chart to represent the various applications of microneedles in the medical field including drug delivery, vaccine and gene delivery, ocular drug delivery, combination therapy, and biomacromolecule delivery [33].

chemical microenvironment rich in various enzymes. Therefore, to make therapeutics more available at the wound bed and also control the distribution of the drug spatially, by having control over the drug content of individual needles, MNA systems are developed. Based on the control temporal release profile, MNAs are classified as passive, active, and smart releases [34]. Researchers have utilized these different strategies to deliver different therapeutics to enhance the healing of the wound process and solve the crucial dysfunctions existing in the chronic wound microenvironments [35].

9.1 Passively delivered biological materials

This method is one of the simplest available methods to carry biologics from MNAs, despite the fact that alteration of release kinetics is not possible when the passive release MNA is in action. However, they can be altered during the development phase of MNAs by changing various components of the system design. Several chronic wound symptoms, such as low vascularization and infection, are addressed using this technique [36]. Fabrication of MNA using an antibiotic agent encapsulated within an MNA structure or an antibacterial material is the straightforward approach to creating antibacterial MNA. Both the concepts mentioned above were achieved by Yi et al. by filling zinc nitrate (Zn^{2+}) into chitosan (CS) MNs, which defeated unloaded CS MNs in the eradication of *S. aureus* and *E. coli*. The worth of piercing the biofilm to eliminate infection was highlighted when the MNAs were capable enough to kill a large number of bacteria compared to a topically applied film with the same

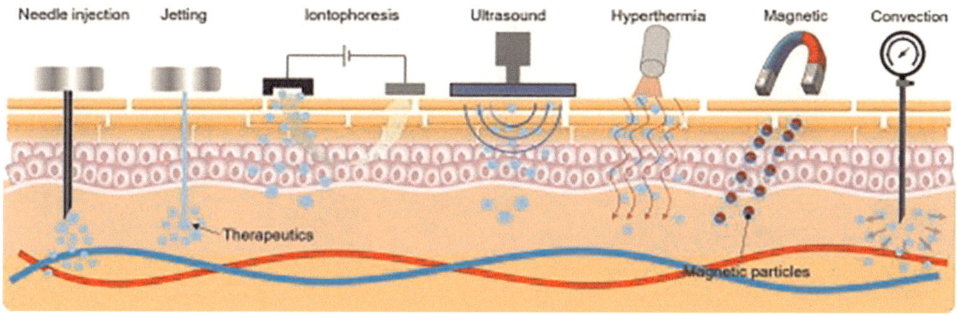

Figure 21.
(A) The different parts of hybrid microneedle including the scaffolding material used for preserving the stem-cell functionality offered by the core-shell structure for facile insertion, (B) the mechanism involved in MNA-based delivery of stem cell action meant for enhanced regeneration [38].

composition [37]. The different parts of the hybrid microneedle including the scaffolding material used for preserving the stem-cell functionality offered by the core-shell structure for facile insertion are shown in **Figure 21A**. **Figure 21B** shows the mechanism involved in MNA-based delivery of stem cell action meant for enhanced regeneration.

9.2 Active system

MNAs that work on passive delivery of biological materials provide effortless and smoothly applicable point of care (POC) systems. It does not adhere to the needs connected with the wound environment, which is dynamic in nature throughout the process of healing. The effect of therapeutics is different at different stages of wound healing. Therapeutics that may improve healing at one stage of healing can prove to be harmful or useless at a different stage. The application of active MNA systems could be a promising alternative to passive MNAs. In this mechanism, the dissolving Gantrez® AN-139 MNA was loaded with photosensitizing methylene blue to perform photodynamic antimicrobial chemotherapy (PACT). In this approach, the photosensitizing drug is activated using light, which releases reactive radicals. The targeted bacteria are broken down by these reactive radicals [39]. The 3D printed SEM image of hollow microneedles is shown in **Figure 22A**. **Figure 22B** shows the smartphone-controlled wireless pumping system that is able to deliver therapeutics on demand.

9.3 MNAs based on smart systems/stimuli-responsive

An additional mechanism in the engineering of systems based on MNA for better healing of the wound is by using smart materials. These smart materials can respond to changes in the environment of the wound. Smart systems are the combination of responsiveness of active systems, which can react to the dynamic requirements of the chronic wound and user simplicity of passive release MNAs. In a recent study of this strategy, the fabrication of MNAs is from a combination of VEGF-loaded NIPAM hydrogel and antibacterial chitosan. NIPAM is temperature sensitive. The release of VEGF from the permeable hydrogel network is triggered by an increase in the temperature of a chronic inflamed wound. The lack of vascularization and bacterial infection are addressed by combining chitosan with VEGF loading. The capability of MNA to kill most of the bacteria in both E. coli and S. aureus cultures was shown in

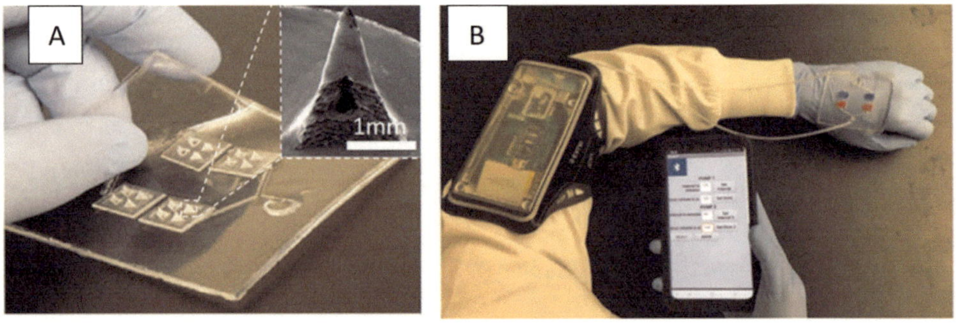

Figure 22.
(A) The MNA integrated with flexible microfluidic patch for drug distribution in the wound bed. Figure shows a 3D printed SEM image hollow microneedles. (B) The smartphone controlled wireless pumping system which is able to deliver the therapeutics on demand [39].

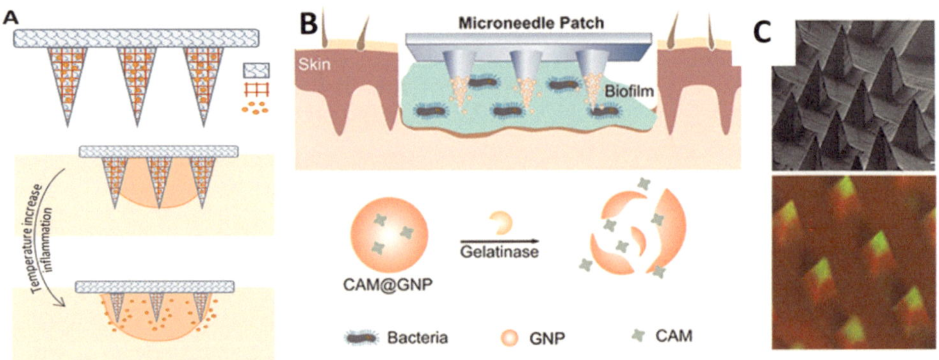

Figure 23.
(A) The mechanism involved in release of VEGF into the wound bed with the increase in temperature during wound inflammation. (B) The mechanism involved in MNA patch action. (C) Fabricated-MNA (top) MNA which is loaded with fluorescent-labelled drugs (bottom) [40].

the antibacterial test. The MNA patch developed was applied to the rats with severely infected wounds, in which it was found that the VEGF-loaded MNA group showed the thickest granulation tissue and the most wound closure. It also demonstrated increased deposition of collagen, angiogenesis, and downregulated inflammatory response.

The MNA systems are also fabricated using bacteria-responsive smart materials to treat infected wounds [40].

Figure 23A shows the mechanism involved in the release of VEGF in the wound bed with the increase in temperature during wound inflammation.

The mechanism involved in the MNA patch is shown in **Figure 23B**. **Figure 23C** shows the fabricated MNA on the top and MNA loaded with florescent loaded drugs in the bottom.

9.4 Mechanically interacting systems

The wound closures are improved by using MNAs and by the physical application of mechanical forces. The MNAs developed are to bring about mechanical interlocking after insertion due to swelling. The mechanism of interlocking by using MNAs helps the process of healing a wound by inducing wound closure and protecting the tissue from mechanical stress. This is achieved using hybrid core-shell structured MNAs consisting of a non-swellable core and a swellable hydrogel shell. After insertion, the ISF is absorbed by the hydrogel, due to which physical entanglement is induced through the swelling of microneedle tips. There has been a significant increase in the resistance against bacterial incursion compared to surgical staples using MNA patches. The application of MNA patches has also limited the scar formation and tissue damage. The use of MNA patches also enhances the mechanical strength of tissues that are healed, which consequently reduces the susceptibility of wound reopening. The mechanism also improves both external and internal wound closure rates compared to suture application in rats. Mechanically self-interlocking needles can hold the MNA in place for a long-term drug delivery which makes them appealing. This strategy can replace the use of sutures on wounds [41].

9.5 Bioinspired design for efficient drug/vaccine coating

Biomimetics is an interdisciplinary scientific field that is aimed to solve complex technological issues. It focuses on the imitation and study of biological systems. The lateral sides of pyramidal MNs are ornamented, with European true bugs structure, facilitating an efficient and directional liquid transport. Two-photon polymerization (TPP) is used to realize this kind of MNs. To prove that these MNs pierce the skin, both *ex vivo* skin tests and *in vivo* tests were performed. The arrays of MNs can be replicated accurately using a micro-molding technique. **Figure 24** shows an image depicting the idea behind biomimetics [42].

9.6 Photon-based smart bandage

Wound healing can be assessed by measuring the pH of the wound. This method is one of the most potential wound healing assessment methods. It indicates the condition and the stage of wound healing. Photons-based smart bandages for assessing wound healing present the first smart wound dressing for pH assessment. This method is based on embedded optical fiber. Optical fibers are pH sensitive and are embedded in gauze fabric and hydrocolloid wound dressing. A fiber-embedded bandage can measure pressure as low as 0.1 kPa and has high linearity in the range of 0–0.3 kPa. This is due to the low Young's modulus of PDMS, which is the component

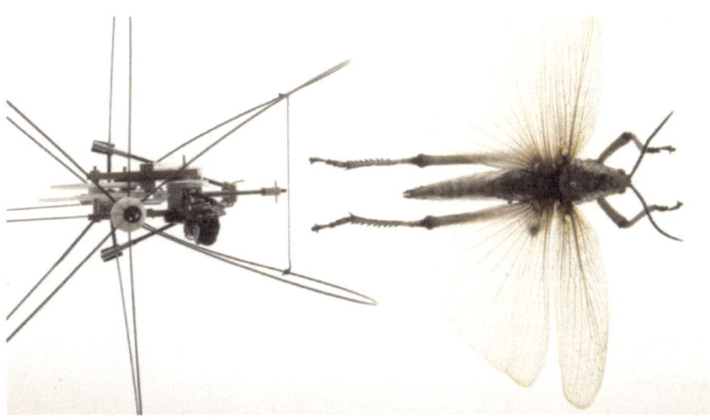

Figure 24.
An image showing the idea behind the concept of biomimetics for the study of biological systems [42].

of the system. The smart bandage, based on optical fiber, is capable of assessment of pressure and pH in the wound region simultaneously [42].

10. Conclusions

In this chapter, we have tried to bring out the understanding of wounds and the healing process, various types of wound healing, their causes, and how today's technology has influenced the rate at which it heals. Microneedle-based drug delivery has played a prominent role in faster wound healing as it is capable of closely monitoring and treating the wound with no physical pain. The research related to microneedle-based wound care management is required to explore more, and we believe that it has a long and promising way to go for the welfare of humanity. Minimally invasive microneedle: a novel approach for drug delivery systems and infected wound care management is making wound healing less painful with microneedles and faster with the appropriate drug usage.

Acknowledgements

The authors of this chapter would like to acknowledge the support of the Indian Institute of Goa, India.

Conflict of interest

The authors declare no conflict of interest.

Abbreviations

ROS	reactive oxygen species
MI	myocardial infraction
NIR	near infrared
GO	graphene oxide
PVA	poly vinyl alcohol
VEGF	vascular endothelial growth factor
MIS	minimally invasive surgery
PDMS	polydimethylsiloxane
FTIR	Fourier transform infrared
US	ultrasound
DDS	drug delivery systems
MNs	microneedles
TPP	two-photon polymerization
MNAs	microneedle array
POC	point of care
Zn	zinc nitrate
CS	chitosan
PACT	photodynamic antimicrobial chemotherapy
VEGF	vascular endothelial growth factor

Author details

Bidhan Pramanick* and Aishwarya G. Patil
IIT Goa, Goa, India

*Address all correspondence to: bidhan@iitgoa.ac.in

References

[1] Broughton G, Janis J, Attinger C. Wound healing: An overview. Plastic and Reconstructive Surgery. 2006;**117** (7S):32

[2] Maria B, Barbul A. General principles of wound healing. Surgical Clinics of North America. 1997;**77**(3):509-528

[3] Velnar T, Bailey T, Smrkolj V. The wound healing process: An overview of the cellular and molecular mechanisms. The Journal of International Medical Research. 2009:1528-1542. PMID: 19930861. DOI: 10.1177/147323000903700531

[4] Samaneh R, Ali Y, Mostafa J, Mahmud NR, Zohre R. Laser Therapy for wound healing: A review of current techniques and mechanisms of action. Ahvaz, Iran: Department of Medical Physics, School of Medicine, Ahvaz Jundishapur University of Medical Sciences. 2015;**8**(2):1121-1127. DOI: 10.13005/bbra/1626

[5] Yadollahpour A, Mostafa J, Samaneh R, Zohreh R. Low Level laser therapy for the Treatment of Chronic Wound: Clinical Considerations. Ahvaz, Iran: Department of Medical Physics, School of Medicine, Ahvaz Jundishapur University of Medical Sciences. 2015;**8** (2):1121-1127.. DOI:10.13005/bjp/866

[6] Damien P. del Valle, San Juan, PR 00901, Injury - Induced Rffectors of Neuropathic Pain. USA: Institute of Neurobiology, University of Puerto Rico; 2019. PMID: 31701439. DOI: 10.1007/s12035-019-01756-w

[7] Badiavas EV, Falanga V. Treatment of chronic wounds with bone marrow–Derived cells. Archives of Dermatology. 2003;**139**(4):510-516. DOI: 10.1001/archderm.139.4.510

[8] Lee JC, Kandula S, Sherber NS. Beyond wet-to-dry: A rational approach to treating chronic wounds. Eplasty. 2009;**9**:e14

[9] Lin L, Pisano AP. Silicon-processed microneedles. Journal of Microelectronic Systems. 1999;**8**(1):78-84. DOI: 10.1109/84.749406

[10] Xie L, Zeng H, Sun J, Qian W. Engineering microneedles for therapy and diagnosis: A survey. Micromachines. 2020;**11**:271

[11] Fan S-L, Lin J-A, Chen S-Y, Lin J-H, Lin H-T, Chen Y-Y, et al. Food. Effects of anthocyanins on the prevention and treatment of cancer. 2016. PMID: 27646173. DOI: 10.1111/bph.13627

[12] Byrne J, Huang H-W, McRae JC, Babaee S, Soltani A, Becker SL, et al. Devices for drug delivery in the gastrointestinal tract: A review of systems physically interacting with the mucosa for enhanced delivery. Advanced Drug Delivery Reviews. 2021;**177**:113926

[13] Chen S, Lu J, You T, Sun D. Metal-organic frameworks for improving wound healing. Coordination Chemistry Reviews. 2021;**439**:213929

[14] Duscher D, Barrera J, Wong VW, Maan ZN, Whittam AJ, Januszyk M, et al. Stem Cells in Wound Healing: The Future of Regenerative Medicine? A Mini-Review. Gerontology. 2016;**62**: 216-225. DOI: 10.1159/000381877

[15] Eaglstein WH, Falanga V. PlumX Metrics. Preclinical safety of negatively charged microspheres (NCMs): Optimization of radiolabeling for in vivo and ex vivo biodistribution studies after

topical administration on full-thickness wounds in a rat model. European Journal of Pharmaceutics and Biopharmaceutics. 2022;**177**:61-67. DOI: 10.1016/S0039-6109(05)70575-2

[16] Robert GF, Banks J. Challenges in the treatment of Chronic Wounds. Advances in Wound Care. 2015;**4**:9. DOI: 10.1089/wound.2015.0635

[17] Sami DG, Heiba HH, Abdellatif A. Wound healing models: A systematic review of animal and non-animal models. Wound Medicine. 2019;**24**(1):8-17

[18] Goldman RJ, Salcido R. More than one way to measure a wound: An overview of tools and techniques. Advances in Skin & Wound Care. 2002;**15**:236-243. PMID: 12368715. DOI: 10.1097/00129334-200209000-00011

[19] Barnum L, Samandari M, Schmidt TA, Tamayol A. Microneedle arrays for the treatment of chronic wounds. Expert Opinion on Drug Delivery. 2020;**17**(12):1767-1780. DOI: 10.1080/17425247.2020.1819787

[20] Khaw PT, Migdal CS. Current techniques in wound healing modulation in glaucoma surgery. Current Opinion in Ophthalmology. 1996;7(2):24-33

[21] Robson MC, Barbul A. Guidelines for the Best Care of Chronic Wounds. Tampa, FL: University of South Florida; 2006;**14**(6):647-648. DOI: 10.1111/j.1524-475X.2006.00173.x

[22] Werdin F, Tennenhaus M, Schaller HE, Rennekampff HO. Evidence-based management strategies for treatment of chronic wounds. Eplasty. 2009;**9**:e19

[23] Singh M, Nuutila K, Kruse C, Robson MC, Caterson E, Eriksson E. Challenging the conventional therapy. Plastic and Reconstructive Surgery. 2015;**136**:524-530

[24] Faraji Rad Z, Prewett PD, Davies GJ. Journal of Nanotechnology. 2021;**12**:1034-1046. DOI: 10.3762/bjnano.12.77

[25] Dabbagh SR, Sarabi MR, Rahbarghazi R, Sokullu E, Yetisen AK, Tasoglu S. 3D-printed microneedles in biomedical applications. iScience. 2021;**24**(1):102012. DOI: 10.1016/j.isci.2020.102012. PMID: 33506186

[26] Kaushik S, Hord AH, Denson DD, Mcallister DV, Smitra S, Allen MG, et al. Lack of pain associated with microfabricated microneedles. Anesthesia & Analgesia. 2001;**92**:502

[27] Plamadeala C, Gosain SR, Hischen F, et al. Bio-inspired microneedle design for efficient drug/vaccine coating. Biomedical Microdevices. 2020;**22**:8

[28] Rzhevskiy AS, Singh TRR, Donnelly RF, Anissimov YG. Microneedles as the technique of drug delivery enhancement in diverse organs and tissues. Journal of Controlled Release. 2018;**270**:184-202

[29] Mizuno Y, Takasawa K, Hanada T, et al. Fabrication of novel-shaped microneedles to overcome the disadvantages of solid microneedles for the transdermal delivery of insulin. Biomedical Microdevices. 2021;**23**:38

[30] Fan Z, Wei Y, Yin Z, Huang H, Liao X, Sun L, et al. Near-infrared light-triggered unfolding microneedle patch for minimally invasive treatment of myocardial ischemia. ACS Applied Materials & Interfaces. 2021;**13**(34):40278-40289. DOI: 10.1021/acsami.1c09658

[31] Park SY, Lee HU, Lee Y-C, Kim GH, Park EC, Han SH, et al. Wound healing potential of antibacterial microneedles loaded with green tea extracts. Materials Science and Engineering. 2014;**42**: 757-762

[32] Chi J, Zhang X, Chen C, Shao C, Zhao Y, Wang Y. Antibacterial and angiogenic chitosan microneedle array patch for promoting wound healing. Bioactive Materials. 2020;**5**(2):253-259

[33] Yin M, Wu J, Deng M, Wang P, Ji G, Wang M, et al. Multifunctional magnesium organic framework-based microneedle patch for accelerating diabetic wound healing. ACS Nano. 2021;**15**(11):17842-17853

[34] Liebl H, Kloth LC. Skin cell proliferation stimulated by microneedles. Journal of the American College of Clinical Wound Specialists. 2012;**4**(1):2-6

[35] Zhao R, Liang H, Clarke E, Jackson C, Xue M. Inflammation in chronic wounds. International Journal of Molecular Sciences. 2016;**17**: 2085

[36] Leal-Junior A, Guo J, Min R, Fernandes A, Frizera A, Marques C. Photonic smart bandage for wound healing assessment. Photonic Research. 2021;**9**:272-280

[37] Konwar A, Kandimalla R, Kalita S, Chowdhury D. Approach to fabricate a compact cotton patch without weaving: A smart bandage material. ACS Sustainable Chemistry & Engineering. 2018;**6**(5):5806-5817. DOI: 10.1021/acssuschemeng.7b03920

[38] Parisi OI, Ruffo M, Scrivano L, Malivindi R, Vassallo A, Puoci F. Smart bandage based on molecularly imprinted polymers (MIPs) for diclofenac controlled release. Pharmaceuticals. 2018;**11**(4):92

[39] de Onzalez AC. Wound Healing—A Literature Review Work. Salvador, BA: Gonçalo Moniz Research Center – Fundação Oswaldo Cruz (CPqGM/Fiocruz); 2016

[40] Charles EH, Loewen-Rodriguez A, Lessem J. Advances in Wound Care. 2012;**1**(3):138-141. PMID:24527294. DOI: 10.1089/wound.2011.0282

[41] Kassal P, Zubak M, Scheipl G, Mohr GJ, Steinberg MD, Steinberg IM. Smart bandage with wireless connectivity for optical monitoring of pH. Sensors and Actuators B: Chemical, Volume. 2017;**246**:455-460

[42] Bjarnsholt T, Kirketerp-Møller K, Jensen PØ, Madsen KG, Phipps R, Krogfelt K, et al. Why chronic wounds will not heal: A novel hypothesis. First published: 2007. DOI: 10.1111/ j.1524-475X.2007.00283.x